Multiple Myeloma

REVLIMID® (lenalidomide) in combination with dexamethasone is indicated for the treatment of multiple myeloma patients who have received at least one prior therapy.

REVLIMID® (lenalidomide) is indicated for the treatment of patients with transfusion-dependent anemia due to Low- or Intermediate-1–risk myelodysplastic syndromes associated with a deletion 5q cytogenetic abnormality, with or without additional cytogenetic abnormalities.

THALOMID® (thalidomide) in combination with dexamethasone is indicated for the treatment of patients with newly diagnosed multiple myeloma. The effectiveness of THALOMID is based on response rates (see CLINICAL STUDIES section). There are no controlled trials demonstrating a clinical benefit, such as an improvement in survival.

THALOMID® (thalidomide) is indicated for the acute treatment of the cutaneous manifestations of moderate to severe erythema nodosum leprosum (ENL). THALOMID® is not indicated as monotherapy for such ENL treatment in the presence of moderate to severe neuritis. THALOMID® is also indicated as maintenance therapy for prevention and suppression of the cutaneous manifestations of ENL recurrence.

TRANSLATIONAL MEDICINE SERIES

1. Prostate Cancer: Translational and Emerging Therapies, *edited by Nancy A. Dawson and W. Kevin Kelly*

2. Breast Cancer: Translational Therapeutic Strategies, *edited by Gary Lyman and Harold Burstein*

3. Lung Cancer: Translational and Emerging Therapies, *edited by Kishan J. Pandya, Julie R. Brahmer, and Manuel Hidalgo*

4. Multiple Myeloma: Translational and Emerging Therapies, *edited by Kenneth C. Anderson and Irene Ghobrial*

Multiple Myeloma

Translational and Emerging Therapies

Edited by

Kenneth C. Anderson
Dana-Farber Cancer Institute, Boston, Massachusetts, USA

Irene M. Ghobrial
Dana-Farber Cancer Institute, Boston, Massachusetts, USA

informa
healthcare

New York London

Informa Healthcare USA, Inc.
52 Vanderbilt Avenue
New York, NY 10017

© 2009 by Informa Healthcare USA, Inc. (hardcover edition published 2008 by Informa Healthcare USA)
Informa Healthcare is an Informa business

No claim to original U.S. Government works
Printed in the United States of America on acid-free paper
10 9 8 7 6 5 4 3 2 1

International Standard Book Number-10: 1-4200-4510-5; 13: 978-1-4200-4510-9 (Hardcover)
International Standard Book Number-10: 1-4398-1819-3; 13: 978-1-4398-1819-0 (Softcover)

Library of Congress Cataloging-in-Publication Data

Multiple myeloma: Translational and emerging therapies / Kenneth C. Anderson, Irene
  Ghobrial, editors.
   p. ; cm. -- (translational medicine series; 4)
   Includes bibliographical references and index
   ISBN-13: 978-1-4200-4510-9 (hardcover : alk. paper)
   ISBN-10: 1-4200-4510-5 (hardcover : alk. paper) 1. Multiple myeloma. I. Anderson,
Kenneth C. II. Ghobrial, Irene. III. Series.
   [DNLM: 1. Multiple Myeloma. WH 540 M9605 2007]

   RC280.B6M852 2007
   616.99'418--dc22   2007023651

Visit the Informa Web site at
www.informa.com

and the Informa Healthcare Web site at
www.informahealthcare.com

Preface

In the past five years, there has been enormous progress in the translation of basic science to clinical practice in multiple myeloma and other plasma cell dyscrasias. Studies on the genetics and pathogenesis of multiple myeloma and its interaction with the bone marrow microenvironment have paved the way for the development of novel therapeutic agents that have demonstrated exciting activity in vitro and in vivo. These agents moved rapidly from the bench to the bedside and were tested in innovative phase I and II clinical trials, followed by pivotal phase III trials, that changed the management of this disease. In the last four years, the Food and Drug Administration has approved four new agents for multiple myeloma based on the rapid translation of basic science to clinical medicine. Moreover, the rapid leaps in elucidating the biology of myeloma and its interaction with the microenvironment have led to an unprecedented number of novel therapeutic agents being tested for this disease, with over twenty new agents in either preclinical or early clinical trials. Indeed, multiple myeloma has become a model disease for the development of novel therapeutic agents.

In designing the current translational book on multiple myeloma and other plasma cell dyscrasias, including primary systemic amyloidosis and Waldenström's macroglobulinemia, we chose to be as inclusive as possible. We wanted a broad representation of genetics, biology, interaction of the malignant cells with their microenvironment, and bone disease in multiple myeloma. We include current treatment options for patients with relapsed or refractory disease, for newly diagnosed, untreated patients, and in clinical trials in early development. We also include advances in translational research in two closely related plasma cell dyscrasias—primary systemic amyloidosis and Waldenström's macroglobulinemia.

The first three chapters discuss the molecular biology, genetics, and cytogenetics of multiple myeloma, as well as molecular mechanisms of growth and resistance of the malignant cells, and current animal models. We have included a chapter on the role of the bone marrow microenvironment in multiple myeloma, including myeloma bone disease and the homing and migration of multiple myeloma cells. The next chapter defines novel therapeutic agents being tested in the preclinical setting and moving forward into clinical practice. This represents the interface between basic science and clinical research. The fourth chapter begins with the clinical long-term follow-up of monoclonal gammopathy and its progression to multiple myeloma. It is followed by an up-to-date assessment of the prognostic factors and classifications of multiple myeloma, which leads to chapters updating therapy for patients with multiple myeloma. These include novel options for therapy in newly diagnosed patients and in patients with relapsed or refractory disease, as well as promising new agents in early phase I and II clinical trials, and immunotherapies in multiple myeloma. Finally, we discuss advances in the biology and therapy of patients with primary systemic amyloidosis and Waldenström's macroglobulinemia.

This book is the first in its category to address the rapid advances in translational research in multiple myeloma and other plasma cell dyscrasias. Its production has required the cooperation of our many contributors. We are grateful to them for providing us with up-to-date chapters that have made this comprehensive work possible. We also appreciate the hard work of our publisher, who helped with the coordination, revisions, and structure of our text. We look forward to further advances in the biology of multiple myeloma and its interaction with the microenvironment, as the rapid translation of basic research to innovative clinical trials will prolong survival and improve the quality-of-life of our patients with multiple myeloma and other plasma cell dyscrasias.

Irene M. Ghobrial
Kenneth C. Anderson

Contents

Contributors

Melissa Alsina H. Lee Moffitt Cancer Center & Research Institute, Tampa, Florida, U.S.A.

Kenneth C. Anderson Department of Medical Oncology, Jerome Lipper Multiple Myeloma Center, Dana-Farber Cancer Institute and Department of Medicine, Harvard Medical School, Boston, Massachusetts, U.S.A.

Daniel R. Carrasco Department of Medical Oncology, Dana-Farber Cancer Institute, Harvard Medical School and Department of Pathology, Brigham and Women's Hospital, Harvard Medical School, Boston, Massachusetts, U.S.A.

Dharminder Chauhan Department of Medical Oncology, Jerome Lipper Multiple Myeloma Center, Dana-Farber Cancer Institute, Harvard Medical School, Boston, Massachusetts, U.S.A.

Meletios A. Dimopoulos Department of Clinical Therapeutics, Alexandra Hospital, University of Athens School of Medicine, Athens, Greece

Ramón García-Sanz Department of Hematology, University Hospital of Salamanca and Center for Cancer Research of Salamanca, Salamanca, Spain

Morie A. Gertz Division of Hematology, Mayo Clinic, Rochester, Minnesota, U.S.A.

Irene M. Ghobrial Department of Medical Oncology, Dana-Farber Cancer Institute, Harvard Medical School, Boston, Massachusetts, U.S.A.

Norma C. Gutiérrez Department of Hematology, University Hospital of Salamanca and Center for Cancer Research of Salamanca, Salamanca, Spain

Jean-Luc Harousseau Hospitalier Universitaire de Nantes, Nantes, France

Teru Hideshima Department of Medical Oncology, Jerome Lipper Multiple Myeloma Center, Dana-Farber Cancer Institute, Harvard Medical School, Boston, Massachusetts, U.S.A.

Alissa Huston James P. Wilmot Cancer Center, University of Rochester Medical Center, Rochester, New York, U.S.A.

Robert A. Kyle Division of Hematology, Mayo Clinic College of Medicine, Rochester, Minnesota, U.S.A.

Xavier Leleu Department of Medical Oncology, Dana-Farber Cancer Institute, Harvard Medical School, Boston, Massachusetts, U.S.A. and Service des Maladies du Sang, CHRU, Lille, France

Constantine S. Mitsiades Department of Medical Oncology, Jerome Lipper Multiple Myeloma Center, Dana-Farber Cancer Institute and Department of Medicine, Harvard Medical School, Boston, Massachusetts, U.S.A

Anne-Sophie Moreau Department of Medical Oncology, Dana-Farber Cancer Institute, Harvard Medical School, Boston, Massachusetts, U.S.A. and Service des Maladies du Sang, CHRU, Lille, France

Nikhil C. Munshi Dana-Farber Cancer Institute, Harvard Medical School and Boston VA Healthcare System, Boston, Massachusetts, U.S.A.

Dheeraj Pelluru Dana-Farber Cancer Institute, Harvard Medical School and Boston VA Healthcare System, Boston, Massachusetts, U.S.A.

Klaus Podar Department of Medical Oncology, Jerome Lipper Multiple Myeloma Center, Dana-Farber Cancer Institute, Harvard Medical School, Boston, Massachusetts, U.S.A.

Rao H. Prabhala Dana-Farber Cancer Institute, Harvard Medical School and Boston VA Healthcare System, Boston, Massachusetts, U.S.A.

Noopur Raje Jerome Lipper Multiple Myeloma Center, Dana-Farber Cancer Institute and Center for Multiple Myeloma, Massachusetts General Hospital, Boston, Massachusetts, U.S.A.

S.Vincent Rajkumar Division of Hematology, Mayo Clinic College of Medicine, Rochester, Minnesota, U.S.A.

Tiffany Richards Department of Lymphoma and Myeloma, The University of Texas M.D. Anderson Cancer Center, Houston, Texas, U.S.A.

Paul Richardson Dana-Farber Cancer Institute, Harvard Medical School, Boston, Massachusetts, U.S.A.

G. David Roodman Bone Biology Center, University of Pittsburgh Medical Center, VA Pittsburgh Healthcare System, Pittsburgh, Pennsylvania, U.S.A.

Jesús F. San Miguel   Department of Hematology, University Hospital of Salamanca and Center for Cancer Research of Salamanca, Salamanca, Spain

Sheeba Thomas   Department of Lymphoma and Myeloma, The University of Texas M.D. Anderson Cancer Center, Houston, Texas, U.S.A.

Giovanni Tonon   Department of Medical Oncology, Dana-Farber Cancer Institute, Harvard Medical School, Boston, Massachusetts, U.S.A.

Donna M. Weber   Department of Lymphoma and Myeloma, The University of Texas M.D. Anderson Cancer Center, Houston, Texas, U.S.A.

1

Xenograft Animal Models for Preclinical Evaluation of Potential Anti-MM Therapeutics: Strengths and Limitations

Constantine S. Mitsiades and Kenneth C. Anderson

*Department of Medical Oncology, Jerome Lipper Multiple Myeloma Center,
Dana-Farber Cancer Institute and Department of Medicine, Harvard Medical School,
Boston, Massachusetts, U.S.A.*

Daniel R. Carrasco

*Department of Medical Oncology, Dana-Farber Cancer Institute, Harvard Medical
School and Department of Pathology, Brigham and Women's Hospital,
Harvard Medical School, Boston, Massachusetts, U.S.A.*

INTRODUCTION

The preclinical evaluation of novel therapeutics for multiple myeloma (MM) relies heavily on in vivo animal models, in which the safety profile and potential anti-MM efficacy of the tested candidate treatments are assessed. Herein, we review the features of some of the key in vivo models that have been applied in the process of development of novel therapeutics for MM. Similar to the preclinical development of therapeutics for solid tumors, subcutaneous xenografts of human MM cell lines into immunocompromised mice have been used extensively in the MM field. However, in view of the role of the bone marrow (BM) microenvironment in proliferation and survival of MM cells [as reviewed in (1)], considerable emphasis in the MM field has been placed on the development of models where MM cells are allowed to form lesions in the bones (2–5). These in vivo models (e.g., the SCID-hu model, the models of the 5T series or the models of diffuse MM lesions in SCID/NOD mice) have provided valuable insight into the pathophysiology of MM and the role of several classes of investigational anti-MM therapeutics which perturb the interactions of MM cells with their local BM milieu. Each of the in vivo models discussed in this review presents us with both advantages and limitations. These aspects have to be taken into account while deciding which model should be applied for the preclinical evaluation of a particular therapeutic agent. These advantages and limitations should also be considered carefully in the interpretation of the results from the preclinical in vivo study of a candidate anti-MM agent.

SUBCUTANEOUS XENOGRAFTS OF MM CELL LINES

In these models, human MM cell lines are injected subcutaneously in immunocompromised (e.g., nude, SCID, or SCID/NOD) mice to allow for formation of palpable tumors (6). In some applications of this model, MM cells are mixed into matrigel and then injected subcutaneously, to facilitate the engraftment of tumor cells (7).

After random assignment of plasmacytoma-bearing mice to drug-treated and control cohorts, treatments of mice with active drugs versus vehicle are initiated. The primary endpoint in these models is the volume of subcutaneous tumors, which can be calculated by various proposed equations (7). The diameter(s) of the tumor, as measured with calipers, are a key determinant for the calculation of tumor burden in these equations. Mice are euthanized when their plasmacytoma crosses a certain predetermined threshold of size (typically a diameter of 2 cm) or when the quality of life of the mouse is deemed to be significantly compromised due to significant weight loss, bleeding, infection, etc.

These models are conceptually and practically identical to those utilized in the field of solid tumors for preclinical evaluation of novel therapeutics. In the MM field, subcutaneous xenograft models have been utilized in the assessment of a very large spectrum of therapeutics, some of which eventually translated into FDA-approved anti-MM medications or in ongoing clinical trials in MM. For instance, proteasome inhibitors [including bortezomib, formerly known as PS-341 (7), and NPI-0052, formerly known as Salinosporamide A (8)], thalidomide and its immunomodulatory derivatives (9) were tested in this model and shown to have anti-MM activity in vivo. Other classes of investigational anti-MM agents that have been tested in this model include the heat shock protein (hsp90) inhibitor IPI-504 (10); the Akt inhibitor perifosine (11); FGF-R3 kinase inhibitors (12,13) or the neutralizing antibody PRO-001 (14); death receptor agonists, such as Apo2L/TRAIL (15); inhibitors of Bcl-2 family members (16), other kinase inhibitors, including VEGF-R kinase inhibitor (17) or p38MAPK inhibitor (18); mTOR inhibitors (19); epothilone (20); or antibodies against targets such as antihuman interleukin-6 receptor (21) or the surface antigen HM1.24 (22).

An advantage of subcutaneous plasmacytoma xenograft models is that the development of MM lesions can be easily monitored and changes in their size can be easily quantified with caliper measurements. Measurements of tumor markers or imaging studies, which are necessary for other models, are not necessary in this case. Furthermore, plasmacytomas can be easily excised to provide samples for in vivo histologic evaluation and molecular profiling studies.

However, in these plasmacytoma models, MM cells are placed in the context of a subcutaneous microenvironment. This is a key limitation of these models because it does not take into account the close relationship of MM cells with the milieu of the BM, where MM cells typically reside and proliferate. There are several examples of conventional antitherapeutics (e.g., dexamethasone, alkylating agents, anthracyclines) which are quite active in vitro against MM cells cultured in isolation, but significantly less active when the MM cells are co-cultured with bone marrow stromal cells (BMSCs) [as reviewed in (1,23)]. Because subcutaneous plasmacytoma xenografts do not involve such MM-BMSCs interactions, it is plausible that an anti-MM therapeutic that demonstrates in vivo activity in these models may not be able to overcome the protective effects of the bone microenvironment. In addition, subcutaneous plasmacytomas can reach large dimensions. However, these often have modest, if not minimal, actual impact on the quality of life of the mouse host, even if they meet the standard criteria for euthanasia of experimental animals. Importantly, these plasmacytomas do not cause any of the characteristic pathophysiologic complications (e.g., bone resorption, spontaneous fractures) associated with the development of MM lesions in the bones, further limiting the relevance of overall survival as an endpoint for evaluation of experimental therapeutics in this model. Taken together, the nonorthotopic location of the xenografted MM cells combined with the dissociation between duration of mouse survival and the pattern of plasmacytoma growth leave room for potential overestimation of the in vivo anti-MM activity of an investigational antitumor agent.

SCID-hu Model

The limitations of conventional subcutaneous xenograft models of MM provided the impetus for application of the MM version of a SCID-hu model. The concept of the SCID-hu mouse was first pioneered in the late 1980s as a heterochimeric small animal model designed to support human hematopoietic differentiation and function in vivo *in* xenograft systems. In the original version of the SCID-hu mouse (24,25), multiple organs of the human hematolymphoid system (including fetal liver, thymus, lymph node, and skin) were successfully engrafted into immunodeficient C.B-17 SCID mouse in order to recapitulate multi-lineage human hematopoiesis in vivo and overcome species-dependent limitations in experimental studies of, e.g., tropism of HIV infection for CD4+ cells of human but not rodent, origin.

Urashima et al. (2) applied the same principle in MM with the surgical implantation in SCID mice of bilateral human fetal bone grafts (SCID-hu mice), which were intended to function as a niche for interaction of human MM cells with a bone microenvironment of human origin. Specifically, mice bearing the human bone grafts received sublethal irradiation and then received, into the BM cavity of these grafts, injections of human MM cell lines. The rationale behind the development of this model in MM was that the interaction of its malignant cells with their local bone microenvironment is so important for the pathophysiology of MM that any in vivo models of this disease should faithfully recapitulate that feature. Importantly, however, the MM-bone microenvironment interaction is mediated by adhesion molecules and cytokines which may function at least in part, in species-dependent manners. For instance, it has been postulated that human MM cells proliferate in response to IL-6 of human origin, but do not respond (or at least do not respond to the same degree) to murine IL-6. In view of these considerations, the SCID-hu MM model emerged as an approach that would allow investigators to evaluate the in vivo behavior of MM cells as they interact with a bone microenvironment of human origin, in a fully species-compatible manner. In the first description of the SCID-hu MM model (2), Urashima et al. observed that injection of as few as 10,000 MM cells into the BM of the human bone graft was sufficient to lead to extensive infiltration of the marrow cavity of the graft with MM cells. The human origin of this neoplastic expansion was confirmed not only through the characteristic histological presentation in the BM, but also by other features including the immunohistochemical identification of human light chain expression in the plasma cells of the human bone graft; the detection of monoclonal human immunoglobulin and human IL-6 in the peripheral blood serum samples of the mice; and the detection of monoclonal Ig light chain deposition in renal tubules. Of note, approximately 12 weeks after injection of human MM cells in one of 2 human bone grafts of the SCID-hu mice, MM cells could be detected in the contralateral, non-MM cell injected, bone graft, while no spread of human MM cells was reported in the murine BM (2).

Since its original description, the SCID-hu MM model has been used extensively to characterize the interaction of human MM cells with the bone microenvironment and for evaluation of various investigational antitumor agents. Yaccoby et al. (26) reported that this model can be utilized to study primary MM cells in vivo; that 80% of primary samples from MM patients can be successfully engrafted in the SCID-hu model and that the implanted human bone often presents with osteolysis, reminiscent of the bone resorption that accompanies the proliferation of MM cells in human patients with the disease (27). In subsequent studies, the group of Yaccoby and Epstein utilized the SCID-hu MM model to report that purified primary CD38(++)CD45(−) myeloma cells consistently (in eight out of nine experiments) grew in the human bone grafts and produced MM and its manifestations. Furthermore, peripheral blood cell preparations that were not depleted of plasma cells grew (in 4 out of 4 cases) and produced myeloma in hosts. In contrast, however, BM or mononuclear cell preparations depleted from plasma cells did not grow or produce myeloma in SCID-hu hosts (28).

The same SCID-hu model (or variations of it) has also been utilized to study the anti-MM activity of thalidomide (29); to characterize the mechanisms whereby human MM cells trigger increased osteoclastogenesis and bone resorption in the bone milieu (30,31). Furthermore this model has been utilized to evaluate the effect of potential anti-MM therapeutics, including not only agents that target the increased bone resorption triggered by MM cells, e.g., RANK-Fc constructs as antagonists of RANKL (30,32); but also small molecule inhibitors, such as the IKK inhibitor MLN120B (33) or the farnesyltransferase inhibitor tipifarnib (34); monocloncal antibodies against CD138 (35) or insulin-like growth factors (36); as well as cytokine superantagonists (37).

In vivo models where MM cells interact with a murine (BM or sub-cutaneous) microenvironment are subject to the concern that cytokines or cell adhesion molecules of the mouse milieu might not interact (optimal) or at all with the human versions of their functional counterparts which are present on human MM cells. A key advantage of the SCID-hu model is that it addresses this concern by allowing human MM cells to interact in vivo with a bone microenvironment of human origin. The ability of the SCID-hu model to overcome such issues of species specificity in tumor-micro-environmental interactions has made this a very useful model for evaluation of characterization of the natural history of MM-associated bone resorption or neovascularization, as well as for evaluation of the anti-MM efficacy of investigational therapeutics. Similar to the subcutaneous models of human plasmacytoma xenografts, the MM cells injected into the SCID-hu model are localized (particularly in the early stages after injection of the MM cells) predominantly in the site of the bone graft. Therefore, sampling of MM-bearing tissue in this model is relatively easy and its analysis can provide a meaningful simulation of MM-bone interactions in patients.

In contrast to subcutaneous plasmacytoma xenograft models, where the size of plasmacytomas is an easily measurable endpoint for the follow-up of MM cell growth in vivo and its response to investigational agents, tumor burden is not as easy to quantify in the SCID-hu model, because the MM cells, at least in the initial phases of their growth, do not grow in the form of a palpable and measurable plasmacytoma, but within the bone graft. Indeed, even after the point where MM cells have completely infiltrated the bone graft and have started to expand beyond the bone graft, the precise tumor volume cannot be reliably estimated on the basis of caliper mea-surements conventionally applied for subcutaneous plasmacytoma xeno-grafts. Instead, a series of serological and biochemical markers are often evaluated in the SCID-hu model, including the quantification in mouse serum samples of levels for human monoclonal immunoglobulin (38); interleukin-6 (IL-6); or its soluble receptor (sIL-6R) (37).

The SCID-hu model has certain limitations, which should be noted, even though they do not and should not negate the scientific value of its advantages. This model does not simulate the diffuse and multi-focal nature of MM lesions. Furthermore, while this is a very good model to study the process of MM-associated bone resorption per se, the pathophysiologic consequences of that resorption, e.g., pathological fractures and their sequelae (such as hind limb paralysis) cannot be evaluated in the SCID-hu model, because the bone graft with its engrafted MM cells is not an essential component of the skeleton, but essentially an appendage to the sub-cutaneous compartment. Consequently, even the complete resorption of the bone fragment by the MM cells can have minimal, if any, functional consequences to the rodent host and its quality of life. These factors confound the interpretation of overall survival data for SCID-hu MM mice and limit the utility of this endpoint for the evaluation of the anti-MM activity of investigational agents.

In addition, the SCID-hu model involves several technically and logistically demanding steps, including the acquisition, processing, and implanting of the human bone grafts in the SCID mice. In principle, the SCID-hu MM model should be amenable to the use of adult human bone tissue. However, at the moment, there are no detailed studies that have formally compared the feasibility of applying the SCID-hu MM model using fetal versus adult human bone grafts. Given the concerns related to research involving human fetal tissues, such studies may become necessary in the near future.

In part because of these considerations, a variation of the original SCID-hu MM model has been proposed by the group of S. Yaccoby, which reported on their experience with the SCID-rab model (39). In that model, instead of introducing in SCID mice subcutaneous implants of fetal human bone grafts, Yaccoby et al. (39) implanted in these mice, rabbit bone fragments, which they directly injected with primary human MM cells: successful engraftment of primary human MM cells occurred in the majority of patient samples (either with unfractionated BM mononuclear cells or with injection of the CD138+ fraction), as evidenced by detection of M-protein isotypes secreted by the respective patients; and osteolytic bone lesions in the rabbit bone graft. Similar to the SCID-hu MM model, primary MM cells injected directly in one bone graft were able to metastasize into another bone graft at a remote site of the same mouse recipient. MM cells derived from patients with extramedullary disease recapitulated that feature by extending their growth beyond the bone graft into contiguous soft tissues (39). The SCID-rab model is one potential approach to bypass the issues related to the availability of fetal bone grafts for use in the SCID-hu MM model. It is notable, though, that more studies will be very useful in ascertaining whether the rabbit bone milieu offers a similarly favorable microenvironment for human MM cells as the human bone milieu.

MODELS OF DIFFUSE MM BONE LESIONS IN SCID/NOD MICE

As its own name implies, MM is a systemic disease with multifocal BM involvement. Therefore for the purpose of anti-MM drug development, it would be ideal to utilize in vivo models which recapitulate the systemic and multifocal nature of MM lesions, and specifically the multi-focal involvement of the skeleton. Subcutaneous plasmacytoma xenograft models or the SCID-hu MM model do not present this feature, because they involve injections of MM cells in very specific singular locations of the body of the experimental animals (i.e., the subcutaneous compartment and the implanted human bone graft, respectively). Instead, the development of diffuse MM lesions in these experimental animals requires injection of the MM cells in the systemic circulation, e.g., by the intravenous or (less frequently) the intracardiac route (40,41). Several studies have indeed documented that human MM cells injected intravenously in immunocompromised mice can engraft in their BM and lead to formation of MM bone lesions with features consistent with those of MM in human patients (3,4,42–51). Some of the first studies of i.v. injection of MM cells into immunocompromised mice utilized the cell line ARH-77, which does lead to formation of osteolytic lesions (52–55), but has subsequently been shown to be a lymphoblastoid EBV+ cell line, rather than a *bona fide* human MM cell line (56). Still, the basic principle that human MM cells injected into the systemic circulation of immunocompromised mice can lead to multifocal MM bone lesions has been validated by multiple labs using several different *bona fide* MM cell lines (3,4,42–51), as well as primary human MM cells (40,41,57). After the early studies with these models of diffuse MM lesions, two main caveats had been voiced, namely the potential incompatibility in the interaction of human MM cells with a murine bone microenvironment and the difficulty of measuring, after the systemic injection of the MM cells in mice, of the tumor burden and its changes over time and with administration of treatment(s). However, these concerns have in large part been addressed.

The concern regarding the homing of human MM cells in a murine BM microenvironment was that the interaction between these two compartments may depend on human MM cells expressing cytokine receptors and adhesion molecules many of which would not cross-react with their functional partners (e.g., cytokines and counterpart adhesion molecules) of murine origin. The reported experience, though, with these models has shown that broad range of bone human *bona fide* MM cell lines can indeed lead to formation of bone lesions in immunocompromised mice. For instance, the JJN-3 MM cell line and its subline JJN-3 T1 led to BM infiltration, radiological signs of osteolysis, histomorphometric evidence of osteoblastopenia, as well as mild hypercalcemia and eventual paralysis of mice (3). Intravenous injection of the KPMM2 cell line, which produces high levels of autocrine IL-6, led to formation of MM lesions in all mice which were predominantly localized in the BM, and led to distinct osteolytic lesions at multiple sites of the skeleton, diffuse decrease in bone density throughout the body, increased levels of ionized plasma calcium, and eventually hind leg paralysis (42). Tail vein injections of the RPMI-8226/ S-GFP (4,47) or MM-1S-GFP/Luc (44) human MM cell lines also lead to development of diffuse skeletal lesions with anatomical distribution and pathophysiological manifestations consistent with the clinical course of MM in human patients. For example, the MM lesions in these models predominantly involved the axial skeleton (e.g., spine, skull, and pelvis), leading to frequent development of paralysis secondary to spinal lesions, while tumor spread to lungs, liver, spleen, or kidney more infrequently. The results that were obtained with a luciferase-expressing MM-1S cell line model were consistent with those obtained subsequently by Wu et al. (51).

Miyakawa et al. (43) performed intravenous injections of the human MM cell line U266 in NOD/SCID/γc null (NOG) mice, leading to hind leg paralysis in all 20 NOG mice tested, infiltration by MM cells of only the BM, without presence of MM cells in other organs, as well as osteolytic lesions in cortical bones and loss of trabecular bones. Interestingly, i.v. injection of the same mouse model with the cell line KMM-1 led to infiltration in BM as well as in the spleen, lung, and liver of mice. (45). Wu et al. (46) reported that intravenous injection of the CAG human MM cell line in SCID/NOD mice led to lesions with anatomical distribution and pathophysiological manifestations in this model were consistent with the clinical course of MM in human patients, i.e., hallmarked by major involvement of the axial skeleton, osteolytic bone lesions captured by both pathology and x-ray examinations (e.g., spine, skull, and pelvis), and frequent development of hind-limb paralysis secondary to spinal lesions, without significant tumor spread to lungs, liver, spleen, or kidney. These findings were also confirmed in a subsequent study (50). Xin et al. (48) reported that female SCID-beige mice injection in their tail vein with KMS-11-luc human MM cells led to typical diffuse multiple skeletal lesions, including skull, pelvis, and spine in the majority of mice. Carlo-Stella et al. (49) also confirmed that i.v. injection of the KMS-11 cell line led to progressive BM infiltration and hind-leg paralysis.

In many of these models, the MM cells (particularly in the advanced stages of its course) also formed lesions in other sites of the body of the mice, e.g., the JJN3 cell line formed lesions in the meninges, liver, and adipose tissue (3); the KPMM2 cell line formed lesions in the lymph nodes (42); the RPMI-8226/S-GFP (4) or MM-1S-GFP/Luc (44) led to infiltration of soft tissues in late stages of the disease; while the KMM-1 cells can also infiltrate the spleen, lung, and liver of mice (45). However, in each one of these studies, the predominant location of MM involvement was the BM. The ability of some human MM cell lines to grow not only in the BM but also at extramedullary sites does not minimize their biological and clinical relevance. In fact, although MM is an osteotropic disease that involves almost exclusively the bone during the early stages of the disease, patients with advanced MM very frequently present with extramedullary involvement. The ability of at least some of these models of diffuse MM lesions to capture extramedullary components of MM is an additional feature that may prove quite beneficial for the development of novel anti-MM therapeutics capable of achieving anti-MM responses even in patients with advanced disease.

These models of diffuse MM lesions in immunocompromised mice have provided valuable insights in the development of novel anti-MM therapeutics, including studies of humanized anti-IL-6 receptor antibody (hPM1) (42); small molecule inhibitors (44) or monoclonal antibodies (51) against IGF-1R; hsp90 inhibitors (47); FGF-R3 kinase inhibitors (48); synthetic epothilone analogs (46); antibodies against CD52 (49); and inhibitor against cyclin-dependent kinase 4/6 (50).

A second concern that had been voiced regards the use of models of diffuse lesions of MM cells related to the difficulty in monitoring the anatomic localization, spatiotemporal progression, and total tumor volume, given the location of the tumors in various locations in internal organs and not in the form of an easily accessible and measurable subcutaneous plasmacytoma. In the earlier versions of this model, X-rays were used to evaluate the degree of bone resorption at sites of MM involvement (54) and measurements of circulating levels of human monoclonal immunoglobulin (s) in the mouse serum were also applied occasionally to evaluate to provide insight into the tumor burden and its changes with treatments (42). However, X-rays do not provide quantitative assessment of tumor burden; are not very sensitive for detection of bone involvement with MM if the associated bone resorption is still in early stages and bone density has not been severely compromised; and do not provide sensitive imaging of tumor involvement in soft tissues. Indeed, as previously mentioned, some MM cells (particularly MM cell lines or primary cells from patients from very advanced disease/extramedullary involvement/plasma cell leukemia) utilized in these models exhibit a tropism for development of extramedullary lesions, which cannot be readily assessed by conventional X-ray imaging. Computerized tomography (CT) and magnetic resonance imaging (MRI) might be considered alternative strategies to address these limitations. However, their cost for pre-clinical studies is still prohibitive.

In view of the limitations of conventional imaging approaches, we adapted the model of diffuse MM bone lesions to include systemic injections of human MM cell lines stably expressing constructs for markers detectable by whole-body fluorescence and/or bioluminescence imaging. For instance, MM cell lines expressing green fluorescent protein (GFP) or its GFP/Luc fusion construct with luciferase (Luc) can be visualized by whole-body fluorescence imaging whereby MM-bearing mice are visualized by near-infrared light, which given the relatively small size of these animals can become detectable with sensitive digital cameras (4,44). Furthermore, MM cell lines expressing Luc or a GFP/Luc fusion construct can be visualized by whole-body bioluminescence imaging. In that modality, MM-bearing mice are anesthetized and injected i.p. with the substrate of luciferase, luciferin. The latter is then distributed through the systemic circulation to the various sites of the body where Luc-expressing tumor cells produce bioluminescence as a result of the interaction of Luc with its substrate. Again, the ability of visible light to penetrate modest lengths of solid tissues combined with the small size of these experimental animals and the use of sensitive charged-couple device (CCD) cameras have allowed the acquisition of whole-body images which provide identification of the sites of luciferase-positive tumor involvement and quantification of the total and site-specific tumor burden (4,44). Both these modalities are noninvasive, can be used safely for the animals, without need for exposure to radiation or additional contrast agents and can be used even in the case of cell lines that produce low levels of monoclonal immunoglobulin or free light chains. Since the first studies that applied fluorescence and bioluminescence imaging in mouse models of MM, several others have applied these imaging modalities in the MM field and confirmed their feasibility and utility (35,46,48,50,51,58,59) in diverse experimental settings.

Another important area of research that has benefited from the use of these models involves the study of clonotypic B-cells in MM patients (40,41,57) and the proposed "myeloma stem cell". Pilarski et al. (40) reported that MM lesions can develop in NOD/SCID mice not only after direct, intraosseous, injection of human MM cells, but also after intra-cardiac (IC) injection of these mice with peripheral blood mononuclear cells from patients with aggressive MM. Indeed, IC injection of PBMCs from patients with aggressive MM led to development in NOD/SCID mice of lytic bone lesions; detection of human Ig in the mouse serum and of human plasma cells in the BM, spleen, and blood of the mice; as well as detection of a high frequency of clonotypic cells in the murine BM. Interestingly, a high frequency of human clonotypic B-cells was detected in the femoral BM even after direct intraosseous injection of human MM cells in the sternum of the mice. These observations were interpreted by the authors to be consistent with ability of MM spread from a primary site of injection to other distant locations in the murine BM. The authors also observed that G-CSF mobilized cells from MM patients with minimal disease, taken at the time of mobilization or after cryopreservation, included MM progenitors, which were identified by virtue of the ability of the corresponding samples to lead to engraftment of clonotypic cells and/or lytic bone disease in mice. Based on these results, the authors concluded that MM progenitors are mobilized into the blood by cyclophosphamide/G-CSF. In subsequent studies, Pilarksi et al. (57) utilized the same SCID/NOD model to evaluate the myelomagenic capabilities of highly purified CD34(+) progenitors from G-CSF-mobilized blood of MM patients. In that study, these samples included, on average, 31% clonotypic MM cells which were reported to be myelomagenic, on the basis of their ability to lead, upon intrasternal injection in SCID/NOD mice, to engraftment of clonotypic cells in the femoral BM and to development of lytic bone lesions at distant skeletal locations.

5T SERIES OF MM MODELS

The 5T series of MM models has been the centerpiece for one of the most prolific lines of in vivo research studies in the MM field over the last 2 decades (59–94). Strictly speaking, the 5T models are not "xenografts" because they do not involve injection of immunocompromised mice with human MM cells. Instead, they involve serial transplantations of murine MM cells arising spontaneously in C57BL/KaLwRij mice in syngeneic recipients. However, this series of models is discussed in this chapter not only because they can address some of the key limitations of *bona fide* MM xenograft models, but also because their use has provided useful results, both in terms of MM pathophysiology and preclinical drug development, in a manner that is complementing the experience obtained with the use of xenograft models.

The 5T series is based on the original observation of J. Radl (95) that C57BL mice of advanced age frequently exhibit an idiopathic paraproteinemia that resembles the development and natural history of human MGUS and eventually human MM. Among the various strains of C57BL mice, C57BL/KaLwRij mice exhibited the highest frequency of this idiopathic paraproteinemia (95). Radl and his group(5) then documented that the clone of cells responsible for this idiopathic paraproteinemia could be further propagated by transplantation of cells from the BM and/or spleen into young, lethally irradiated and, equally as well, into nonirradiated C57BL/KaLwRij recipients.

The two main versions of 5T models utilized in recent studies are the 5T2MM and the 5T33MM models. These models share some common features, including the similar pattern of expression of adhesion molecules such as LFA-1, CD44, VLA-4, and VLA-5 (83), likely reflecting their common derivation, but also some notable differences, including shorter time to BM infiltration by 5T33MM cells (which occurs within 2 weeks compared to 9 weeks for the 5T2MM cells); as well as more consistent development of osteolytic lesions by the 5T2MM model (77); a tendency of 5T33MM cells to home not only in the BM, but also in the spleen and liver;

and a general observation that 5T2MM MM cells are less aggressive in vivo than 5T33 MM cells (83).

The 5T models have been the focus of studies that have provided insight into the role of OPG and RANK/RANKL interactions in MM bone disease (60); the role of bisphosphonates in affecting the extent of MM bone disease (62,63,94); and the role of cell adhesion molecules in MM cell proliferation and/or homing (64,65,70,74,75). In addition, 5T models have been used for the study of several aspects of MM pathophysiology, including the role of chemokines in MM cell homing in vivo (66,96,97); the process of MM-associated neoangiogenesis (67,68); the normoxic versus hypoxic status of BM microenvironment (98); and the role of matrix metalloproteinases in MM pathophysiology (68). Furthermore, these models have been the basis for studies of the anti-MM properties of various agents including erythropoietin (71), all-trans retinoic acid (72); glucolipid synthase inhibitor P4 (81); bisphosphonates (99); IGF-1R kinase inhibitor (100); and HMG-CoA reductase inhibitor (101).

The syngeneic nature of interaction of the MM cells with the microenvironment of the host is a key advantage of the 5T models. The concern that human MM cells xenografted in murine models would not interact optimally with adhesion molecules and cytokines of the host milieu does not apply in the 5T models. Furthermore, the mouse recipients of the syngeneic tumor cells are immunocompetent, unlike all aforementioned human MM xenograft models. Therefore, 5T models are suitable for studies of immunotherapeutic strategies, which cannot be readily addressed in SCID-hu or other xenograft models in immunocompromised mice.

An understandable limitation of the 5T models is that, unlike the SCID-hu model, they do not provide insight into in vivo interactions of human MM cells with the human bone microenvironment. Furthermore, the limited number of 5T cell lines currently available does not capture the full spectrum of genetic heterogeneity of human MM (85,92). Nonetheless, this consideration does not neutralize the utility of the 5T models, which could conceivably be complemented in the future by the development of more 5T cell lines in order to encompass a broader part of the genetic spectrum of MM. These 5T cell lines could be derived either as sublines of the original 5T2MM or 5T33MM [e.g., as in the study of Libouban et al. (102) who developed the 5THL cell line, a more aggressive derivative cell line generated by successive passaging of 5T2MM cells in C57BL/KaLwRij mice] or by *de novo* development of new 5T cell lines by a process similar to the original establishment of the 5T2MM or 5T33MM cells by Radl and his colleagues.

LAGλ-1 MODELS

Campbell et al. (103) recently described another approach to develop models of human MM tumors growing in immunodeficient mice. In this model, fresh whole core BM biopsies obtained from 33 MM patients were engrafted into the hind-limb muscles of SCID mice. Human Ig was detected in the majority (28 of 33) of mice and 3 of them grew palpable tumors with morphological and immunophenotypic features of MM. Campbell et al. then performed intramuscular passage of these cells and were able to achieve development of plasma cell tumors. One of these models, termed LAG*l*-1, was generated from an IgG-*l*-producing tumor and could lead to formation of MM lesions after injection of its cells by intramuscular, subcutaneous, or intravenous administration. This LAG*l*-1 was tested for its in vivo response to established anti-MM agents, such as bortezomib, melphalan, and doxorubicin. LAG*l*-1 tumor-bearing mice responded to high doses of bortezomib and low doses of doxorubicin, but not to low-dose bortezomib or conventional doses of melphalan (consistent with the clinical resistance of the corresponding patient to this alklylator).

FUTURE PERSPECTIVES

This review highlighted the experience that has been generated in the MM field with the use of some of the key xenograft models (or the syngeneic 5T series) that have been utilized for preclinical drug development and pathophysiological studies for this disease. Each of these models has different strengths and limitations, but they share the common feature that the biological behavior of the resulting MM tumors is determined to a very large extent by the biological features of the human (or murine, in the case of the 5T series of models) MM cells injected into the mouse recipients. Therefore, it is important to emphasize that all these models, which essentially involve transplantation of established MM cells to MM-free murine recipients, are distinct from genetic mouse models for spontaneous establishment of MM or related plasma cell dyscrasias. While extensive efforts have been made for several years now to develop genetic mouse models for spontaneous establishment of MM or related plasma cell dyscrasias (104–107), these studies yielded mostly models of B-cell neoplasias with features compatible with earlier stages of the B-cell lineages, rather than typical MM.

However, this void in the MM field is being addressed by recent advances which include a transgenic mouse model in which the spliced form of the plasma cell differentiation factor XBP-1 (XBP-1s) is targeted to the B cell lineage under the control of the IgH promoter and enhancer elements (pEμ) (108). This pEμXBP-1s model is prone to development of MM. Indeed, by one year of age, a significant proportion of the pEμXBP-1s transgenic mice present with a clinical and histopathologic picture similar to human MM, including marked elevation of serum IgM and IgG in the majority of transgenic mice; expansion of the plasma cell population in the BM; development of plasmacytic tumors resembling human MGUS or MM; and eventual development of bone lytic lesions. Despite the long latency and low penetrance of the transformed phenotype, this model would be of value in investigating the genetic lesions responsible for the progression from MGUS to MM.

In another model reported by Sebag et al. (109), c-myc is activated in postgerminal B cells of C57Bl6/J mice by somatic hypermutation. These mice (Vk*myc) spontaneously develop monoclonal gammopathies and plasma cell expansion in the BM (but not secondary lymphoid organs, and exhibit monoclonal paraproteinemia; BM infiltration with plasma cells that have low proliferative index; anemia; and decreased bone mineral density. Interestingly, these mice are responsive to drugs commonly used to treat MM (melphalan, dexamethasone, and bortezomib). These novel models may provide useful insights in the pathophysiology of MM and function as useful tools for the evaluation of novel therapeutics for this disease, in a mutually complementing fashion with existing xenograft models, building on their respective strengths and addressing some of their limitations.

ACKNOWLEDGMENTS

This work is supported by the Multiple Myeloma Research Foundation (MMRF) and a National Cancer Institute SPORE grant Career Developmental Award (CSM). C.S.M is a Special Fellow of the Leukemia and Lymphoma Society. D.R.C is supported by a Kimmel Award.

The authors apologize in advance for the inability, due to space limitations, to reference all studies relevant to the scope of this article.

REFERENCES

1. Mitsiades CS, Mitsiades N, Munshi NC, Anderson KC. Focus on multiple myeloma. Cancer Cell 2004; 6:439–44.
2. Urashima M, Chen BP, Chen S, et al. The development of a model for the homing of multiple myeloma cells to human bone marrow. Blood 1997; 90: 754–65.
3. Hjorth-Hansen H, Seifert MF, Borset M, et al. Marked osteoblastopenia and reduced bone formation in a model of multiple myeloma bone disease in severe combined immunodeficiency mice. J Bone Miner Res 1999; 14:256–63.
4. Mitsiades CS, Mitsiades NS, Bronson RT, et al. Fluorescence imaging of multiple myeloma cells in a clinically relevant SCID/NOD in vivo model: biologic and clinical implications. Cancer Res 2003; 63:6689–96.
5. Radl J, De Glopper ED, Schuit HR, Zurcher C. Idiopathic paraproteinemia. II. Transplantation of the paraprotein-producing clone from old to young C57BL/KaLwRij mice. J Immunol 1979; 122:609–13.
6. Tong AW, Huang YW, Zhang BQ, Netto G, Vitetta ES, Stone MJ. Heterotransplantation of human multiple myeloma cell lines in severe combined immunodeficiency (SCID) mice. Anticancer Res 1993; 13:593–7.

7. LeBlanc R, Catley LP, Hideshima T, et al. Proteasome inhibitor PS-341 inhibits human myeloma cell growth in vivo and prolongs survival in a murine model. Cancer Res 2002; 62:4996–5000.

8. Chauhan D, Hideshima T, Anderson KC. A novel proteasome inhibitor NPI-0052 as an anticancer therapy. Br J Cancer 2006; 95:961–5.

9. Lentzsch S, Rogers MS, LeBlanc R, et al. S-3-Amino-phthalimido-glutarimide inhibits angiogenesis and growth of B-cell neoplasias in mice. Cancer Res 2002; 62:2300–5.

10. Sydor JR, Normant E, Pien CS, et al. Development of 17-allylamino-17-demethoxygeldanamycin hydroquinone hydrochloride (IPI-504), an anti-cancer agent directed against Hsp90. Proc Natl Acad Sci USA 2006; 103: 17408–13.

11. Hideshima T, Catley L, Yasui H, et al. Perifosine, an oral bioactive novel alkylphospholipid, inhibits Akt and induces in vitro and in vivo cytotoxicity in human multiple myeloma cells. Blood 2006; 107:4053–62.

12. Trudel S, Ely S, Farooqi Y, et al. Inhibition of fibroblast growth factor receptor 3 induces differentiation and apoptosis in t(4; 14) myeloma. Blood 2004; 103:3521–8.

13. Trudel S, Li ZH, Wei E, et al. CHIR-258, a novel, multitargeted tyrosine kinase inhibitor for the potential treatment of t(4; 14) multiple myeloma. Blood 2005; 105:2941–8.

14. Trudel S, Stewart AK, Rom E, et al. The inhibitory anti-FGFR3 antibody, PRO-001, is cytotoxic to t(4; 14) multiple myeloma cells. Blood 2006; 107: 4039–46.

15. Mitsiades CS, Treon SP, Mitsiades N, et al. TRAIL/Apo2L ligand selectively induces apoptosis and overcomes drug resistance in multiple myeloma: therapeutic applications. Blood 2001; 98:795–804.

16. Trudel S, Stewart AK, Li Z, et al. The Bcl-2 family protein inhibitor, ABT-737, has substantial antimyeloma activity and shows synergistic effect with dexamethasone and melphalan. Clin Cancer Res 2007; 13:621–9.

17. Podar K, Tonon G, Sattler M, et al. The small-molecule VEGF receptor inhibitor pazopanib (GW786034B) targets both tumor and endothelial cells in multiple myeloma. Proc Natl Acad Sci USA 2006; 103:19478–83.

18. Navas TA, Nguyen AN, Hideshima T, et al. Inhibition of p38alpha MAPK enhances proteasome inhibitor-induced apoptosis of myeloma cells by modulating Hsp27, Bcl-X(L), Mcl-1 and p53 levels in vitro and inhibits tumor growth in vivo. Leukemia 2006; 20:1017–27.

19. Yan H, Frost P, Shi Y, et al. Mechanism by which mammalian target of rapamycin inhibitors sensitize multiple myeloma cells to dexamethasone-induced apoptosis. Cancer Res 2006; 66:2305–13.

20. Lin B, Catley L, LeBlanc R, et al. Patupilone (epothilone B) inhibits growth and survival of multiple myeloma cells in vitro and in vivo. Blood 2005; 105: 350–7.

21. Suzuki H, Yasukawa K, Saito T, et al. Anti-human interleukin-6 receptor antibody inhibits human myeloma growth in vivo. Eur J Immunol 1992; 22: 1989–93.

22. Ozaki S, Kosaka M, Harada M, Nishitani H, Odomi M, Matsumoto T. Radioimmunodetection of human myeloma xenografts with a monoclonal

antibody directed against a plasma cell specific antigen, HM1.24. Cancer 1998; 82:2184–90.

23. Hideshima T, Bergsagel PL, Kuehl WM, Anderson KC. Advances in biology of multiple myeloma: clinical applications. Blood 2004; 104:607–18.

24. Namikawa R, Kaneshima H, Lieberman M, Weissman IL, McCune JM. Infection of the SCID-hu mouse by HIV-1. Science 1988; 242:1684–6.

25. McCune JM, Namikawa R, Kaneshima H, Shultz LD, Lieberman M, Weissman IL. The SCID-hu mouse: murine model for the analysis of human hematolymphoid differentiation and function. Science 1988; 241:1632–9.

26. Yaccoby S, Barlogie B, Epstein J. Primary myeloma cells growing in SCID-hu mice: a model for studying the biology and treatment of myeloma and its manifestations. Blood 1998; 92:2908–13.

27. Epstein J, Yaccoby S. The SCID-hu myeloma model. Methods Mol Med 2005; 113:183–90.

28. Yaccoby S, Epstein J. The proliferative potential of myeloma plasma cells manifest in the SCID-hu host. Blood 1999; 94:3576–82.

29. Yaccoby S, Johnson CL, Mahaffey SC, Wezeman MJ, Barlogie B, Epstein J. Antimyeloma efficacy of thalidomide in the SCID-hu model. Blood 2002; 100: 4162–8.

30. Pearse RN, Sordillo EM, Yaccoby S, et al. Multiple myeloma disrupts the TRANCE/ osteoprotegerin cytokine axis to trigger bone destruction and promote tumor progression. Proc Natl Acad Sci USA 2001; 98:11581–6.

31. Yaccoby S, Pearse RN, Johnson CL, Barlogie B, Choi Y, Epstein J. Myeloma interacts with the bone marrow microenvironment to induce osteoclasto-genesis and is dependent on osteoclast activity. Br J Haematol 2002; 116: 278–90.

32. Sordillo EM, Pearse RN. RANK-Fc: a therapeutic antagonist for RANK-L in myeloma. Cancer 2003; 97:802–12.

33. Hideshima T, Neri P, Tassone P, et al. MLN120B, a novel IkappaB kinase beta inhibitor, blocks multiple myeloma cell growth in vitro and in vivo. Clin Cancer Res 2006; 12:5887–94.

34. Zhu K, Gerbino E, Beaupre DM, et al. Farnesyltransferase inhibitor R115777 (Zarnestra, Tipifarnib) synergizes with paclitaxel to induce apoptosis and mitotic arrest and to inhibit tumor growth of multiple myeloma cells. Blood 2005; 105:4759–66.

35. Tassone P, Goldmacher VS, Neri P, et al. Cytotoxic activity of the maytansinoid immunoconjugate B-B4-DM1 against CD138+ multiple mye-loma cells. Blood 2004; 104:3688–96.

36. Araki K, Sangai T, Miyamoto S, et al. Inhibition of bone-derived insulin-like growth factors by a ligand-specific antibody suppresses the growth of human multiple myeloma in the human adult bone explanted in NOD/SCID mouse. Int J Cancer 2006; 118:2602–8.

37. Tassone P, Neri P, Burger R, et al. Combination therapy with interleukin-6 receptor superantagonist Sant7 and dexamethasone induces antitumor effects in a novel SCID-hu in vivo model of human multiple myeloma. Clin Cancer Res 2005; 11:4251–8.

38. Tassone P, Gozzini A, Goldmacher V, et al. In vitro and in vivo activity of the maytansinoid immunoconjugate huN901-N2'-deacetyl-N2'-(3-mercapto-

1-oxopropyl)-maytansine against CD56+ multiple myeloma cells. Cancer Res 2004; 64:4629–36.

39. Yata K, Yaccoby S. The SCID-rab model: a novel in vivo system for primary human myeloma demonstrating growth of CD138-expressing malignant cells. Leukemia 2004; 18:1891–7.

40. Pilarski LM, Hipperson G, Seeberger K, Pruski E, Coupland RW, Belch AR. Myeloma progenitors in the blood of patients with aggressive or minimal disease: engraftment and self-renewal of primary human myeloma in the bone marrow of NOD SCID mice. Blood 2000; 95:1056–65.

41. Pilarski LM, Seeberger K, Coupland RW, et al. Leukemic B cells clonally identical to myeloma plasma cells are myelomagenic in NOD/SCID mice. Exp Hematol 2002; 30:221–8.

42. Tsunenari T, Koishihara Y, Nakamura A, et al. New xenograft model of multiple myeloma and efficacy of a humanized antibody against human interleukin-6 receptor. Blood 1997; 90:2437–44.

43. Miyakawa Y, Ohnishi Y, Tomisawa M, et al. Establishment of a new model of human multiple myeloma using NOD/SCID/gammac(null) (NOG) mice. Biochem Biophys Res Commun 2004; 313:258–62.

44. Mitsiades CS, Mitsiades NS, McMullan CJ, et al. Inhibition of the insulin-like growth factor receptor-1 tyrosine kinase activity as a therapeutic strategy for multiple myeloma, other hematologic malignancies, and solid tumors. Cancer Cell 2004; 5:221–30.

45. Dewan MZ, Watanabe M, Terashima K, et al. Prompt tumor formation and maintenance of constitutive NF-kappaB activity of multiple myeloma cells in NOD/SCID/gammacnull mice. Cancer Sci 2004; 95:564–8.

46. Wu KD, Cho YS, Katz J, et al. Investigation of antitumor effects of synthetic epothilone analogs in human myeloma models in vitro and in vivo. Proc Natl Acad Sci USA 2005; 102:10640–5.

47. Mitsiades CS, Mitsiades NS, McMullan CJ, et al. Antimyeloma activity of heat shock protein-90 inhibition. Blood 2006; 107:1092–100.

48. Xin X, Abrams TJ, Hollenbach PW, et al. CHIR-258 is efficacious in a newly developed fibroblast growth factor receptor 3-expressing orthotopic multiple myeloma model in mice. Clin Cancer Res 2006; 12:4908–15.

49. Carlo-Stella C, Guidetti A, Di Nicola M, et al. CD52 antigen expressed by malignant plasma cells can be targeted by alemtuzumab in vivo in NOD/SCID mice. Exp Hematol 2006; 34:721–7.

50. Baughn LB, Di Liberto M, Wu K, et al. A novel orally active small molecule potently induces G1 arrest in primary myeloma cells and prevents tumor growth by specific inhibition of cyclin-dependent kinase 4/6. Cancer Res 2006; 66:7661–7.

51. Wu KD, Zhou L, Burtrum D, Ludwig DL, Moore MA. Antibody targeting of the insulin-like growth factor I receptor enhances the anti-tumor response of multiple myeloma to chemotherapy through inhibition of tumor proliferation and angiogenesis. Cancer Immunol Immunother 2007; 56: 343–57.

52. Huang YW, Richardson JA, Tong AW, Zhang BQ, Stone MJ, Vitetta ES. Disseminated growth of a human multiple myeloma cell line in mice with severe combined immunodeficiency disease. Cancer Res 1993; 53:1392–6.

53. Alsina M, Boyce BF, Mundy GR, Roodman GD. An in vivo model of human multiple myeloma bone disease. Stem Cells 1995; 13(Suppl 2):48–50.
54. Alsina M, Boyce B, Devlin RD, et al. Development of an in vivo model of human multiple myeloma bone disease. Blood 1996; 87:1495–501.
55. Bellamy WT, Mendibles P, Bontje P, et al. Development of an orthotopic SCID mouse–human tumor xenograft model displaying the multidrug-resistant phenotype. Cancer Chemother Pharmacol 1996; 37:305–16.
56. Drexler HG, Matsuo Y, MacLeod RA. Persistent use of false myeloma cell lines. Hum Cell 2003; 16:101–5.
57. Pilarski LM, Belch AR. Clonotypic myeloma cells able to xenograft myeloma to nonobese diabetic severe combined immunodeficient mice copurify with CD34(+) hematopoietic progenitors. Clin Cancer Res 2002; 8:3198–204.
58. Tassone P, Neri P, Carrasco DR, et al. A clinically relevant SCID-hu in vivo model of human multiple myeloma. Blood 2005; 106:713–16.
59. Alici E, Konstantinidis KV, Aints A, Dilber MS, Abedi-Valugerdi M. Visualization of 5T33 myeloma cells in the C57BL/KaLwRij mouse: establishment of a new syngeneic murine model of multiple myeloma. Exp Hematol 2004; 32:1064–72.
60. Heath DJ, Vanderkerken K, Cheng X, et al. An osteoprotegerin-like peptidomimetic inhibits osteoclastic bone resorption and osteolytic bone disease in myeloma. Cancer Res 2007; 67:202–8.
61. Potter M. Neoplastic development in plasma cells. Immunol Rev 2003; 194: 177–95.
62. Libouban H, Moreau MF, Basle MF, Bataille R, Chappard D. Increased bone remodeling due to ovariectomy dramatically increases tumoral growth in the 5T2 multiple myeloma mouse model. Bone 2003; 33:283–92.
63. Croucher PI, Shipman CM, Van Camp B, Vanderkerken K. Bisphosphonates and osteoprotegerin as inhibitors of myeloma bone disease. Cancer 2003; 97: 818–24.
64. Asosingh K, Vankerkhove V, Van Riet I, Van Camp B, Vanderkerken K. Selective in vivo growth of lymphocyte function-associated antigen-1-positive murine myeloma cells. Involvement of function-associated antigen-1-mediated homotypic cell-cell adhesion. Exp Hematol 2003; 31:48–55.
65. Asosingh K. Migration, adhesion and differentiation of malignant plasma cells in the 5T murine model of myeloma. Verh K Acad Geneeskd Belg 2003; 65:127–34.
66. Vanderkerken K, Vande Broek I, Eizirik DL, et al. Monocyte chemoattractant protein-1 (MCP-1), secreted by bone marrow endothelial cells, induces chemo-attraction of 5T multiple myeloma cells. Clin Exp Metastasis 2002; 19:87–90.
67. Van Valckenborgh E, De Raeve H, Devy L, et al. Murine 5T multiple myeloma cells induce angiogenesis in vitro and in vivo. Br J Cancer 2002; 86: 796–802.
68. Van Valckenborgh E, Bakkus M, Munaut C, et al. Upregulation of matrix metalloproteinase-9 in murine 5T33 multiple myeloma cells by interaction with bone marrow endothelial cells. Int J Cancer 2002; 101:512–18.
69. Menu E, Braet F, Timmers M, Van Riet I, Van Camp B, Vanderkerken K. The F-actin content of multiple myeloma cells as a measure of their migration. Ann N Y Acad Sci 2002; 973:124–36.

70. Asosingh K, Menu E, Van Valckenborgh E, et al. Mechanisms involved in the differential bone marrow homing of CD45 subsets in 5T murine models of myeloma. Clin Exp Metastasis 2002; 19:583–91.
71. Mittelman M, Neumann D, Peled A, Kanter P, Haran-Ghera N. Erythropoietin induces tumor regression and antitumor immune responses in murine myeloma models. Proc Natl Acad Sci USA 2001; 98:5181–6.
72. Henry JM, Morley AA, Sykes PJ. Purging of myeloma cells using all-trans retinoic acid in a mouse model. Exp Hematol 2001; 29:315–21.
73. Bakkus MH, Asosingh K, Vanderkerken K, et al. Myeloma isotype-switch variants in the murine 5T myeloma model: evidence that myeloma IgM and IgA expressing subclones can originate from the IgG expressing tumour. Leukemia 2001; 15:1127–32.
74. Asosingh K, Gunthert U, De Raeve H, Van Riet I, Van Camp B, Vanderkerken K. A unique pathway in the homing of murine multiple myeloma cells: CD44v10 mediates binding to bone marrow endothelium. Cancer Res 2001; 61:2862–5.
75. Asosingh K, De Raeve H, Croucher P, et al. in vivo homing and differentiation characteristics of mature (CD45–) and immature (CD45+) 5T multiple myeloma cells. Exp Hematol 2001; 29:77–84.
76. Vanderkerken K, Van Camp B, De Greef C, Vande Broek I, Asosingh K, Van Riet I. Homing of the myeloma cell clone. Acta Oncol 2000; 39: 771–6.
77. Vanderkerken K, De Greef C, Asosingh K, et al. Selective initial in vivo homing pattern of 5T2 multiple myeloma cells in the C57BL/KalwRij mouse. Br J Cancer 2000; 82:953–9.
78. Oyajobi BO, Deng JH, Dallas SL, Jenson HB, Mundy GR, Gao SJ. Absence of herpesvirus DNA sequences in the 5T murine model of human multiple myeloma. Br J Haematol 2000; 109:413–19.
79. Asosingh K, Radl J, Van Riet I, Van Camp B, Vanderkerken K. The 5TMM series: a useful in vivo mouse model of human multiple myeloma. Hematol J 2000; 1:351–6.
80. Vanderkerken K, Asosingh K, Braet F, Van Riet I, Van Camp B. Insulin-like growth factor-1 acts as a chemoattractant factor for 5T2 multiple myeloma cells. Blood 1999; 93:235–41.
81. Manning LS, Radin NS. Effects of the glucolipid synthase inhibitor, P4, on functional and phenotypic parameters of murine myeloma cells. Br J Cancer 1999; 81:952–8.
82. Zhu D, van Arkel C, King CA, et al. Immunoglobulin VH gene sequence analysis of spontaneous murine immunoglobulin-secreting B-cell tumours with clinical features of human disease. Immunology 1998; 93: 162–70.
83. Vanderkerken K, De Raeve H, Goes E, et al. Organ involvement and phenotypic adhesion profile of 5T2 and 5T33 myeloma cells in the C57BL/KaLwRij mouse. Br J Cancer 1997; 76:451–60.
84. Vanderkerken K, Goes E, De Raeve H, Radl J, Van Camp B. Follow-up of bone lesions in an experimental multiple myeloma mouse model: description of an in vivo technique using radiography dedicated for mammography. Br J Cancer 1996; 73:1463–5.

85. van den Akker TW, Radl J, Franken-Postma E, Hagemeijer A. Cytogenetic findings in mouse multiple myeloma and Waldenström's macroglobulinemia. Cancer Genet Cytogenet 1996; 86:156–61.

86. Bradley TR, Kriegler AB, Verschoor SM, Tzelepis SM, Cooper IA. Interaction between a murine myeloma cell line and bone marrow stromal cells. Exp Hematol 1996; 24:307–9.

87. Manning LS, Chamberlain NL, Leahy MF, Cordingley FT. Assessment of the therapeutic potential of cytokines, cytotoxic drugs and effector cell populations for the treatment of multiple myeloma using the 5T33 murine myeloma model. Immunol Cell Biol 1995; 73:326–32.

88. Turner JH, Claringbold PG, Manning LS, O'Donoghue HL, Berger JD, Glancy RJ. Radiopharmaceutical therapy of 5T33 murine myeloma by sequential treatment with samarium-153 ethylenediaminetetramethylene phosphonate, melphalan, and bone marrow transplantation. J Natl Cancer Inst 1993; 85:1508–13.

89. Manning LS, Berger JD, O'Donoghue HL, Sheridan GN, Claringbold PG, Turner JH. A model of multiple myeloma: culture of 5T33 murine myeloma cells and evaluation of tumorigenicity in the C57BL/KaLwRij mouse. Br J Cancer 1992; 66:1088–93.

90. Croese JW, Vissinga CS, Boersma WJ, Radl J. Immune regulation of mouse 5T2 multiple myeloma. I. Immune response to 5T2 MM idiotype. Neoplasma 1991; 38:457–66.

91. Croese JW, Van den Enden-Vieveen MH, Radl J. Immune regulation of 5T2 mouse multiple myeloma. II. Immunological treatment of 5T2 MM residual disease. Neoplasma 1991; 38:467–74.

92. Radl J, Punt YA, van den Enden-Vieveen MH, et al. The 5T mouse multiple myeloma model: absence of c-myc oncogene rearrangement in early transplant generations. Br J Cancer 1990; 61:276–8.

93. Croese JW, Vas Nunes CM, Radl J, van den Enden-Vieveen MH, Brondijk RJ, Boersma WJ. The 5T2 mouse multiple myeloma model: characterization of 5T2 cells within the bone marrow. Br J Cancer 1987; 56:555–60.

94. Radl J, Croese JW, Zurcher C, et al. Influence of treatment with APD-bisphosphonate on the bone lesions in the mouse 5T2 multiple myeloma. Cancer 1985; 55:1030–40.

95. Radl J, Hollander CF, van den Berg P, de Glopper E. Idiopathic paraproteinaemia. I. Studies in an animal model—the ageing C57BL/KaLwRij mouse. Clin Exp Immunol 1978; 33:395–402.

96. Menu E, De Leenheer E, De Raeve H, et al. Role of CCR1 and CCR5 in homing and growth of multiple myeloma and in the development of osteolytic lesions: a study in the 5TMM model. Clin Exp Metastasis 2006; 23:291–300.

97. Menu E, Asosingh K, Indraccolo S, et al. The involvement of stromal derived factor 1alpha in homing and progression of multiple myeloma in the 5TMM model. Haematologica 2006; 91:605–12.

98. Asosingh K, De Raeve H, de Ridder M, et al. Role of the hypoxic bone marrow microenvironment in 5T2MM murine myeloma tumor progression. Haematologica 2005; 90:810–17.

99. Croucher PI, De Hendrik R, Perry MJ, et al. Zoledronic acid treatment of 5T2MM-bearing mice inhibits the development of myeloma bone disease:

evidence for decreased osteolysis, tumor burden and angiogenesis, and increased survival. J Bone Miner Res 2003; 18:482–92.

100. Menu E, Jernberg-Wiklund H, Stromberg T, et al. Inhibiting the IGF-1 receptor tyrosine kinase with the cyclolignan PPP: an in vitro and in vivo study in the 5T33MM mouse model. Blood 2006; 107:655–60.

101. Edwards CM, Mueller G, Roelofs AJ, et al. Apominetrade mark, an inhibitor of HMG-CoA-reductase, promotes apoptosis of myeloma cells in vitro and is associated with a modulation of myeloma in vivo. Int J Cancer 2007; 120: 1657–63.

102. Libouban H, Moreau MF, Basle MF, Bataille R, Chappard D. Selection of a highly aggressive myeloma cell line by an altered bone microenvironment in the C57BL/KaLwRij mouse. Biochem Biophys Res Commun 2004; 316: 859–66.

103. Campbell RA, Manyak SJ, Yang HH, et al. LAGlambda-1: a clinically relevant drug resistant human multiple myeloma tumor murine model that enables rapid evaluation of treatments for multiple myeloma. Int J Oncol 2006; 28:1409–17.

104. Kovalchuk AL, Kim JS, Park SS, et al. IL-6 transgenic mouse model for extraosseous plasmacytoma. Proc Natl Acad Sci USA 2002; 99:1509–14.

105. Chiarle R, Gong JZ, Guasparri I, et al. NPM-ALK transgenic mice spontaneously develop T-cell lymphomas and plasma cell tumors. Blood 2003; 101:1919–27.

106. Cheung WC, Kim JS, Linden M, et al. Novel targeted deregulation of c-Myc cooperates with Bcl-X(L) to cause plasma cell neoplasms in mice. J Clin Invest 2004; 113:1763–73.

107. Kim JS, Han SS, Park SS, McNeil N, Janz S. Plasma cell tumour progression in iMycEmu gene-insertion mice. J Pathol 2006; 209:44–55.

108. Carrasco DR, Sukhdeo K, Protopopova M, et al. The stress differentiation and stress response factor XBP-1 drives multiple myeloma pathogenesis. Cancer Cell 2007; 11(4):349–60.

109. Sebag M, Stewart K, Palmer S, Kremer R, Bergsagel PL, Chesi M. A novel transgenic mouse model of multiple myeloma reliably predicts drug response. Blood 2006; 108.

2

The Role of the Bone Marrow Microenvironment in the Pathogenesis of Multiple Myeloma

Teru Hideshima

Department of Medical Oncology, Jerome Lipper Multiple Myeloma Center, Dana-Farber Cancer Institute, Harvard Medical School, Boston, Massachusetts, U.S.A.

Noopur Raje

Jerome Lipper Multiple Myeloma Center, Dana-Farber Cancer Institute, Harvard Medical School and Center for Multiple Myeloma, Massachusetts General Hospital, Boston, Massachusetts, U.S.A.

INTRODUCTION

The bone marrow microenvironment plays a crucial role in multiple myeloma (MM) cell pathogenesis. Specifically, growth advantage, survival, and drug resistance of MM cells can be modulated by various subsets of bone marrow (BM) cell components including BM stromal cells (BMSCs), osteoclasts (OCLs), osteoblasts (OBLs), and vascular endothelial cells. Recognition of the biologic significance of the BM microenvironment as a potential target for novel therapeutics has derived several promising approaches. For example, novel agents including thalidomide, its immuno-modulatory derivatives lenalidomide/Revlimid®, and proteasome inhibitor bortezomib/Velcade® are directed at molecular targets not only in MM cells but also in its BM milieu, and have already achieved promising results both in preclinical and clinical studies.

THE ROLE OF THE BM MICROENVIRONMENT IN MM

The interaction of MM cells with extracellular matrix (ECM) proteins and BM stromal cells (SCs), osteoblasts, osteoclasts, endothelial cells, as well as factors in the BM milieu (cytokines, angiogenesis) plays a crucial role in MM pathogenesis and drug resistance (1–4). The BM microenvironment is composed of heterogeneous cellular components: hematopoietic stem cells; progenitor and precursor cells; immune cells; erythrocytes; BMSCs; BM endothelial cells (ECs); as well as osteoclasts and osteoblasts. These cells not only physically interact with MM cells, but also secrete growth and/or antiapoptotic factors such as interleukin (IL)-6, insulin-like growth factor (IGF)-1, vascular endothelial growth factor (VEGF), and tumor necrosis factor (TNF)-α (2–7).

Within the BM microenvironment, several proliferative/antiapoptotic signaling cascades are activated in MM cells: phosphatidylinositol-3 kinase (PI3K)/Akt; IκB kinase (IKK)/nuclear factor κ-B (NFκB); Ras/Raf/mitogen-activated protein kinase (MAPK) kinase (MEK)/extracellular signal-related kinase (ERK); and Janus kinase (JAK) 2/signal transducers and activators of transcription (STAT)-3 (Fig. 1, Table 1). These signaling cascades mediate: cytoplasmic sequestration of many transcription factors; upregulation of cyclin D and antiapoptotic Bcl-2 family members; as well as augmentation of telomerase activity (2,8). Importantly, these molecular events are triggered by both MM cell adherence to BMSCs and by cytokines

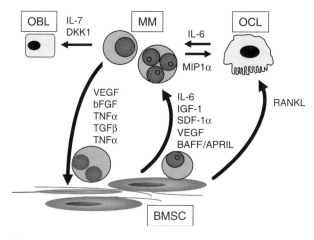

Figure 1 Cytokines and growth factors in the multiple myeloma (MM) bone marrow (BM) milieu. MM cells secrete VEGF, bFGF, TNF-α, TGF-β, and MIP-1α. BMSCs secrete IL-6, VEGF, SDF-1α, BAFF/APRIL, and RANKL. Importantly, cytokines secreted from either MM cells or bone marrow stromal cells (BMSCs) further augment cytokine secretion. For example, TNF-α, VEGF, and TGF-β from MM cells enhance IL-6 secretion from BMSCs. IL-7 and DKK1 From MM cells inhibit osteoblastogenesis. MIP-1α and RANKL trigger osteoclast formation, thereby promoting bone destruction in MM. Osteoclasts also produce IL-6, inducing MM cell growth. *Abbreviations*: OBL, osteoblast; OCL, osteoclast.

Table 1   Differential Effects of Cytokines on Signaling Cascades

Cytokines	p42/44 MAPK	JAK2/STAT3	PI3-K/Akt
IL-6	+	+	+
IGF-1	+	−	+
VEGF	+	−	+
SDF-1α	+	−	+
BAFF	+	−	+

secreted from BMSCs (9–11). Cytokines secreted from MM cells and BMSCs and other cells in turn further augment cytokine secretion from these cells.

Novel, biologically-based treatments target not only the MM cell, but also MM cell–host interactions, cytokines, and their sequelae in the BM milieu. Proteasome inhibitor bortezomib/Velcade® (12–15), as well as thalidomide and its immunomodulatory derivative (IMiD) lenalidomide/Revlimid (16,17), are examples of such agents targeting the tumor cell in its BM milieu which can achieve responses even in refractory, relapsed MM. Preclinical and clinical studies already suggest that these therapies can overcome resistance to conventional therapies, with great promise to improve patient outcome in MM (11,18).

CELL COMPONENTS IN THE BM MICROENVIRONMENT

Bone Marrow Stromal Cells

The interactions of MM cells with the BM microenvironment activates a pleiotropic cascade of proliferative/antiapoptotic signaling cascades: PI3K/Akt (also known as protein kinase B); NF-κB; Ras/Raf/MEK/ERK; and JAK 2/signal transducers and activators of transcription (STAT) 3 (Fig. 1). Downstream sequelae include: cytoplasmic sequestration of many transcription factors (i.e., FKFR); upregulation of cell cycle regulating proteins (i.e., cyclin D) and antiapoptotic proteins, i.e., Bcl-2, Bcl-xL, Mcl-1); and increased activity of telomerase (10) (Fig. 2). These molecular events are triggered either directly, via cell adhesion molecule-mediated interactions of MM cells with BMSCs and ECM; or indirectly, by growth factors released by BMSCs and/or MM cells. Many growth factors also induce pleiotropic effects by stimulating osteoclastogenesis (IL-6, IL-1, VEGF, SDF-1α, MIP-1α) or modulating adhesion molecule profiles on MM cells and BMSCs (TNF-α) (10). Importantly, this growth factor circuit between MM cells and BMSCs in the BM milieu promotes MM cell growth, survival, and migration, contributing to both MM progression and resistance to conventional therapies. Thus, targeting these growth factors can provide the basis for novel treatment strategies.

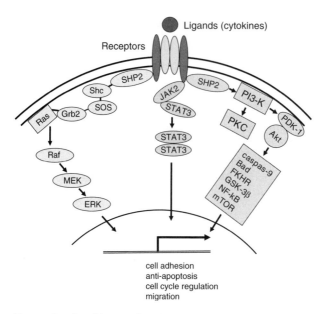

Figure 2 Cytokine-mediated signaling cascades in MM. IL-6 triggers Ras/Raf/ MEK/ERK–mediated proliferation; activates JAK2/STAT3 signaling promoting MM cell survival by regulating Bcl-XL and/or Mcl-1 protein expression; and activates PI3-K/Akt signaling, thereby promoting anti-apoptosis and drug resistance in MM cells. Importantly, these signaling cascades triggered by IL-6 may reduce the effectiveness of conventional chemotherapeutic agents against MM cells in the BM milieu. IGF-1, VEGF, BAFF/APRIL trigger Ras/Raf/MEK/ERK and PI3-K/Akt, but not JAK2/STAT3 signaling.

These bidirectional MM cell–BM interactions have important clinical sequelae including enhanced osteoclastogenesis resulting in osteolytic lesions; as well as MM cell resistance to conventional chemotherapeutic agents, even in the absence of genetic lesions that confer constitutive resistance (12). Importantly, genetic lesions in monoclonal gammopathy of undetermined significance (MGUS)/MM may not only confer enhanced proliferative capacity and/or increased resistance to apoptosis, but also modulate the ability of MM cells to interact with their BM milieu. For example, MM cells with t(14;16) translocations overexpress the transcription factor c-maf which transactivates the cyclin D2 promoter, thereby enhancing MM cell proliferation as well as enhancing β7-integrin expression and tumor cell adhesion to BMSCs (19). Hyperdiploidy renders MM cells uniquely dependent on the BM microenvironment, which induces cyclin D1 overexpression despite absence of Ig translocations (20). These cases highlight the biological significance of specific genetic lesions and pathways mediating MM-microenvironmental interactions.

Bone Marrow Endothelial Cells

Bone marrow endothelial cells (BMECs) are involved in the initial homing of MM cells to the BM stromal compartment, conversely, medullary angiogenesis in active MM is driven by the paracrine activation of BMEC by angiogenic cytokines (i.e., VEGF, FGF) and proteases secreted by myeloma cells, fibroblasts, and osteoclasts. The adhesion between MM cells and BMSCs upregulates many cytokines that have angiogenic activity. In MM cells, these angiogenic factors may also be produced constitutively as a result of oncogene activation and/or genetic mutations. Bone marrow angiogenesis is sustained by VEGF, basic fibroblast growth factor (bFGF), and matrix metalloproteinases (MMPs) secreted by MM cells (21). Conversely, BMECs secrete growth factors, including VEGF and bFGF, promoting MM cell growth in the BM milieu. Importantly, these autocrine and/or paracrine loops in the BM milieu mediate progression of MM. Angiogenesis promotes MM tumor cell growth by enhancing delivery of oxygen and nutrients, removing catabolites, and associated secretion of growth factors for tumor cells from endothelial cells.

Clinical progression of several hematological cancers including non-Hodgkin's lymphomas, lymphoblastic leukemia, B-cell chronic lymphocytic leukemia and acute myeloid leukemia is correlated with the degree of angiogenesis. It has also been demonstrated that BM angiogenesis is a hallmark of MM progression and correlates with disease activity. The level of BM angiogenesis, as assessed by grading and/or microvessel density (MVD), is consistently increased in patients with active MM as compared with those with inactive disease or monoclonal gammopathy of undetermined significance (MGUS). Moreover, within MM, increased MVD in patient BM specimens parallels disease progression and correlates with poor prognosis (21), and BM MVD at diagnosis is an important prognostic factor for survival of patients who undergo autologous transplantation as frontline therapy. BM neovascularization can be also targeted by novel agents. For example, empiric use of thalidomide therapy in MM was based on its antiangiogenic effects, providing further evidence of the role of angiogenesis in MM progression (22). Thalidomide inhibits secretion of VEGF, bFGF, and hepatocyte growth factor (HGF) as well as proliferation and capillarogenesis in patient BMECs (23–25).

Osteoclast

The increase of osteoclast activation and formation is mainly involved in the development of osteolytic bone lesions that characterize MM patients. It is well known that MM cells enhance osteoclast activity (26,27). Specifically, the osteclastgenesis is increased adjacent to MM cells, which results in enhanced bone resorption. However, the biologic mechanisms involved in the pathogenesis of MM-induced bone disease are not totally understood.

Two major factors produced by stromal-osteoblastic cells regulate bone resorption: osteoprotegerin (OPG) and receptor activator of NF-κB ligand (RANKL). OPG is a member of the TNF receptor family, which binds to the ligand for RANK and inhibits bone resorption. RANKL stimulates osteoclast differentiation and activity, whereas OPG inhibits these processes (28,29). BMSCs secrete OPG, which prevents excessive activation of osteoclasts by serving as a decoy receptor and competing with RANK for binding to RANKL. Blockade of RANKL binding to RANK receptor by either a soluble form of the RANK receptor or OPG inhibits osteoclast maturation and bone destruction in a mouse MM model (30); in contrast, ligation of vascular cell adhesion molecule 1 (VCAM-1) on BMSCs via α4β1 integrin on MM cells decreases secretion of OPG and increases expression of RANKL, thereby promoting osteolysis (31,32) (Fig. 1). Furthermore, OPG may function as a paracrine survival factor in MM in the BM microenvironment (33). Importantly, myeloma cells affect the OPG/RANKL ratio in the BM environment, promoting bone disease (34).

The interaction of RANK on osteoclasts with RANKL on osteoblasts and BMSCs, as well as macrophage inflammatory protein-1α (MIP-1α) secreted by MM cells, play important roles in mediating bone destruction in MM (35). MIP-1 α is a potent inducer of osteoclast formation, independently of RANKL, and enhances both RANKL- and IL-6-stimulated osteoclast formation (36). Levels of MIP-1α in patient BM plasma are elevated and correlate with osteolytic lesions. Moreover, blocking expression of MIP-1α using antisense oligonucleotide decreases bone destruction and adherence to BM stromal cells, as well as MM tumor burden in a murine model of MM (36). Importantly, osteoclasts produce a variety of factors that stimulate growth of MM cells, including IL-6 (37). These findings suggest that paracrine loops between osteoclasts and MM cells confer MM cell growth, as well as bone destruction, in the BM milieu. Moreover, the direct production of the MIP-1α by MM cells, in combination with the RANKL induction in BMSCs in response to MM cells, are critical in osteoclast activation and osteoclastogenesis (38). A recent study demonstrated that MIP-1α utilizes either CCR1 or CCR5 for its effects on OCL formation and MM cells, and that blocking either CCR1 or CCR5 inhibits OCL formation and MM cell adhesion to stromal cells (39). Most recently, requirement of p38 MAPK in osteoclast formation via modulation of IL-11, RANKL, and MIP-1α has also been demonstrated (40). Chondroitin synthase 1 has been shown to be a key molecule in cell–osteoclast interactions (41).

Osteoblast

In addition to activated osteclastgenesis, lower activity of osteoblasts may also contribute to osteolytic lesion in MM patients. The formation and differentiation of osteoblastic cells from mesenchymal stem cells require the activity and function of the transcription factor Runx2/Cbfa1 (42–44). The effect of MM cells on Runx2/Cbfa1 activity appears to be primarily mediated by cell-to-cell contact between MM cells and osteoprogenitor cells. This cell-to-cell contact involves interactions between very late antigen-4 (VLA-4) on MM cells and VCAM-1 on osteoblast progenitors, as demonstrated by the capacity of a neutralizing anti-VLA-4 antibody to reduce the inhibitory effects of MM cells on Runx2/Cbfa1 activity (45).

Soluble factors may also contribute to the inhibitory effects of MM cells on osteoblast differentiation and Runx2/Cbfa1 activity. Canonical Wingless-type (Wnt) signaling pathway has recently been shown to play an important role in osteoblast differentiation. Dickkopf 1 (DKK1) is a Wnt inhibitor, and BM-biopsy specimens show detectable DKK1 in MM cells. Moreover, elevated DKK1 levels in MM plasma and peripheral blood from patients with MM are associated with focal bone lesions. Importantly, recombinant human DKK1 or BM serum containing elevated levels of DKK1 inhibits the differentiation of osteoblast precursor cells in vitro, suggesting that production of DKK1 is an inhibitor of osteoblast differentiation (46) (Fig. 1).

Although IL-3 has been shown to stimulate osteoclast activity, a recent study has reported that IL-3 inhibited basal and bone morphogenic protein-2 (BMP-2)-stimulated osteoblast formation, without affecting cell growth. In contrast, anti-IL-3 Ab blocks this effect, suggesting that IL-3 plays a role in the bone destructive process in MM by inhibiting osteoblast formation (47). Besides DKK1, MM cell lines and patient MM cells constitutively produce a soluble Wnt inhibitor Frizzled-related protein 2 (sFRP-2), which significantly suppresses osteoblast differentiation (48). We have previously shown that TGF-β from MM cells augment IL-6 secretion from BMSCs (49). Similarly, TGF-β also enhances IL-6 secretion from osteoblasts (50). Importantly, OPG and OPGL produced by stromal-osteoblastic cells have a critical role in regulation of osteoblastogenesis. HGF can be produced by MM cells, and high concentrations of HGF are often found in MM patient BM. There is a negative correlation between HGF and bone specific alkaline phosphatase, a marker of osteoblast activity, in sera from MM patients. Moreover, HGF can directly inhibit osteoblastogenesis in vitro (51). Of note, osteoblasts can be activated by proteasome inhibitors (52–54).

BIOLOGIC IMPACT OF CELL ADHESION OF MM CELLS TO THE BM COMPONENTS

The homing of MM cells to the BM is mediated by the interaction of MM cells and BMSCs via adhesion molecules. Adhesion molecules mediate both homotypic and heterotypic adhesion of MM cells to either ECM proteins or BMSCs. Adhesion molecules CD44, VLA-4, (CD49d), VLA-5 (CD49e), leukocyte function-associated antigen-1 (LFA-1, CD11a), neuronal adhesion molecule (NCAM, CD56), intercellular adhesion molecule (ICAM-1, CD54), syndecan-1 (CD138), and MPC-1 mediate homing of MM cells to the BM. Specifically, tumor cells bind to ECM proteins, i.e., via syndecan-1 and VLA-4 on MM cells to type I collagen and fibronectin, respectively, and to BMSCs, i.e., via VLA-4 on MM cells to VCAM-1 (CD106) on BMSCs. This MM cell adherence to BMSCs not only localizes tumor cells in the BM microenvironment, but also has important functional sequelae. Elevated serum soluble syndecan-1 correlates with increased tumor cell mass, decreased metalloproteinase-9 activity, and poor prognosis (55). Furthermore, adhesion of MM cells via syndecan-1 to collagen induces matrix metalloproteinase-1, thereby promoting bone resorption and tumor invasion. Moreover, binding via VLA-4 on MM cells to the fibronectin upregulates $p27^{Kip1}$ and other genetic changes in tumor cells, which confer cell adhesion-mediated drug resistance (CAM-DR) (1,56–58).

Adhesion of MM cells to BMSCs (i.e., via VLA-4 on MM cells to VCAM-1 on BMSCs) triggers NFκB-dependent transcription and secretion of IL-6 in BMSCs; conversely, inhibition of NFκB activity abrogates this response (5,59). Importantly, binding via VLA-4 on MM cells to the ECM protein fibronectin triggers up-regulation of $p27^{Kip1}$ and other genetic changes conferring CAM-DR. Moreover, MM cells localized in the BM milieu secrete cytokines such as TNF-α, TGF-β, and VEGF, which further up-regulate IL-6 secretion from BMSCs (9,49,59,60). NFκB mediates expression of many adhesion molecules expressed on both MM cells and BMSCs. Activation of NFκB by cell adhesion and cytokines (i.e., TNF-α) increases binding of MM cells to BMSCs, which in turn upregulates IL-6 transcription and secretion in BMSCs (59). Specifically, interaction of CD40–CD40L (CD40 ligand) upregulates adhesion molecules (i.e., LFA-1, VLA-4), translocating nuclear Ku86/Ku70 to the cell membrane, where it augments adhesion, thereby increasing IL-6 and VEGF secretion in BMSCs (61). Conversely, blocking interaction of CD40 and CD40L by anti-CD40 antibodies SGN-40 or CHIR-12.12 inhibits MM cell adhesion to fibronectin and BMSCs, decreasing IL-6 and VEGF secretion from BMSCs (62,63). Novel agents proteasome inhibitors, thalidomide, and IMiDs can overcome CAM-DR and the growth advantage conferred by the BM, and therefore hold great promise to overcome conventional drug resistance and improve patient outcome (18).

ROLE OF GROWTH FACTORS IN THE BM MILIEU

IL-6

IL-6 was originally described as a factor that induced differentiation of normal B cells to plasma cells and promoted MM cell growth (64). Specifically, reports support an autocrine IL-6-mediated growth mechanism in MM, since some MM cells and derived cell lines both produce and respond to IL-6 in vitro (64). Autocrine IL-6 production is associated with a highly malignant phenotype, high proliferative index, and resistance to drug-induced apoptosis (65). IL-6 has been implicated in both autocrine and paracrine growth of MM cells within the BM milieu. Importantly, serum IL-6 and IL-6 receptors are prognostic factors in MM and reflect the proliferative fraction of MM cells within patients (66,67).

IL-6 is a potent survival and antiapoptotic factor in MM cells *via* activation of at least 3 major signaling cascades. The first step of IL-6-mediated signaling is triggered by IL-6 binding to IL-6R/gp80, which subsequently induces phosphorylation and homodimerization of gp130 (68). After gp130 phosphorylation, three major signaling cascades including Ras/Raf/MEK/ERK, JAK2/STAT3, and PI3K/Akt pathway are activated. IL-6-induced proliferation is mediated by activation of Ras/Raf/MEK/ERK signaling cascade (69,70). Survival of MM cells triggered by IL-6 is conferred via JAK2/STAT3 signaling by up-regulating downstream antiapoptotic Bcl-XL and Mcl-1 protein expression (71). Mcl-1 is essential for the survival of human MM cells in vitro (72) and is overexpressed in tumor cells in patients with relapsed or poor prognosis MM (73), suggesting JAK2/STAT3 signaling cascade as a novel therapeutic target in MM. PI3K/Akt signaling mediates cell growth through its effects on mammalian target of rapamycin (mTOR)/p70 S6 kinase pathway, and modulates cell cycle and proliferation both via its direct activity on cyclin-dependent kinase inhibitors $p21^{WAF1/Cip1}$ and $p27^{Kip1}$, as well as indirectly by affecting the levels of p53 and cyclin D1. Akt is also a major factor which inhibits proapoptotic proteins Bad and caspase-9, as well as modulates p53, NFκB, and telomerase (74,75) (Table 1, Fig. 2). Specifically, dexamethasone-induced apoptosis is completely blocked by IL-6 via Akt activation (8).

Importantly, most IL-6 in the BM milieu is secreted by BMSCs, and its transcription and secretion in BMSCs are further augmented both by binding of tumor cells to BMSCs (76) and by secretion of cytokines (TNF-α, VEGF, and TGF-β) within the BM microenvironment (77). We have shown that both MM cell adhesion and TNF -induced IL-6 secretion in BMSCs is mediated via NFκB activation (5); conversely, inhibition of NFκB activity by specific IκB kinase inhibitor downregulates IL-6 secretion from BMSCs and related tumor cell growth (78). Of note, novel agents including proteasome inhibitor bortezomib and immunomodulatory agent lenalidomide can abrogate the growth, survival, and drug resistance induced by IL-6 and thereby overcome conventional drug resistance (12,16).

Insulin-Like Growth Factor-1

Insulin-like growth factor-1 (IGF-1) is a multifunctional peptide that regulates cell proliferation, differentiation, and apoptosis (79–83). In the circulation, IGF-1 binds predominantly to the main IGF binding protein, IGFBP-3. Although several studies suggest that high concentrations of circulating IGF-1 are associated with an increased risk of several cancers, the direct relationship of serum IGF-1 level and prognosis in MM has not yet been clarified.

Recent studies have delineated the biologic sequelae of IGF-1 in MM cells. IGF-1 mediates MM cell growth and survival in MM cells both in vitro (80,84) and in vivo (81). In contrast to IL-6, IGF-1 activates only Ras/Raf/MEK/ERK and PI3K/Akt signaling, but not JAK2/STAT3 pathways, via type1 IGF receptor (85) (Table 1, Fig. 2). IGF-1 stimulates sustained activation of PI3K/Akt (more potent than IL-6) and NFκB; induces phosphorylation of FKHR transcription factor; upregulates a series of intracellular antiapoptotic proteins including FLIP, survivin, cIAP-2, A1/Bfl-1, and XIAP; thereby decreasing drug sensitivity of MM cells (80). The antiapoptotic effect of IGF-1 has also been studied using an in vitro model system of MM cells in the BM milieu. Like IL-6, IGF-1 inhibits dexamethasone-induced apoptosis in MM cells by activation of ERK and PI3K/Akt signaling pathways (77). IGF-1 also attenuates anti-MM activity of other antitumor drugs, including cytotoxic chemotherapy and proteasome inhibitors (81).

Vascular Endothelial Growth Factor

VEGF is a known angiogenic factor not only in solid tumors, but also in hematologic malignancies (86). In MM, VEGF is produced both by MM cells and BMSCs (87,88) and may account, at least in part, for the increased angiogenesis observed in MM patient BM. Although MVD in the BM in MM patients correlates with progression of disease, direct evidence linking VEGF level and prognosis in MM patients is not firmly established (89).

Our recent studies show that some MM cell lines and patient cells express VEGF receptor Flt-1, and that VEGF triggers its phosphorylation, ERK activation, and proliferation (87,88), which can be neutralized by either antibody to VEGF or the VEGF receptor tyrosine kinase inhibitors (90,91). We have shown that VEGF upregulates Mcl-1 expression in MM cell lines and MM patient cells; conversely, pan-VEGF inhibitor abrogates VEGF induced-upregulation of Mcl-1, associated with decreased proliferation and induction of apoptosis (92). In MM, migration is necessary for tumor cell homing to the BM, expansion within the BM microenvironment, and egress into the peripheral blood. VEGF-induced migration of MM cells is associated with PI3K-dependent protein kinase C (PKC) α activation and is abrogated by bisindolylmaleimide or neutralizing antibody to VEGF (88). VEGF also triggers Src-dependent phosphorylation of caveolin-1, which is required for p130^{Cas} phosphorylation and MM cell migration. These direct effects of VEGF on tumor cells, coupled with its induction of cytokines (i.e., IL-6) and angiogenesis in the BM milieu, provide the framework for targeting VEGF in treatment strategies.

Tumor Necrosis Factor-α

Circulating tumor necrosis factor-α (TNF-α) levels are higher in MM patients with overt bone disease, whose osteoblasts constitutively over-express Fas, DR4/DR5 complex as receptors for TNF-related apoptosis-inducing ligand and intercellular adhesion molecule-1 (ICAM-1) (93). Although TNF-α secreted by tumor cells does not induce significant growth or drug resistance in MM cells, TNF-α is the most potent inducer of NFκB activation and IL-6 secretion from BMSCs (59). NFκB is a transcriptional factor which regulates transcription of a number of cytokines, chemokines, cell adhesion molecules, as well as antiapoptotic and cellular growth control proteins (94).

NFκB is typically a heterodimer composed of p50 (NFκB1) and p65 (RelA) subunits, and its activity is regulated by association with IκB family proteins (typically IκBα). After stimulation by TNF-α, IκBα protein is phosphorylated by IκB kinase (IKK), typically IKKβ. Phosphorylated IκBα is subsequently ubiquitinated and degraded by the 26S proteasome, thereby inducing p50/p65 NFκB nuclear translocation to modulate gene transcription, including adhesion molecules (95,96). TNF-α therefore upregulates adhesion molecules on both MM cells and BMSCs, thereby increasing binding of MM cells and resultant induction of IL-6 transcription and secretion in BMSCs, and CAM-DR (97). Novel agents targeting TNF-α signaling, including thalidomide and IMiDs (98), may act, at least in part, by inhibiting NFκB activity. Recent studies demonstrated that expression of the osteoblast differentiation factor RUNX2/Cbfa1 can be inhibited by TNF-α (99).

Fibroblast Growth Factor

MM cells express and secrete fibroblast growth factor (FGF), a potent angiogenic cytokine which contributes to the increased angiogenic potential of BM plasma cells in progressive MM (21). BMSCs from MM patients and control subjects express high-affinity FGF receptors R1 through R4. Importantly, stimulation of BMSCs with bFGF induces a time- and dose-dependent increase in IL-6 secretion; in turn, stimulation with IL-6 enhances bFGF expression and secretion by MM cell lines, as well as patient MM cells (100). These data suggest paracrine interaction of IL-6 and bFGF between MM and BMSCs triggering not only neovascularization, but also MM cell growth and survival, in the BM microenvironment. In MM, dysregulation of FGF receptor 3 (FGFR3) by the t(4;14) translocation is a primary event in 10–20% MM patients and confers poor prognosis (101).

Recent studies have demonstrated that FGFR3 inhibitors induce cytotoxicity in primary MM tumor cells with t(4;14) (102,103), and clinical trials of FGFR3 inhibitor therapies are now under way.

Stromal Cell–Derived Factor-1α

Chemokines play an important role in lymphocyte trafficking and homing. Stromal cell–derived factor-1α (SDF-1α) is a ligand of CXCR4 and mediates migration of normal hematopoietic stem cells. We and others found that both MM cell lines and patient tumor cells express CXCR4. We have also shown SDF-1α in BM plasma from patients with MM and in supernatants from MM patient BMSCs. Interestingly, Gazitt et al (104) reported that levels of both SDF-1α and surface expression of CXCR4 significantly decrease on MM cells in four consecutive apheresis collections, compared with premobilization BM specimens. Of note, SDF-1α expression is regulated, at least in part, by TGF-β. SDF-1α promotes proliferation, induces migration, and protects against dex-induced apoptosis in MM cells (105). SDF-1α triggered signaling cascade was first reported in hematopoietic progenitor cells, in which it activated Jak2 and tyrosine phosphorylation of focal adhesion proteins and migration (106). In MM cells, SDF-1α activates MAPK, PI3-K/Akt, and NF-κB (105) (Table 1, Fig. 2). Within the BM microenvironment, SDF-1α upregulates secretion of VEGF in BMSCs, thereby promoting tumor cell growth, survival, drug resistance, migration and protects against dex-induced apoptosis (107).

Wnt

Wnts comprise a family of secreted proteins that interact with receptors, consisting of a Frizzled (Fz) family member alone or complexed with LDL receptor-related proteins (LRP5/6). Wnt signaling regulates various developmental processes and can lead to malignant formation. Intracellularly, the Wnt signaling cascade blocks degradation of β-catenin by proteasomes, thereby leading to accumulation of β-catenin in the cytoplasm (108). In MM, a canonical Wnt signaling pathway is activated following treatment with Wnt-3a, associated with accumulation of β-catenin. Wnt-3a treatment further led to significant morphological changes in MM cells, accompanied by rearrangement of the actin cytoskeleton. Derksen et al. demonstrated that MM cells overexpress β-catenin, including its N-terminally unphosphorylated form, consistent with active β-catenin/T cell factor-mediated transcription. Further accumulation and nuclear localization of β-catenin, and/or increased cell proliferation, was achieved by stimulation of Wnt signaling with either Wnt-3a, LiCl, or the constitutively active mutant of β-catenin (109). Importantly, MM cells in BM-biopsy specimens contained detectable DKK1, a negative regulator of Wnt signaling cascade and a target of the β-catenin/TCF pathway. Moreover, elevated DKK1 levels in BM plasma and peripheral blood from patients with MM correlated with the DKK1 gene-expression patterns and were associated with the presence of focal bone lesions (46).

Transforming Growth Factor-β

Transforming growth factor-β (TGF-β) is secreted by MM cells and triggers IL-6 secretion in BMSCs, thereby augmenting paracrine IL-6 related tumor cell growth in the BM milieu (49). TGF-β secreted by MM cells likely also contributes to the immunodeficiency characteristic of MM by down-regulating B cells, T cells, and natural killer cells, without similarly inhibiting the growth of MM cells. Our recent studies demonstrated that TGF-β receptor tyrosine kinase inhibitor SD-208 significantly inhibits not only transcription, but also secretion, of both IL-6 and VEGF from BMSCs triggered by either TGF-β1 or adhesion of MM cells to BMSCs. Moreover, SD-208 decreased tumor cell growth triggered by MM cell adhesion to BMSCs, suggesting that TGF-β mediates, at least in part, MM cell growth, survival, drug resistance, and migration in the BM milieu (110).

Notch

Notch is a transmembrane protein that plays a critical role in the determination of cellular differentiation pathways. Although its importance in the development of mesenchymal tissues has been suggested, its role in MM cells has not been clarified. Moreover, the effect of Notch signaling in promoting MM cell growth is still unclear. Signaling induced by interaction between the receptor Notch and its ligand (delta-1, Jagged-1 and Jagged-2) plays an important role in cell fate determination in vertebrates. Notch receptors and their ligand Jagged-1 are highly expressed both on MM cell lines and primary MM cells. Ligand-induced Notch signaling promotes MM cell growth, suggesting that this interaction contributes to MM pathogenesis in vivo (111). However, another study reported that overexpression of Notch-1 in Notch-1(-) U266 MM cells upregulates p21^{WAF1} and induces growth arrest, protecting against drug-induced apoptosis (112). Moreover, Notch-induced growth arrest and apoptosis has also been demonstrated in B cells, as well as MM cells (113). Interestingly, IL-6 secretion from BMSC was blocked in vitro by interference with anti-Notch-1 monoclonal antibodies (114), suggesting that inhibition of Notch signaling may block antiapoptotic effect of IL-6 in the BM milieu.

B-Cell Activating Factor

B-cell activating factor (BAFF) (also known as BLyS) is a TNF family member cytokine which is essential for B cell generation and maintenance

(115,116). Three receptors have been identified that bind to BAFF: transmembrane activator, calcium modulator, and cyclophilin ligand interactor (TACI); B cell maturation Ag (BCMA); and BAFF-R. MM cells express these three receptors (117). In the BM milieu, BAFF is secreted from BMSCs and osteoclast (118,119), which can be augmented by MM cell adhesion (118). Importantly, BAFF promotes MM cell proliferation and inhibits Dex-induced apoptosis (120,121). A recent study has shown an increase in adhesion of MM cells to BMSCs, which is primarily mediated via activation of Akt and NF-κB signaling (118).

Other Cytokines

A variety of other cytokines including IL-1β, IL-11, IL-15, IL-21, and leukemia inhibitory factor 1 have been reported to play a role in MM pathogenesis (77). These growth factors can be targeted in novel treatment strategies. In fact, novel therapies including proteasome inhibitor bortezomib/Velcade as well as thalidomide and its analog lenalidomide/ Revlimid, target not only MM cells but also their BM microenvironment (10,11,122).

CONCLUSION

A new treatment paradigm is evolving in MM based upon using novel agents to target not only the MM cells, but also the MM cell–host interaction and BM milieu. These novel agents, used alone or in combination with conventional or other novel agents, offer great promise to improve patient outcome. Importantly, genomic and proteomic evaluation of MM cells from patients treated on clinical protocols with these novel agents will define the molecular mechanisms of tumor cell sensitivity versus resistance, thereby providing the framework for developing next generation more selective and potent, as well as less toxic, targeted MM therapies.

REFERENCES

1. Damiano JS, Cress AE, Hazlehurst LA, Shtil AA, Dalton WS. Cell adhesion mediated drug resistance (CAM-DR): role of integrins and resistance to apoptosis in human myeloma cell lines. Blood 1999; 93:1658–67.
2. Akiyama M, Hideshima T, Hayashi T, et al. Cytokines modulate telomerase activity in a human multiple myeloma cell line. Cancer Res 2002; 62:3876–82.
3. Chauhan D, Li G, Hideshima T, Podar K, et al. Blockade of ubiquitin-conjugating enzyme CDC34 enhances anti-myeloma activity of bortezomib/ proteasome inhibitor PS-341. Oncogene 2004; 23:3597–602.
4. Hideshima T, Catley L, Yasui H, et al. Perifosine, an oral bioactive novel alkylphospholipid, inhibits Akt and induces in vitro and in vivo cytotoxicity in human multiple myeloma cells. Blood 2006; 107:4053–62.

5. Chauhan D, Uchiyama H, Akbarali Y, et al. Multiple myeloma cell adhesion-induced interleukin-6 expression in bone marrow stromal cells involves activation of NF-kB. Blood 1996; 87:1104–12.
6. Chauhan D, Catley L, Li G, et al. A novel orally active proteasome inhibitor induces apoptosis in multiple myeloma cells with mechanisms distinct from Bortezomib. Cancer Cell 2005; 8:407–19.
7. Catley L, Tai YT, Shringarpure R, et al. Proteasomal degradation of topoisomerase I is preceded by c-Jun NH2-terminal kinase activation, Fas up-regulation, and poly(ADP-ribose) polymerase cleavage in SN38-mediated cytotoxicity against multiple myeloma. Cancer Res 2004; 64:8746–53.
8. Hideshima T, Nakamura N, Chauhan D, Anderson KC. Biologic sequelae of interleukin-6 induced PI3-K/Akt signaling in multiple myeloma. Oncogene 2001; 20:5991–6000.
9. Dankbar B, Padro T, Leo R, et al. Vascular endothelial growth factor and interleukin-6 in paracrine tumor-stromal cell interactions in multiple myeloma. Blood 2000; 95:2630–6.
10. Hideshima T, Bergsagel PL, Kuehl WM, Anderson KC. Advances in biology of multiple myeloma: clinical applications. Blood 2004; 104:607–18.
11. Mitsiades CS, Mitsiades N, Munshi NC, Anderson KC. Focus on multiple myeloma. Cancer Cell 2004; 6:439–44.
12. Hideshima T, Richardson P, Chauhan D, et al. The proteasome inhibitor PS-341inhibits growth, induces apoptosis, and overcomes drug resistance in human multiple myeloma cells. Cancer Res 2001; 61:3071–6.
13. Richardson PG, Barlogie B, Berenson J, et al. A phase 2 study of bortezomib in relapsed, refractory myeloma. N Engl J Med 2003; 348:2609–17.
14. Richardson PG, Sonneveld P, Schuster MW, et al. Bortezomib or high-dose dexamethasone for relapsed multiple myeloma. N Engl J Med 2005; 352: 2487–98.
15. Richardson PG, Briemberg H, Jagannath S, et al. Frequency, characteristics, and reversibility of peripheral neuropathy during treatment of advanced multiple myeloma with bortezomib. J Clin Oncol 2006; 24:3113–20.
16. Hideshima T, Chauhan D, Shima Y, et al. Thalidomide and its analogues overcome drug resistance of human multiple myeloma cells to conventional therapy. Blood 2000; 96:2943–50.
17. Richardson PG, Blood E, Mitsiades CS, et al. A randomized phase 2 study of lenalidomide therapy for patients with relapsed or relapsed and refractory multiple myeloma. Blood 2006; 108:3458–64.
18. Hideshima T. Anderson KC. Molecular mechanisms of novel therapeutic approaches for multiple myeloma. Nat Rev Cancer 2002; 2:927–37.
19. Hurt EM, Wiestner A, Rosenwald A, et al. Overexpression of c-maf is a frequent oncogenic event in multiple myeloma that promotes proliferation and pathological interactions with bone marrow stroma. Cancer Cell 2004; 5:191–9.
20. Bergsagel PL, Kuehl WM, Zhan F, Sawyer J, Barlogie B, Shaughnessy J Jr. Cyclin D dysregulation: an early and unifying pathogenic event in multiple myeloma. Blood 2005; 106:296–303.
21. Vacca A, Ribatti D, Presta M, et al. Bone marrow neovascularization, plasma cell angiogenic potential, and matrix metalloproteinase-2 secretion parallel progression of human multiple myeloma. Blood 1999; 93:3064–73.

22. Singhal S, Mehta J, Desikan R, et al. Antitumor activity of thalidomide in refractory multiple myeloma. N Engl J Med 1999; 341:1565–71.
23. Vacca A, Ria R, Semeraro F, et al. Endothelial cells in the bone marrow of patients with multiple myeloma. Blood 2003; 102:3340–8.
24. Vacca A, Scavelli C, Montefusco V, et al. Thalidomide downregulates angiogenic genes in bone marrow endothelial cells of patients with active multiple myeloma. J Clin Oncol 2005; 23:5334–46.
25. Ribatti D. Vacca A. Novel therapeutic approaches targeting vascular endothelial growth factor and its receptors in haematological malignancies. Curr Cancer Drug Targets 2005; 5:573–8.
26. Mundy GR, Raisz LG, Cooper RA, Schecter GP, Salmon SE. Evidence for the secretion of an osteoclast stimulating factor in myeloma. N Engl J Med 1974; 291:1041–6.
27. Yaccoby S, Pearse RN, Johnson CL, Barlogie B, Choi Y, Epstein J. Myeloma interacts with the bone marrow microenvironment to induce osteoclastogenesis and is dependent on osteoclast activity. Br J Haematol 2002; 116: 278–90.
28. Sezer O, Heider U, Zavrski I, Kuhne CA, Hofbauer LC. RANK ligand and osteoprotegerin in myeloma bone disease. Blood 2003; 101:2094–8.
29. Hofbauer LC. Schoppet M. Clinical implications of the osteoprotegerin/RANKL/RANK system for bone and vascular diseases. JAMA 2004; 292: 490–5.
30. Croucher PI, Shipman CM, Lippitt J, et al. Osteoprotegerin inhibits the development of osteolytic bone disease in multiple myeloma. Blood 2001; 98: 3534–40.
31. Michigami T, Shimizu N, Williams PJ, et al. Cell–cell contact between marrow stromal cells and myeloma cells via VCAM-1 and α4β1-integrin enhances production of osteoclast-stimulating activity. Blood 2000; 96: 1953–60.
32. Pearse RN, Sordillo EM, Yaccoby S, et al. Multiple myeloma disrupts the TRANCE/osteoprotegerin cytokine axis to trigger bone destruction and promote tumor progression. Proc Natl Acad Sci USA 2001; 98:11581–6.
33. Shipman CM. Croucher PI. Osteoprotegerin is a soluble decoy receptor for tumor necrosis factor-related apoptosis-inducing ligand/Apo2 ligand and can function as a paracrine survival factor for human myeloma cells. Cancer Res 2003; 63:912–16.
34. Giuliani N, Bataille R, Mancini C, Lazzaretti M, Barille S. Myeloma cells induce imbalance in the osteoprotegerin/osteoprotegerin ligand system in the human bone marrow environment. Blood 2001; 98:3527–33.
35. Roodman GD. Pathogenesis of myeloma bone disease. Blood Cells Mol Dis 2004; 32:290–2.
36. Choi SJ, Oba Y, Gazitt Y, et al. Antisense inhibition of macrophage inflammatory protein 1-α blocks bone destruction in a model of myeloma bone disease. J Clin Invest 2001; 108:1833–41.
37. Roodman GD, Kurihara N, Ohsaki Y, et al. Interleukin 6. A potential autocrine/paracrine factor in Paget's disease of bone. J Clin Invest 1992; 89: 46–52.

38. Giuliani N, Colla S, Rizzoli V. New insight in the mechanism of osteoclast activation and formation in multiple myeloma: focus on the receptor activator of NF-κB ligand (RANKL). Exp Hematol 2004; 32:685–91.
39. Oba Y, Lee JW, Ehrlich LA, Chung HY, et al. MIP-1α utilizes both CCR1 and CCR5 to induce osteoclast formation and increase adhesion of myeloma cells to marrow stromal cells. Exp Hematol 2005; 33:272–8.
40. Nguyen AN, Stebbins EG, Henson M, et al. Normalizing the bone marrow microenvironment with p38 inhibitor reduces multiple myeloma cell proliferation and adhesion and suppresses osteoclast formation. Exp Cell Res 2006; 312:1909–23.
41. Yin L. Chondroitin synthase 1 is a key molecule in myeloma cell–osteoclast interactions. J Biol Chem 2005; 280:15666–72.
42. Ducy P, Zhang R, Geoffroy V, Ridall AL, Karsenty G. Osf2/Cbfa1: a transcriptional activator of osteoblast differentiation. Cell 1997; 89:747–54.
43. Karsenty G, Ducy P, Starbuck M, et al. Cbfa1 as a regulator of osteoblast differentiation and function. Bone 1999; 25:107–8.
44. Giuliani N, Rizzoli V, Roodman GD. Multiple myeloma bone disease: pathophysiology of osteoblast inhibition. Blood 2006; 108:3992–6.
45. Giuliani N, Colla S, Morandi F, et al. Myeloma cells block RUNX2/CBFA1 activity in human bone marrow osteoblast progenitors and inhibit osteoblast formation and differentiation. Blood 2005; 106:2472–83.
46. Tian E, Zhan F, Walker R, et al. The role of the Wnt-signaling antagonist DKK1 in the development of osteolytic lesions in multiple myeloma. N Engl J Med 2003; 349:2483–94.
47. Ehrlich LA, Chung HY, Ghobrial I, et al. IL-3 is a potential inhibitor of osteoblast differentiation in multiple myeloma. Blood 2005; 106:1407–14.
48. Oshima T, Abe M, Asano J, et al. Myeloma cells suppress bone formation by secreting a soluble Wnt inhibitor, sFRP-2. Blood 2005; 106:3160–5.
49. Urashima M, Ogata A, Chauhan D, et al. Transforming growth factor β1: differential effects on multiple myeloma versus normal B cells. Blood 1996; 87:1928–38.
50. Franchimont N, Rydziel S, Canalis E. Transforming growth factor-β increases interleukin-6 transcripts in osteoblasts. Bone 2000; 26:249–53.
51. Standal T, Abildgaard N, Fagerli UM, et al. HGF inhibits BMP-induced osteoblastogenesis: possible implications for the bone disease of multiple myeloma. Blood 2006; 109:3024–30.
52. Murray, EJ1, Bentley GV, Grisanti MS, Murray SS. The ubiquitin-proteasome system and cellular proliferation and regulation in osteoblastic cells. Exp Cell Res 1998; 242:460–9.
53. Garrett IR, Chen D, Gutierrez G, et al. Selective inhibitors of the osteoblast proteasome stimulate bone formation in vivo and in vitro. J Clin Invest 2003; 111:1771–82.
54. Heider U, Kaiser M, Muller C, et al. Bortezomib increases osteoblast activity in myeloma patients irrespective of response to treatment. Eur J Haematol 2006; 77:233–8.
55. Yang Y, Yaccoby S, Liu W, et al. Soluble syndecan-1 promotes growth of myeloma tumors in vivo. Blood 2002; 100:610–17.

56. Damiano JS. Dalton WS. Integrin-mediated drug resistance in multiple myeloma. Leuk Lymphoma 2000; 38:71–81.

57. Hazlehurst LA, Damiano JS, Buyuksal I, Pledger WJ, Dalton WS. Adhesion to fibronectin via beta1 integrins regulates p27^{kip1} levels and contributes to cell adhesion mediated drug resistance (CAM-DR). Oncogene 2000; 19:4319–27.

58. Hazlehurst LA, Enkemann SA, Beam CA, et al. Genotypic and phenotypic comparisons of de novo and acquired melphalan resistance in an isogenic multiple myeloma cell line model. Cancer Res 2003; 63:7900–6.

59. Hideshima T, Chauhan D, Schlossman RL, Richardson PR, Anderson KC. Role of TNF-α in the pathophysiology of human multiple myeloma: therapeutic applications. Oncogene 2001; 20:4519–27.

60. Gupta D, Treon SP, Shima Y, et al. Adherence of multiple myeloma cells to bone marrow stromal cells upregulates vascular endothelial growth factor secretion: therapeutic applications. Leukemia 2001; 15:1950–61.

61. Urashima M, Chauhan D, Uchiyama H, Freeman GJ, Anderson KC. CD40 ligand triggered interleukin-6 secretion in multiple myeloma. Blood 1995; 85: 1903–12.

62. Tai YT, Catley LP, Mitsiades CS, et al. Mechanisms by which SGN-40, a humanized anti-CD40 antibody, induces cytotoxicity in human multiple myeloma cells: clinical implications. Cancer Res 2004; 64:2846–52.

63. Tai YT, Li X, Tong X, et al. Human anti-CD40 antagonist antibody triggers significant antitumor activity against human multiple myeloma. Cancer Res 2005; 65:5898–906.

64. Kawano M, Hirano T, Matsuda T, et al. Autocrine generation and requirement of BSF-2/IL-6 for human multiple myelomas. Nature 1988; 332:83–5.

65. Frassanito MA, Cusmai A, Iodice G, Dammacco F. Autocrine interleukin-6 production and highly malignant multiple myeloma: relation with resistance to drug-induced apoptosis. Blood 2001; 97:483–9.

66. Bataille R, Jourdan M, Zhang XG, Klein B. Serum levels of interleukin 6, a potent myeloma cell growth factor, as a reflect of disease severity in plasma cell dyscrasias. J Clin Invest 1989; 84:2008–11.

67. Pulkki K, Pelliniemi TT, Rajamaki A, Tienhaara A, Laakso M, Lahtinen R. Soluble interleukin-6 receptor as a prognostic factor in multiple myeloma. Br J Haematol 1996; 92:370–4.

68. Taga T, Hibi M, Hirata Y, et al. Interleukin-6 triggers the association of its receptor with a possible signal transducer, gp130. Cell 1989; 58:573–81.

69. Ogata A, Chauhan D, Teoh G, et al. Interleukin-6 triggers cell growth via the ras-dependent mitogen-activated protein kinase cascade. J Immunol 1997; 159:2212–21.

70. Ogata A, Chauhan D, Urashima M, Teoh G, Treon SP, Anderson KC. Blockade of mitogen-activated protein kinase cascade signaling in interleukin-6 independent multiple myeloma cells. Clin Cancer Res 1997; 3: 1017–22.

71. Catlett-Falcone R, Landowski TH, Oshiro MM, et al. Constitutive activation of STAT-3 signaling confers resistance to apoptosis in human U266 myeloma cells. Immunity 1999; 10:105–15.

72. Zhang B, Potyagaylo V, Fenton RG. IL-6-independent expression of Mcl-1 in human multiple myeloma. Oncogene 2003; 22:1848–59.
73. Wuilleme-Toumi S, Robillard N, Gomez P, et al. Mcl-1 is overexpressed in multiple myeloma and associated with relapse and shorter survival. Leukemia 2005; 19:1248–52.
74. Akiyama M, Hideshima T, Hayashi T, et al. Nuclear factor-κB p65 mediates tumor necrosis factor alpha-induced nuclear translocation of telomerase reverse transcriptase protein. Cancer Res 2003; 63:18–21.
75. Cantley LC. The phosphoinositide 3-kinase pathway. Science 2002; 296: 1655–7.
76. Uchiyama H, Barut BA, Mohrbacher AF, Chauhan D, Anderson KC. Adhesion of human myeloma-derived cell lines to bone marrow stromal cells stimulates IL-6 secretion. Blood 1993; 82:3712–20.
77. Hideshima T, Podar K, Chauhan D, Anderson KC. Cytokines and signal transduction. Best Pract Res Clin Haematol 2005; 18:509–24.
78. Hideshima T, Chauhan D, Richardson P, et al. NF-kB as a therapeutic target in multiple myeloma. J Biol Chem 2002; 277:16639–47.
79. Ogawa M, Nishiura T, Oritani K, et al. Cytokines prevent dexamethasone-induced apoptosis via the activation of mitogen-activated protein kinase and phosphatidylinositol 3-kinase pathways in a new multiple myeloma cell line. Cancer Res 2000; 60:4262–9.
80. Mitsiades CS, Mitsiades N, Poulaki V, et al. Activation of NF-kB and upregulation of intracellular anti-apoptotic proteins via the IGF-1/Akt signaling in human multiple myeloma cells: therapeutic implications. Oncogene 2002; 21:5673–83.
81. Mitsiades CS, Mitsiades NS, McMullan CJ, et al. Inhibition of the insulin-like growth factor receptor-1 tyrosine kinase activity as a therapeutic strategy for multiple myeloma, other hematologic malignancies, and solid tumors. Cancer Cell 2004; 5:221–30.
82. Pollak MN. Insulin-like growth factors and neoplasia. Novartis Found Symp 2004; 262:84–98.
83. Menu E, Jernberg-Wiklund H, Stromberg T, et al. Inhibiting the IGF-1 receptor tyrosine kinase with the cyclolignan PPP: an in vitro and in vivo study in the 5T33MM mouse model. Blood 2006; 107:655–60.
84. Jelinek DF, Witzig TE, Arendt BK. A role for insulin-like growth factor in the regulation of IL-6-responsive human myeloma cell line growth. J Immunol 1997; 159:487–96.
85. Qiang YW, Kopantzev E, Rudikoff S. Insulinlike growth factor-I signaling in multiple myeloma: downstream elements, functional correlates, and pathway cross-talk. Blood 2002; 99:4138–46.
86. Podar K. Anderson KC. The pathophysiological role of VEGF in hematological malignancies: therapeutic implications. Blood 2005; 105:1383–95.
87. Podar K, Tai YT, Davies FE, et al. Vascular endothelial growth factor triggers signaling cascades mediating multiple myeloma cell growth and migration. Blood 2001; 98:428–35.
88. Podar K, Tai YT, Lin BK, et al. Vascular endothelial growth factor-induced migration of multiple myeloma cells is associated with β 1 integrin- and

phosphatidylinositol 3-kinase-dependent PKC alpha activation. J Biol Chem 2002; 277:7875–81.

89. Ria R, Roccaro AM, Merchionne F, Vacca A, Dammacco F, Ribatti D. Vascular endothelial growth factor and its receptors in multiple myeloma. Leukemia 2003; 17:1961–6.

90. Podar K, Catley LP, Tai YT, et al. GW654652, the pan-inhibitor of VEGF receptors, blocks the growth and migration of multiple myeloma cells in the bone marrow microenvironment. Blood 2004; 103:3474–9.

91. Podar K, Tonon G, Sattler M, et al. The small-molecule VEGF receptor inhibitor pazopanib (GW786034B) targets both tumor and endothelial cells in multiple myeloma. Proc Natl Acad Sci USA 2006; 103:19478–83.

92. Le Gouill S, Podar K, Amiot M, et al. VEGF induces MCL-1 upregulation and protects multiple myeloma cells against apoptosis. Blood 2004; 104: 2886–92.

93. Silvestris F, Cafforio P, Calvani N, Dammacco F. Impaired osteoblastogenesis in myeloma bone disease: role of upregulated apoptosis by cytokines and malignant plasma cells. Br J Haematol 2004; 126:475–86.

94. Karin M. Mitogen activated protein kinases as targets for development of novel anti-inflammatory drugs. Ann Rheum Dis 2004; 63 Suppl 2:ii62–4.

95. Karin M, Cao Y, Greten FR, Li ZW. NF-κB in cancer: from innocent bystander to major culprit. Nat Rev Cancer 2002; 2:301–10.

96. Karin M. Lin A. NF-κB at the crossroads of life and death. Nat Immunol 2002; 3:221–7.

97. Landowski TH, Olashaw NE, Agrawal D, Dalton WS. Cell adhesion-mediated drug resistance (CAM-DR) is associated with activation of NF-κB (RelB/p50) in myeloma cells. Oncogene 2003; 22:2417–21.

98. Chauhan D, Pandey PTH, Treon S, et al. SHP2 mediates the protective effect of interleukin-6 against dexamethasone-induced apopotosis in multiple myeloma cells. J Biol Chem 2000; 275:27845–50.

99. Gilbert L, He X, Farmer P, et al. Expression of the osteoblast differentiation factor RUNX2 (Cbfa1/AML3/Pebp2α A) is inhibited by tumor necrosis factor-α. J Biol Chem 2002; 277:2695–701.

100. Bisping G, Leo R, Wenning D, et al. Paracrine interactions of basic fibroblast growth factor and interleukin-6 in multiple myeloma. Blood 2003; 101: 2775–83.

101. Chang H, Stewart AK, Qi XY, Li ZH, Yi QL, Trudel S. Immuno-histochemistry accurately predicts FGFR3 aberrant expression and t(4;14) in multiple myeloma. Blood 2005; 106:353–5.

102. Trudel S, Li ZH, Wei E, et al. CHIR-258, a novel, multitargeted tyrosine kinase inhibitor for the potential treatment of t(4;14) multiple myeloma. Blood 2005; 105:2941–8.

103. Trudel S, Stewart AK, Rom E, et al. The inhibitory anti-FGFR3 antibody, PRO-001, is cytotoxic to t(4;14) multiple myeloma cells. Blood 2006; 107: 4039–46.

104. Gazitt Y. Akay C. Mobilization of myeloma cells involves SDF-1/CXCR4 signaling and downregulation of VLA-4. Stem Cells 2004; 22:65–73.

105. Hideshima T, Chauhan D, Hayashi et al. The biological sequelae of stromal cell-derived factor-1α in multiple myeloma. Mol Cancer Ther 2002; 1:539–44.

106. Zhang XF, Wang JF, Matczak E, Proper JA, Groopman JE. Janus kinase 2 is involved in stromal cell-derived factor-1α-induced tyrosine phosphorylation of focal adhesion proteins and migration of hematopoietic progenitor cells. Blood 2001; 97:3342–8.

107. Neuhaus T, Stier S, Totzke G, et al. Stromal cell-derived factor 1α (SDF-1α) induces gene-expression of early growth response-1 (Egr-1) and VEGF in human arterial endothelial cells and enhances VEGF induced cell proliferation. Cell Prolif 2003; 36:75–86.

108. Qiang YW, Endo Y, Rubin JS, Rudikoff S. Wnt signaling in B-cell neoplasia. Oncogene 2003; 22:1536–45.

109. Derksen PW, Tjin E, Meijer HP, et al. Illegitimate WNT signaling promotes proliferation of multiple myeloma cells. Proc Natl Acad Sci USA 2004; 101: 6122–7.

110. Hayashi T, Hideshima T, Nguyen AN, et al. TGF-β receptor I kinase inhibitor downregulates cytokine secretion and multiple myeloma cell growth in the bone marrow microenvironment. Clin Cancer Res 2004; 10:7540–6.

111. Jundt F, Probsting KS, Anagnostopoulos I, et al. Jagged1-induced Notch signaling drives proliferation of multiple myeloma cells. Blood 2004; 103: 3511–15.

112. Nefedova Y, Cheng P, Alsina M, Dalton WS, Gabrilovich DI. Involvement of Notch-1 signaling in bone marrow stroma-mediated de novo drug resistance of myeloma and other malignant lymphoid cell lines. Blood 2004; 103: 3503–10.

113. Zweidler-McKay PA, He Y, Xu L, et al. Notch signaling is a potent inducer of growth arrest and apoptosis in a wide range of B-cell malignancies. Blood 2005; 106:3898–906.

114. Houde C, Li Y, Song L, et al. Overexpression of the NOTCH ligand JAG2 in malignant plasma cells from multiple myeloma patients and cell lines. Blood 2004; 104:3697–704.

115. Mackay F. Browning JL. BAFF: a fundamental survival factor for B cells. Nat Rev Immunol 2002; 2:465–75.

116. Mackay F, Schneider P, Rennert P, Browning J. BAFF AND APRIL: a tutorial on B cell survival. Annu Rev Immunol 2003; 21:231–64.

117. Novak AJ, Darce JR, Arendt BK, et al. Expression of BCMA, TACI, and BAFF-R in multiple myeloma: a mechanism for growth and survival. Blood 2004; 103:689–94.

118. Tai YT, Li XF, Breitkreutz I, et al. Role of B-cell-activating factor in adhesion and growth of human multiple myeloma cells in the bone marrow microenvironment. Cancer Res 2006; 66:6675–82.

119. Abe M, Kido S, Hiasa M, et al. BAFF and APRIL as osteoclast-derived survival factors for myeloma cells: a rationale for TACI-Fc treatment in patients with multiple myeloma. Leukemia 2006; 20:1313–15.

120. Klein B, Tarte K, Jourdan M, et al. Survival and proliferation factors of normal and malignant plasma cells. Int J Hematol 2003; 78:106–13.

121. Moreaux J, Legouffe E, Jourdan E, et al. BAFF and APRIL protect myeloma cells from apoptosis induced by interleukin 6 deprivation and dexamethasone. Blood 2004; 103:3148–57.
122. Yasui H, Hideshima T, Richardson PG, Anderson KC. Novel therapeutic strategies targeting growth factor signalling cascades in multiple myeloma. Br J Haematol 2006; 132:385–97.

3

Myeloma Bone Disease

Alissa Huston

James P. Wilmot Cancer Center, University of Rochester Medical Center, Rochester, New York, U.S.A.

G. David Roodman

Bone Biology Center, University of Pittsburgh Medical Center, VA Pittsburgh Healthcare System, Pittsburgh, Pennsylvania, U.S.A.

INTRODUCTION

Multiple myeloma (MM) represents the second most common hematological malignancy with an incidence of 4/100,000 individuals (1). There were approximately 16,000 new cases of MM and 11,000 deaths in 2005 alone (2). MM represents a severely debilitating and essentially fatal neoplastic disease of B-cell origin. One of the major sources of morbidity and mortality for patients with MM results from osteolytic bone lesions throughout the axial skeleton which develop in over 70–80% of patients (3). These lesions are frequently associated with severe and debilitating bone pain, and pathologic fractures can occur in up to 60% of patients (4). Bataille and colleagues have demonstrated that there is a balance between bone destruction and new bone formation, as shown in bone biopsies from patients with MM (5). In more advanced disease this balance is lost, resulting in bone destruction and the development of osteolytic lesions (5). The mechanism involved is increased osteoclast activity and bone destruction which develops adjacent to MM cells, yet not in areas of normal bone marrow. Furthermore new bone formation, which would normally develop at sites of prior bone destruction, is absent with evidence of apoptotic osteoblasts (6). The lack of new bone formation explains why nuclear medicine bone scans can severely underestimate the degree of bone destruction in patients with MM. The bone lesions that develop rarely heal, even when patients are in a complete remission. As a consequence of increased bone destruction, nearly 15% of patients develop hypercalcemia. Overall, the combination of hypercalcemia, pathologic fractures, potential nerve compression, and severe bone pain frequently results in a significant degree of morbidity and mortality for patients with myeloma (7).

ROLE OF OSTEOCLASTS

The bone marrow microenvironment plays a pivotal role in the development of MM bone disease. Multiple factors are produced by both the MM cells and neighboring stromal cells within the microenvironment which interact to shift the delicate balance towards increased bone destruction and decreased new bone formation. There are several factors implicated in this complex process, and those produced by MM cells in vivo which are felt to be responsible for the increased osteoclast activity (thus increased bone destruction) include: receptor activator of NF-κB ligand (RANKL), macrophage inflammatory protein-1α (MIP-1α), interleukin-3 (IL-3), and interleukin-6 (IL-6) (Fig. 1) (8–11).

Receptor Activator of NF-κB Ligand

RANK ligand is a member of the tumor necrosis factor (TNF) family and serves a major role in the increased osteoclastogenesis implicated in MM bone disease. MM cell binding to neighboring stromal cells within the bone marrow of patients with MM results in increased RANKL expression.

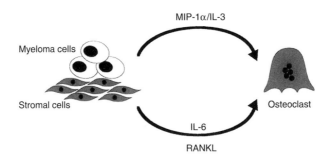

Figure 1   Model of osteoclast activation in multiple myeloma. Lines ending with arrows indicate activating effects. Production of macrophage inflammatory protein-1α (MIP-1α) by myeloma cells results in osteoclast formation and activation. MIP-1α enhances the adhesive interactions between myeloma cells and neighboring stromal cells, increasing the expression of interleukin-6 (IL-6) and receptor activator of NF-κB ligand (RANKL), leading to osteoclast activation. Interleukin-3 (IL-3), also produced by myeloma cells, further induces osteoclast formation. This interplay of factors results in increased bone destruction and tumor burden.

This leads to an increase in osteoclast activity through the binding of RANKL to its receptor, on osteoclast precursor cells, which further promotes their differentiation (12). RANKL is also involved in inhibition of osteoclast apoptosis. Although the precise mechanism is not entirely elucidated, recent evidence points towards a decrease in Fas (a death receptor which mediates apoptosis) and Fas-mediated apoptosis (13). RANKL is also expressed by T-lymphocytes within the bone marrow microenvironment of MM. The mechanism postulated is that MM cells release a soluble factor which upregulates RANKL expression on T-lymphocytes, thereby resulting in enhanced bone destruction (14). Interleukin-7 (IL-7) is involved in this process, since neutralizing antibody to IL-7 has been shown to inhibit RANKL production by T cells. There is controversy regarding whether MM cells directly produce RANKL. Evidence has pointed towards direct production of RANKL by MM cells (15,16); however, other investigators have not been able to detect RANKL in either MM cell lines or patient samples (14,17).

Osteoprotegerin (OPG) is a soluble decoy receptor for RANKL which is produced by stromal cells within the bone marrow and balances RANKL's role and activity in osteoclast activation. Osteoclast activation and bone destruction is further enhanced due to a decline in OPG production. This decrease results from interactions between MM cells and neighboring bone marrow stromal cells. When OPG levels fall, there is increased binding of RANKL to its receptor, further enhancing osteoclast activity (18). Giuliani et al. have demonstrated imbalance between OPG and RANKL levels in the bone marrow microenvironment of MM patients (19). Their work showed that RANKL was not expressed by MM cells, and that these cells produced only low amounts of OPG. However, when human MM cells were cocultured with bone marrow stromal cells, RANKL protein and mRNA expression was upregulated whereas OPG production was downregulated. Pearse et al. evaluated MM bone marrow biopsy specimens and showed upregulation of RANKL and low expression of OPG compared to normal control samples (20). These studies, taken together with those of other investigators (21), demonstrate an imbalance between the levels of RANKL and OPG expression in MM promoting osteoclastogenesis and osteoclast activation.

Importantly, Croucher et al. demonstrated, in a murine model of MM, that inhibition of osteolytic bone destruction by administration of OPG resulted in decreased tumor burden (22,23). Moreover, in a xenograft model where patient primary MM cells are injected into human fetal bone rudiments in severe combined immunodeficiency mice, both bone resorption and tumor burden can be decreased by treatment with either a RANKL inhibitor (RANK-Fc) or bisphosphonate therapy (23,24). Therefore, inhibition of RANKL may both inhibit bone destruction and decrease tumor burden in patients with MM (25).

Macrophage Inflammatory Protein-1α

The chemokine MIP-1α was initially identified by Roodman et al. in samples from MM bone marrow in patients with extensive bone disease and subsequently found to be an important factor in osteoclastogenesis (10,26). In approximately 70% of patients with MM, levels of MIP-1α mRNA and protein from bone marrow were discovered to be increased (8). In contrast, MIP-1α levels have been identified as being slightly increased in approximately 21% of patients with other hematological malignancies and not elevated in normal control samples. Osteoclast formation from human bone marrow cultures can also be induced with recombinant human MIP-1α (8), and a neutralizing antibody to MIP-1α in these same cultures treated with MM patient marrow plasma inhibits the increased osteoclast formation. However, there has been no observed change in osteoclast formation from control samples following anti-MIP-1α treatment. Abe et al. showed that elevated levels of MIP-1α were identified in 15/20 patient samples (15). A correlation has been identified between levels of MIP-1α and bone lesions, as demonstrated in 16/18 MM patients with bone lesions who expressed elevated levels of MIP-1α (17). The above data indicates that elevated MIP-1α levels are present in bone marrow samples from patients with active MM, but not in samples from patients with other hematologic disorders or normal control samples. This data underscores the important role of MIP-1α in patients with active MM (25).

The conclusion that MIP-1α was overexpressed in MM cells and not other hematologic malignancies suggested a regulatory abnormality in the expression of MIP-1α in MM. The MIP-1α promoter contains two AML-1 sites, and an imbalance exists between the forms (AML-1A and AML-1B) of the AML-1 transcription factor expression in MM cells (27). AML-1B drives the transcription of genes regulated by AML-1, and AML-1A is a truncated form of AML-1B that inhibits the binding of AML-1B to AML-1 transcription factor binding sites. AML-1B expression levels are higher or equal to AML-1A in normal cells. However, MM cells expressing high levels of MIP-1α also demonstrated higher levels of AML-1A than AML-1B. MIP-1α production was enhanced in MM cells transfected with AML-1A, but was decreased after transfection with AML-1B. Other genes regulated by AML-1, including interleukin-3 (IL-3) and IL-7, were also increased in marrow plasma from patients with MM. Both IL-3 and IL-7 have significant effects on both osteoclast formation and the inhibition of bone formation in MM.

In vivo studies using murine models of MM bone disease have demonstrated an important in vivo role for MIP-1α. In a SCID model, human MM cells stably transfected with an antisense construct to MIP-1α were implanted into mice. Both tumor burden (as measured by immunoglobulin levels used as a surrogate for disease burden) and bone destruction were markedly decreased, as compared to mice implanted with MM cells expressing high levels of MIP-1α (28). Thus, MIP-1α has a profound effect on bone destruction and tumor growth in MM (28,29). Oyajobi et al. (30,31) further reported that murine 5TGM1 MM cells produced MIP-1α. They demonstrated that treatment of mice implanted with 5TGM1 MM cells with a neutralizing antibody to MIP-1α blocked both bone destruction and decreased tumor burden. These studies demonstrate that blocking MIP-1α could have significant effects upon both bone destruction and tumor growth in MM. As a result, therapeutic agents to target MIP-1α are under development for further clinical evaluation.

MIP-1α is important in osteoclast development, as well as in enhancing the MM cell and stromal cell adhesive interactions (32). When MM cells and bone marrow stromal cells interact, both RANKL and IL-6 production are increased leading to enhanced bone destruction (33). Inhibition of MIP-1α has further been associated with a decrease in the adherent capabilities of MM cells when cocultured with stromal cell lines. The effects of MM cell and stromal cell interactions were evaluated following MIP-1α blockade on a transformed MM cell line. Specifically, Choi et al. (29) transfected the MM cell line ARH-77, with an antisense construct to MIP-1α or empty vector (EV) and noted a decrease in adherence to the ST2 stromal cell line in the antisense transfected cells. The integrins VLA-4 ($\alpha_4\beta_1$) and VLA-5 ($\alpha_5\beta_1$) have been shown to be involved in MM cell adherence to stromal cells (34,35); therefore, mRNA levels were measured for both the antisense and EV transfected MM cells. Levels of $\alpha_4\beta_1$ were similar between the two transfected cell lines; however, a decline in mRNA expression levels for $\alpha_5\beta_1$ was observed, which could be increased by the addition of MIP-1α (29).

Stewart's group (36) reported that patients with a t(4;14) chromosomal translocation have constitutively active fibroblast growth factor 3 (FGFR3) receptor producing high levels of MIP-1α. MIP-1α was found to be a downstream target of FGFR3 and RAS/MAPK signaling, suggesting a possible therapeutic strategy of MIP-1α blockade, particularly in patients expressing the chromosomal translocation t(4:14), and an adverse prognosis (37).

Overall, MIP-1α is a potent osteoclast activating factor, enhances the growth of MM cells, plays an important role in MM cell homing and adhesion, and is associated with poor prognosis (25).

Interleukin-3

Marrow plasma from patients with MM was found to have significantly elevated levels of IL-3 as compared to normal controls (11). Up to 40% of patients with MM have been found to have elevated levels of IL-3 in the peripheral blood, and 75% of bone marrow from patients with MM have elevated IL-3 mRNA and protein levels (10). Median observed levels of IL-3 in MM patients were 66.4 ± 12 pg/ml, as compared to 22.1 ± 8.2 pg/ml in healthy controls (11). Serum derived from MM patients with elevated IL-3 levels also stimulates the growth of MM cell lines dependent on IL-6 (38). Osteoclast formation can be induced by IL-3 at levels similar to those observed from MM patient samples, and inhibition of osteoclast formation can be induced through blocking IL-3 (11). IL-3 further enhances the effects of RANKL and MIP-1α on osteoclast growth and development, and directly stimulates the growth of MM cells (11). Osteoclast-like cells can be induced when IL-3 is added to murine bone marrow cultures, evidenced by development of multinucleated cells staining positive for tartrate resistant acid-phosphatase (a marker enzyme of osteoclasts) (39). IL-3 appears to be an osteoclast stimulatory factor in MM through increasing the number and activity of osteoclasts, thus resulting in further bone destruction (25).

Interleukin-6

IL-6 is thought to play a more controversial role in MM. It remains uncertain if increased levels of IL-6 correlate with disease status (10,40). In patients with osteolytic lesions, levels of IL-6 have been observed to be elevated as compared to patients with MM and no lytic lesions or those with monoclonal gammopathy of undetermined significance (MGUS) (41). Levels of IL-6 derived from bone marrow samples, but not peripheral blood, have been correlated with markers of bone turnover, including C-terminal propeptide of pro-collagen I, C-terminal telopeptide of pro-collagen I, and bone specific alkaline phosphatase (42). The fact that IL-6 levels from bone marrow, but not peripheral blood, were correlated with bone turnover markers supports the importance of locally acting factors within the bone marrow microenvironment being important in the development of bone destruction in MM (12).

   Most studies support the notion that IL-6 production is from neighboring cells within the bone marrow microenvironment following contact with MM cells, including osteoblasts, osteoclasts, and stromal cells. What is not clear, although suggested by some, is whether MM cells directly produce IL-6 (41). Sati et al. (41) demonstrated by fluorescent in situ hybridization (FISH) techniques the presence of IL-6 in plasma cells from human bone marrow in patients with MM and MGUS, but not in normal controls. Coculture experiments of both human osteoblasts and osteoclasts with MM cells have also demonstrated an increased production of IL-6 (43,44). In both studies, the effects of IL-6 production appeared to be increased when there was direct cell-to-cell contact between the MM cells and osteoblasts or osteoclasts. However, increased IL-6 could still be observed when conditioned media from MM cells was cultured with osteoblasts, suggesting a role for a soluble factor; however, the same effects were abolished when transwell inserts were used to separate MM cells from osteoclasts. Increased IL-6 appears to enhance the growth of MM cells and inhibit MM cell apoptosis (44,45). While the precise role of IL-6 remains under debate, IL-6 production by osteoclasts may increase MM tumor burden, thereby resulting in enhanced bone destruction (25).

ROLE OF OSTEOBLASTS

Several factors are felt to be responsible for the suppressed osteoblast activity observed in MM; however, their precise role is just beginning to be identified. Some of these markers include: IL-3, dickkopf 1 (DKK1), secreted frizzled-related protein-2 and IL-7 (Fig. 2) (46–49). Certain factors (DKK1 and sFRP-2) appear to affect the Wnt signaling pathway, critical for osteoblast differentiation (50), while others (IL-3 and IL-7) do not appear to directly affect this signaling pathway. These are soluble inhibitors of signaling pathways which affect osteoblast differentiation and not osteoblast survival, suggesting that their inhibitory effects should be reversible when MM cells are no longer present (25).

Interleukin-3

IL-3 enhances the effects of MIP-1α and TNF-α on osteoblasts and is involved in suppressing osteoblast differentiation (11). Ehrlich et al. reported that primary mouse and human marrow stromal cells treated with

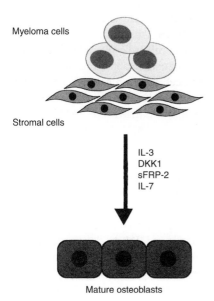

Figure 2 Model of osteoblast suppression in multiple myeloma. Line ending with a bar indicates inhibitory effect. Interleukin-3 (IL-3), dickkopf 1 (DKK1), secreted frizzled-related protein-2 (sFRP-2), and interleukin-7 (IL-7) are all produced by myeloma cells. DKK1 and sFRP-2 target the Wnt signaling pathway (critical to osteoblast differentiation from stromal cells), whereas IL-3 and IL-7 are not thought to directly affect this signaling pathway. The combined actions result in osteoblast inhibition, leading to a decrease in bone formation.

IL-3 inhibited basal and bone morphogenic protein-2 (BMP-2) stimulated osteoblast formation in a dose-dependent manner, without any effects on cell growth (46). Furthermore, osteoblast differentiation was inhibited by marrow plasma from MM patients with high IL-3 levels, which was reversed by anti-IL-3. Preosteoblast development into mature osteoblasts was also inhibited by IL-3 at concentrations similar to those observed in patients with MM. Osteoblast-like cell lines were not inhibited by IL-3. An increase in the number of CD45$^+$/CD11b$^+$ monocyte/macrophage hematopoietic cells was induced by IL-3 in primary stromal cell cultures. CD45$^+$ cell depletion abolished the inhibitory effects of IL-3 on osteoblasts (46), whereas reconstituting the cultures with CD45$^+$ cells restored IL-3's osteoblast inhibitory activity, suggesting an indirect mechanism of IL-3's osteoblast inhibitory activity (46). IL-3 therefore appears to play a dual role in the bone destructive process in MM through direct stimulation of osteoclasts and indirect inhibition of osteoblast formation (25).

Dickkopf 1

A soluble inhibitor of the Wnt signaling pathway, DKK1, is produced by osteoblasts and plays a critical role in osteoblast differentiation (48,49). Tian et al. (49) reported that DKK1 may be important in osteoblast suppression in myeloma.: DKK1 was secreted by MM cells, and in vitro studies in a murine mesenchymal stem cell line demonstrated that marrow plasma from MM patients with more than 12 ng/ml of DKK1 inhibited osteoblast differentiation. DKK1 levels were also observed to be elevated in mature plasma cells, but not in immature or plasmablastic variants. Furthermore, a high correlation of DKK1 gene expression levels with the extent of bone disease was demonstrated in MM patients. In contrast, other investigators have found DKK1 not to be expressed by MM cells (48,49), no evidence of upregulation following MM cell binding to preosteoblasts, and an absence of blockade on the inhibitory effects of MM cell lines on human osteoblast differentiation when treated with antibody to DKK1. A more recent study by Politou et al. (51) measured levels of DKK1 in patients with MM before and after autologous stem cell transplantation, patients with MGUS, and in normal individuals. Levels of DKK1 were elevated in patients with MM as compared to either those with MGUS or normal controls. A sustained decrease in levels following autologous stem cell transplantation correlated with a normalization of markers of bone turnover, suggesting a return of osteoblast activity (51). Recently, Yaccoby and coworkers demonstrated that treating SCID mice implanted with rabbit bone rudiments containing primary myeloma cells with an antibody to DKK1 decreased bone destruction, increased bone formation, and decreased tumor growth (52).

Although DKK1 appears to be important in osteoblast suppression in MM, its precise role in myeloma bone disease remains unclear (25).

Secreted Frizzled-Related Protein-2

Oshima et al. (48) have reported that MM cells secrete a different soluble inhibitor of the Wnt signaling pathway, sFRP-2, also involved in osteoblast suppression. Conditioned media from MM cell lines and primary MM cells suppressed in vitro mineralization and blocked alkaline phosphatase activity induced by BMP-2 treatment of osteoblasts. The MM cell lines used in these experiments produced sFRP-2, but not DKK1. Further observations demonstrated expression of sFRP-2 from MM cells derived from patients with advanced bone disease. Experiments depleting sFRP-2 from MM cell conditioned media resulted in a loss of osteoblast inhibitory activity. However, other investigators have not found increased levels of sFRP-2 in myeloma patients, as observed with DKK1 (47). The role of the Wnt signaling pathway inhibitors in MM bone disease remains controversial and provides an important area of further research (25).

Interleukin-7

Giuliani et al. (47) reported an increase in IL-7 in human MM marrow plasma samples, and observed an inhibitory activity of IL-7 on osteoblast differentiation of early human osteoblast precursors (colony-forming unit fibroblast [CFU-F]) and more differentiated osteoblast precursors (colony-forming unit osteoblast [CFU-OB]) (47). Conversely, a neutralizing antibody to IL-7 was able to reverse the inhibition of human osteoblast differentiation by MM cell lines and primary MM cells. IL-7 could also inhibit in vitro bone nodule formation by osteoblast precursors and block the binding of CBAF1/RUNX2 DNA, critical for osteoblast differentiation, as demonstrated by electrophoretic mobility shift assays (29). Gene and protein expression levels of the IL-7 receptor have been identified at high levels in both human stromal cell lines and primary stromal cell samples (53). From these experiments, IL-7 appears to be a potent inhibitor of osteoblast differentiation in MM and a potential target for reversing the severe osteoblast suppression observed (25).

ADDITIONAL CYTOKINES

In MM, several other cytokines affecting the growth of MM cells and the activity of osteoclasts or osteoblasts have been identified including hepatocyte growth factor (HGF), insulin-like growth factor, interleukin-1, and TNF-α (7). This chapter will further focus on two of these, HGF and TNF-α.

Hepatocyte Growth Factor

HGF exerts proliferative and anti-apoptotic effects on MM cells, and is associated with osteoclast activation. In patients with MM, measurement of HGF levels were reported to be significantly elevated and to correlate with more advanced disease (54–56). HGF is known to be produced by both MM cell lines and primary MM cells, and is an inducer of angiogenesis through downstream signaling via the cyclooxygenase-2 (COX-2) pathway (54,57). Levels of HGF have been correlated with increases in TNF-α and IL-6, both being potent stimulators of osteoclast activity. In cell culture experiments of MM cells with human osteoblast-like cells, HGF induced interleukin-11 (IL-11) secretion, with a decrease in IL-11 observed following treatment with anti-HGF. There was also an observed increase in the amount of HGF secreted when MM cells and osteoblasts were in direct contact, versus when contact was inhibited by a membrane insert. IL-11 is important both as a stimulator of osteoclastogenesis, as well as an inhibitor of osteoblast activity (58,59). The induction of IL-11 through HGF may be an important factor in furthering the bone destruction in MM, and targeting HGF through either COX-2 inhibition or direct inhibition of the HGF receptor (c-met) represents a novel therapeutic strategy for MM bone disease.

Tumor Necrosis Factor-α

Although its precise role has not been fully defined, TNF-α has been implicated in MM bone disease. Elevated plasma TNF-α levels have been identified in MM patients with advanced bone disease and osteolytic lesions, as compared to those without evidence of bone disease, or patients with MGUS (60). Bone marrow samples from patients were also found to contain elevated levels of TNF-α; however, direct correlations between levels and markers of bone metabolism or histomorphometry were not done (42). A role of TNF-α in directly stimulating osteoclastogenesis has been established; however, the mechanisms by which it mediates MM bone disease remains to be fully defined (25).

THERAPEUTIC OPTIONS

Bisphosphonates

The mainstay of therapy for MM-induced bone lesions has been bisphosphonate therapy. Bisphosphonate (pamidronate, zoledronic acid, ibandronate) therapy results in a decrease in the number of skeletal related events (SREs) and an improvement in pain related to MM bone disease. It also induces MM cell apoptosis (61). Previous studies have demonstrated a correlation between markers of bone turnover (urinary N-telopeptide/creatinine [NTX], serum NTX, serum bone specific alkaline phosphatase [BALP]) and clinical response: a decline in these specific markers predicts for therapeutic response (62). Bisphosphonates may have improved the outcome of patients with MM bone disease; however, they have not changed overall survival rates (unless used in combination with myeloma therapy). Although the SRE rate is observed to have decreased following treatment, it is only by a factor of 50% (63,64). There are also serious adverse risks associated with the use of bisphosphonates including the development of renal failure, nephrotic syndrome, or osteonecrosis of the jaw (65,66). Therefore, there remains an important need to understand the mechanisms involved in the development of MM bone disease in order to identify novel therapeutic targets (25).

Denosumab

Recently work on denosumab (Amgen), a fully human monoclonal antibody against RANKL, was evaluated in women with postmenopausal osteoporosis, as well as in patients with MM or bone metastases from breast cancer. Initial studies demonstrated that a single dose of denosumab resulted in a dose-dependent, rapid, and sustained decline in markers of bone turnover (urinary N-telopeptide/creatinine [NTX], serum NTX, serum bone specific alkaline phosphatase [BALP]) (67). Further studies identified an increase in bone mineral density, observed following a year of therapy, with results similar to those observed in studies using oral bisphosphonate therapy (68). A safety study conducted in patients with MM or bone metastases from breast cancer comparing denosumab to pamidronate also demonstrated similar sustained suppression in markers of bone turnover (as in the initial postmenopausal studies) lasting up to 84 days (69). Currently, there are several trials underway evaluating denosumab as a potential single-agent therapy in MM bone disease.

CONCLUSION

Bone disease resulting from MM represents a major source of morbidity for patients. Bisphosphonates have been the mainstay of therapy for many years, with notable improvements in SREs, bone pain, and disease burden. Newer agents, such as denosumab, are being developed to improve upon the success of bisphosphonate therapy. As newer therapies become available which extend the survival of MM patients, understanding the mechanisms within the bone marrow microenvironment responsible for suppressed bone formation becomes critical. Thus, studies delineating the mechanisms responsible for the severe osteoblast suppression and osteoclast activation, along with the effects of anabolic agents on MM bone disease, should lead to novel therapies that can ameliorate or prevent the suppression of osteoblast function and improve the overall quality of life of patients with myeloma (25).

REFERENCES

1. Kyle RA, Therneau TM, Rajkumar SV, et al. Incidence of multiple myeloma in Olmsted County, Minnesota: trend over 6 decades. Cancer 2004; 101(11): 2667–74.

2. Edwards BK, Brown ML, Wingo PA, et al. Annual report to the nation on the status of cancer, 1975–2002, featuring population-based trends in cancer treatment. J Natl Cancer Inst 2005; 97(19):1407–27.

3. Callander NS, Roodman GD. Myeloma bone disease. Semin Hematol 2001; 38 (3):276–85.

4. Melton LJ, III, Kyle RA, Achenbach SJ, et al. Fracture risk with multiple myeloma: a population-based study. J Bone Miner Res 2005; 20(3):487–93.

5. Bataille R, Chappard D, Marcelli C, et al. Mechanisms of bone destruction in multiple myeloma: the importance of an unbalanced process in determining the severity of lytic bone disease. J Clin Oncol 1989; 7(12):1909–14.

6. Taube T, Beneton MN, McCloskey EV, et al. Abnormal bone remodelling in patients with myelomatosis and normal biochemical indices of bone resorption. Eur J Haematol 1992; 49(4):192–8.

7. Roodman GD. Pathogenesis of myeloma bone disease. Blood Cells Mol Dis 2004; 32(2):290–2.

8. Gunn WG, Conley A, Deininger L, et al. A crosstalk between myeloma cells and marrow stromal cells stimulates production of DKK1 and IL-6: a potential role in the development of lytic bone disease and tumor progression in multiple myeloma stem. Cells 2005.

9. Giuliani N, Colla S, Rizzoli V. New insight in the mechanism of osteoclast activation and formation in multiple myeloma: focus on the receptor activator of NF-kappaB ligand (RANKL). Exp Hematol 2004; 32(8):685–91.

10. Choi SJ, Cruz JC, Craig F, et al. Macrophage inflammatory protein 1-alpha is a potential osteoclast stimulatory factor in multiple myeloma. Blood 2000; 96(2): 671–5.

11. Lee JW, Chung HY, Ehrlich LA, et al. IL-3 expression by myeloma cells increases both osteoclast formation and growth of myeloma cells. Blood 2004; 103(6):2308–15.

12. Ehrlich LA, Roodman GD. The role of immune cells and inflammatory cytokines in Paget's disease and multiple myeloma. Immunol Rev 2005; 208: 252–66.

13. Wu X, Pan G, McKenna MA, et al. RANKL regulates Fas expression and Fas-mediated apoptosis in osteoclasts. J Bone Miner Res 2005; 20(1): 107–16.

14. Giuliani N, Colla S, Sala R, et al. Human myeloma cells stimulate the receptor activator of nuclear factor-kappa B ligand (RANKL) in T lymphocytes: a potential role in multiple myeloma bone disease. Blood 2002; 100(13):4615–21.

15. Sezer O, Heider U, Jakob C, et al. Immunocytochemistry reveals RANKL expression of myeloma cells. Blood 2002; 99(12):4646–47; author reply 4647.

16. Farrugia AN, Atkins GJ, To LB, et al. Receptor activator of nuclear factor-kappaB ligand expression by human myeloma cells mediates osteoclast formation in vitro and correlates with bone destruction in vivo. Cancer Res 2003; 63(17):5438–45.

17. Pearse RN, Sordillo EM, Yaccoby S, et al. Multiple myeloma disrupts the TRANCE/osteoprotegerin cytokine axis to trigger bone destruction and promote tumor progression. Proc Natl Acad Sci USA 2001; 98(20): 11581–6.

18. Teoh G, Anderson KC. Interaction of tumor and host cells with adhesion and extracellular matrix molecules in the development of multiple myeloma. Hematol Oncol Clin North Am 1997; 11(1):27–42.
19. Still K, Phipps RJ, Scutt A. Effects of risedronate, alendronate, and etidronate on the viability and activity of rat bone marrow stromal cells in vitro. Calcif Tissue Int 2003; 72(2):143–50.
20. Nagashima M, Sakai A, Uchida S, et al. Bisphosphonate (YM529) delays the repair of cortical bone defect after drill-hole injury by reducing terminal differentiation of osteoblasts in the mouse femur. Bone 2005; 36(3):502–11.
21. Vanderkerken K, Van Camp B, De Greef C, et al. Homing of the myeloma cell clone. Acta Oncol 2000; 39(7):771–6.
22. Vanderkerken K, Goes E, De Raeve H, et al. Follow-up of bone lesions in an experimental multiple myeloma mouse model: description of an in vivo technique using radiography dedicated for mammography. Br J Cancer 1996; 73(12):1463–5.
23. Menu E, Asosingh K, Van Riet I, et al. Myeloma cells (5TMM) and their interactions with the marrow microenvironment. Blood Cells Mol Dis 2004; 33 (2):111–19.
24. Epstein J, Yaccoby S. The SCID-hu myeloma model. Methods Mol Med 2005; 113:183–90.
25. Huston A, Roodman GD. Role of the microenvironment in multiple myeloma bone disease. Future Oncol 2006; 2(3):371–8.
26. Han JH, Choi SJ, Kurihara N, et al. Macrophage inflammatory protein-1alpha is an osteoclastogenic factor in myeloma that is independent of receptor activator of nuclear factor kappaB ligand. Blood 2001; 97(11):3349–53.
27. Choi SJ, Oba T, Callander NS, et al. AML-1A and AML-1B regulation of MIP-1alpha expression in multiple myeloma. Blood 2003; 101(10):3778–83.
28. Alsina M, Boyce B, Devlin RD, et al. Development of an in vivo model of human multiple myeloma bone disease. Blood 1996; 87(4):1495–501.
29. Choi SJ, Oba Y, Gazitt Y, et al. Antisense inhibition of macrophage inflammatory protein 1-alpha blocks bone destruction in a model of myeloma bone disease. J Clin Invest 2001; 108(12):1833–41.
30. Oyajobi BO, Franchin G, Williams PJ, et al. Dual effects of macrophage inflammatory protein-1alpha on osteolysis and tumor burden in the murine 5TGM1 model of myeloma bone disease. Blood 2003; 102(1):311–19.
31. Oyajobi BO, Mundy GR. Receptor activator of NF-kappaB ligand, macrophage inflammatory protein-1alpha, and the proteasome: novel therapeutic targets in myeloma. Cancer 2003; 97(3 Suppl):813–17.
32. Vidriales MB and Anderson KC. Adhesion of multiple myeloma cells to the bone marrow microenvironment: implications for future therapeutic strategies. Mol Med Today 1996; 2(10):425–31.
33. Roodman GD, Choi SJ. MIP-1 alpha and myeloma bone disease. Cancer Treat Res 2004; 118:83–100.
34. Robledo MM, Sanz-Rodriguez F, Hidalgo A, et al. Differential use of very late antigen-4 and -5 integrins by hematopoietic precursors and myeloma cells to adhere to transforming growth factor-beta1-treated bone marrow stroma. J Biol Chem 1998; 273(20):12056–60.

35. Michigami T, Shimizu N, Williams PJ, et al. Cell–cell contact between marrow stromal cells and myeloma cells via VCAM-1 and alpha(4)beta(1)-integrin enhances production of osteoclast-stimulating activity. Blood 2000; 96(5): 1953–60.

36. Masih-Khan E, Trudel S, Heise C, et al. MIP-1alpha (CCL3) is a downstream target of FGFR3 and RAS-MAPK signaling in multiple myeloma. Blood 2006; 108(10):3465–71.

37. Keats JJ, Reiman T, Maxwell CA, et al. In multiple myeloma, t(4; 14)(p16; q32) is an adverse prognostic factor irrespective of FGFR3 expression. Blood 2003; 101(4):1520–9.

38. Merico F, Bergui L, Gregoretti MG, et al. Cytokines involved in the progression of multiple myeloma. Clin Exp Immunol 1993; 92(1):27–31.

39. Barton BE, Mayer R. IL-3 induces differentiation of bone marrow precursor cells to osteoclast-like cells. J Immunol 1989; 143(10):3211–16.

40. Solary E, Guiguet M, Zeller V, et al. Radioimmunoassay for the measurement of serum IL-6 and its correlation with tumour cell mass parameters in multiple myeloma. Am J Hematol 1992; 39(3):163–71.

41. Sati HI, Apperley JF, Greaves M, et al. Interleukin-6 is expressed by plasma cells from patients with multiple myeloma and monoclonal gammopathy of undetermined significance. Br J Haematol 1998; 101(2):287–95.

42. Abildgaard N, Glerup H, Rungby J, et al. Biochemical markers of bone metabolism reflect osteoclastic and osteoblastic activity in multiple myeloma. Eur J Haematol 2000; 64(2):121–9.

43. Karadag A, Oyajobi BO, Apperley JF, et al. Human myeloma cells promote the production of interleukin 6 by primary human osteoblasts. Br J Haematol 2000; 108(2):383–90.

44. Abe M, Hiura K, Wilde J, et al. Osteoclasts enhance myeloma cell growth and survival via cell-cell contact: a vicious cycle between bone destruction and myeloma expansion Blood 2004; 104(8):2484–91.

45. Anderson KC, Jones RM, Morimoto C, et al. Response patterns of purified myeloma cells to hematopoietic growth factors. Blood 1989; 73(7):1915–24.

46. Ehrlich LA, Chung HY, Ghobrial I, et al. IL-3 is a potential inhibitor of osteoblast differentiation in multiple myeloma. Blood 2005; 106(4):1407–14.

47. Giuliani N, Colla S, Morandi F, et al. Myeloma cells block RUNX2/CBFA1 activity in human bone marrow osteoblast progenitors and inhibit osteoblast formation and differentiation. Blood 2005; 106(7):2472–83.

48. Oshima T, Abe M, Asano J, et al. Myeloma cells suppress bone formation by secreting a soluble Wnt inhibitor, sFRP-2. Blood 2005; 106(9):3160–5.

49. Tian E, Zhan F, Walker R, et al. The role of the Wnt-signaling antagonist DKK1 in the development of osteolytic lesions in multiple myeloma. N Engl J Med 2003; 349(26):2483–94.

50. Canalis E, Deregowski V, Pereira RC, et al. Signals that determine the fate of osteoblastic cells. J Endocrinol Invest 2005; 28(8 Suppl):3–7.

51. Politou MC, Heath DJ, Rahemtulla A, et al. Serum concentrations of Dickkopf-1 protein are increased in patients with multiple myeloma and reduced after autologous stem cell transplantation. Int J Cancer 2006; 119(7): 1728–31.

52. Yaccoby S, Ling W, Zhan F, et al. Antibody-based inhibition of DKK1 suppresses tumor-induced bone resorption and multiple myeloma growth in-vivo. Blood 2007; 109(5):2106–11.

53. Iwata M, Graf L, Awaya N, et al. Functional interleukin-7 receptors (IL-7Rs) are expressed by marrow stromal cells: binding of IL-7 increases levels of IL-6 mRNA and secreted protein. Blood 2002; 100(4):1318–25.

54. Sengupta S, Sellers LA, Cindrova T, et al. Cyclooxygenase-2-selective nonsteroidal anti-inflammatory drugs inhibit hepatocyte growth factor/scatter factor-induced angiogenesis. Cancer Res 2003; 63(23):8351–9.

55. Iwasaki T, Hamano T, Ogata A, et al. Clinical significance of vascular endothelial growth factor and hepatocyte growth factor in multiple myeloma. Br J Haematol 2002; 116(4):796–802.

56. Derksen PW, de Gorter DJ, Meijer HP, et al. The hepatocyte growth factor/ Met pathway controls proliferation and apoptosis in multiple myeloma. Leukemia 2003; 17(4):764–74.

57. Borset M, Hjorth-Hansen H, Seidel C, et al. Hepatocyte growth factor and its receptor c-met in multiple myeloma. Blood 1996; 88(10):3998–4004.

58. Alexandrakis MG, Passam FH, Sfiridaki A, et al. Elevated serum concentration of hepatocyte growth factor in patients with multiple myeloma: correlation with markers of disease activity. Am J Hematol 2003; 72(4):229–33.

59. Hjertner O, Torgersen ML, Seidel C, et al. Hepatocyte growth factor (HGF) induces interleukin-11 secretion from osteoblasts: a possible role for HGF in myeloma-associated osteolytic bone disease. Blood 1999; 94(11):3883–8.

60. Silvestris F, Cafforio P, Calvani N, et al. Impaired osteoblastogenesis in myeloma bone disease: role of upregulated apoptosis by cytokines and malignant plasma cells. Br J Haematol 2004; 126(4):475–86.

61. Gordon S, Helfrich MH, Sati HI, et al. Pamidronate causes apoptosis of plasma cells in vivo in patients with multiple myeloma. Br J Haematol 2002; 119 (2):475–83.

62. Vinholes JJ, Purohit OP, Abbey ME, et al. Relationships between biochemical and symptomatic response in a double-blind randomised trial of pamidronate for metastatic bone disease. Ann Oncol 1997; 8(12):1243–50.

63. Berenson JR, Lichtenstein A, Porter L, et al. Efficacy of pamidronate in reducing skeletal events in patients with advanced multiple myeloma. Myeloma Aredia Study Group. N Engl J Med 1996; 334(8):488–93.

64. Petcu EB, Schug SA, Smith H. Clinical evaluation of onset of analgesia using intravenous pamidronate in metastatic bone pain. J Pain Symptom Manage 2002; 24(3):281–4.

65. Markowitz GS, Appel GB, Fine PL, et al. Collapsing focal segmental glomerulosclerosis following treatment with high-dose pamidronate. J Am Soc Nephrol 2001; 12(6):1164–72.

66. Desikan R, Veksler Y, Raza S, et al. Nephrotic proteinuria associated with high-dose pamidronate in multiple myeloma. Br J Haematol 2002; 119(2): 496–9.

67. Bekker PJ, Holloway DL, Rasmussen AS, et al. A single-dose placebo-controlled study of AMG 162, a fully human monoclonal antibody to RANKL, in postmenopausal women. J Bone Miner Res 2004; 19(7):1059–66.

68.   McClung MR LE, Bolognese MA, et al. AMG 162 increases bone mineral density (BMD) within 1 month in postmenopausal women with low BMD. J Bone Miner Res 2004; 19(Supp 1):S20 (Abstract 1072).

69.   Body JJ, Facon T, Coleman RE, et al. A study of the biological receptor activator of nuclear factor-kappaB ligand inhibitor, denosumab, in patients with multiple myeloma or bone metastases from breast cancer. Clin Cancer Res 2006; 12(4):1221–8.

4

Niches Within the Multiple Myeloma Bone Marrow Microenvironment

**Klaus Podar, Irene Ghobrial, Teru Hideshima,
Dharminder Chauhan, and Kenneth C. Anderson**

*Department of Medical Oncology, Jerome Lipper Multiple Myeloma Center,
Dana-Farber Cancer Institute, Harvard Medical School, Boston,
Massachusetts, U.S.A.*

INTRODUCTION

The bone marrow (BM) microenvironment consists of hematopoietic and nonhematopoietic cells, as well as an extracellular and liquid compartment organized in a complex architecture of sub-microenvironments ("niches") within the protective coat of mineralized bone. Niches are physical entities composed of stromal cells which maintain hematopoietic cell (e.g., hematopoietic stem cell, HSC) quiescence, maintenance, expansion, and survival, as well as enable their migration. These processes are mediated both *via* direct cell-cell contact as well as release of soluble factors. Under physiologic conditions the cellular, extracellular, and liquid compartments are highly organized by cell-cell and cell-matrix interactions within a regulative liquid milieu, thereby supporting normal hematopoiesis. The conduit between this "encapsulated chamber" and the peripheral circulation is a complex system of vasculature.

It is now well established that the BM microenvironment plays a pivotal pathophysiologic role in multiple myeloma (MM). In MM, the balanced homeostasis between the cellular, the extracellular, and the liquid compartment within the BM is disrupted. Specifically, the BM microenvironment is impacted by tumor cells characteristically causing immune suppression and lytic bone lesions; conversely, the BM provides signals which influence the behavior of MM cells, e.g., tumor cell growth, survival, migration, and drug resistance. Angiogenesis, normally tightly regulated by pro- and antiangiogenic molecules, is also altered in MM, with increased BM microvascular density (MVD) correlated with disease progression and poor prognosis. Importantly, the therapeutic success of novel agents, e.g., bortezomib and lenalidomide, even in relapsed/refractory disease is, at least in part, due to their activity against BM microenvironment- derived effects on MM cells. Deeper insights into the architecture of the BM micro-environment and molecular interactions between its distinct compartments will help to identify new therapeutic strategies to re-establish BM home-ostasis and improve MM patient outcome.

INTERACTION OF MM CELLS WITH OTHER CELLULAR COMPONENTS AND THE EXTRACELLULAR MATRIX OF THE BM MICROENVIRONMENT

The BM constitutes a microenvironment required for differentiation, maintenance, expansion, and development of drug resistance of MM cells. It is composed of (1) a heterogeneous population of cells; (2) the insoluble extracellular matrix (ECM); as well as (3) a variety of cytokines, growth factors, and hormones within a liquid milieu highly enriched for calcium salts. Cells represented within the BM microenvironment include hemato-poietic stem cells; endothelial cells; stromal cells (e.g., fibroblasts, adipo-cytes, and immune cells such as macrophages and T lymphocytes); as well as cells involved in bone homeostasis (chondroclasts, osteoclasts, and osteo-blasts), which are tightly associated with strong adhesive ECM proteins (e.g., fibronectin, collagen, laminin, proteoglycans, and glycosaminogly-cans). Cell-cell as well as cell-ECM interactions are regulated *via* several families of surface receptors including integrins, cadherins, selectins, syn-decans, and the immunoglobulin superfamily of cell adhesion molecules; as well as a multitude of cytokines, growth factors, and hormones and their respective receptors. In MM pathogenesis, MM cell binding to stromal cells supports tumor cell proliferation, survival, and drug resistance. Specifically, cell–cell adhesion mediated by various adhesion molecules (e.g., VLA-4, ICAM-1) stimulates MM cell growth and survival both directly by induction of signaling cascades downstream of the surface molecules, as well as indirectly by autocrine and paracrine cytokine/growth factor production and secretion.

MM cells typically express β1 (CD29)-integrins including very late activating antigen-4 and -5 (VLA-4, VLA-5) (1,2), as well as integrin αvβ3 (3,4). β1-integrins mediate MM cell adhesion to endothelial cells, BMSCs, as well as ECM proteins fibronectin and laminin, thereby enhancing MM cell growth and survival and conferring protection against drug- induced apoptosis. These sequelae are due to cell–cell contact as well as nuclear factor κB (NFκB)-dependent transcription and secretion of IL-6, a major

MM growth, survival, and drug resistance factor (5,6). Importantly, MM cell adhesion to fibronectin also protects tumor cells from DNA damaging drugs (e.g., anthracyclines and alkylating agents) by induction of cell-adhesion mediated drug resistance (CAM-DR), a reversible G1-arrest with increased p27kip1 levels (2,7). $\alpha v\beta 3$-integrin-mediated binding of MM cells to vitronectin and fibronectin stimulate production and release of urokinase-type plasminogen activator, metalloproteinase-2, and metalloproteinase-9, thereby promoting tumor cell invasion and spreading (3).

Based on these findings, ongoing studies are evaluating compounds which alter adhesive interaction of MM cells with cells in the BM microenvironment and ECM, in order to induce MM cell death and apoptosis. These agents have great promise to enhance efficacy of anticancer therapy by overcoming conventional drug-resistance.

CYTOKINES, GROWTH FACTORS AND THEIR IMPACT ON MM CELL GROWTH, SURVIVAL, AND MIGRATION WITHIN THE BM MICROENVIRONMENT

Tumor cells activate the stroma by producing and secreting cytokines and growth factors, matrix metalloproteinases (MMPs), as well as specific ECM components, thereby reducing the expression of endogenous tissue inhibitors of metalloproteinases (TIMP). Specifically, activated stroma triggers the paracrine and aurocrine production and secretion of a variety of cytokines and growth factors into the MM BM microenvironment including: interleukin-6 (IL-6), insulin-like growth factor-1 (IGF-1), vascular endothelial growth factor (VEGF), tumor necrosis factor-α (TNF-α), stromal derived factor-1α (SDF-1α), tumor growth factor-β (TGF-β), basic fibroblast growth factor (bFGF), MIP-1α, stem cell factor (SCF), hepatocyte growth factor scatter factor (HGF), IL-1β, IL-3, IL-10, IL-15, and IL-21; as well as Ang-1 and matrix metalloproteinases, e.g., MMP-2 and MMP-9. In addition, our own studies recently also established a role of B-cell-activating factor (BAFF) in localization and survival of MM cells in the BM microenvironment (8). These signals contribute to MM pathogenesis by both directly triggering tumor cell responses and indirectly modifying the tumor microenvironment. Specifically, they support tumor growth and expansion directly as well as indirectly by inducing functional defects of nontumor cells, e.g., increasing tumor-angiogenesis (9).

IL-6 is the major growth and survival factor in MM cells, which also confers drug (e.g., dexamethasone) resistance. Since IL-6 plays a pivotal role in hematopoietic stem cell differentiation, its potential role in clonal development of MM is suggested. Production and secretion of IL-6 by cells within the BM microenvironment is tightly regulated. Specifically, adherence of MM cells to BMSCs induces NFκB-dependent IL-6 production and secretion by BM cells, resulting in significantly increased MM cell proliferation. In addition, IL-6 stimulates paracrine and autocrine production and secretion of the VEGF, the key regulator of physiologic and pathologic angiogenesis by MM cells and BMSCs which, in turn stimulates production and secretion of IL-6 in BM stromal cells (6,10,11). Both IL-6 and VEGF secretion are also induced by CD40 activation of tumor cells (12,13) or other cytokines present in the BM microenvironment, including TNF-α (14) and IL-1 (15,16). Another mechanism regulating VEGF expression in MM cells is exemplified by c-maf- driven expression of integrin β7, which enhances adhesion to BM stroma and thereby increases VEGF production (17). Therefore, besides hypoxia/Hif-1α, a variety of mechanisms are regulating VEGF expression in the BM microenvironment.

In addition to its role as an essential regulator of physiologic endothelial cell growth, permeability, and migration in vitro and in vivo, VEGF is a pivotal factor in hematopoiesis affecting the differentiation of multiple lineages (18–21). Specifically, VEGF mediates hematopoietic stem cell survival and repopulation *via* an autocrine loop, whereas angiogenesis is regulated *via* a paracrine VEGF loop (21). In addition, VEGF: inhibits maturation of dendritic cells through inhibition of NFκB activation (22); increases both osteoclastic bone-resorbing activity and osteoclast chemotaxis (23); induces migration, parathyroid hormone (PTH)-dependent cAMP accumulation, and alkaline phosphatase in osteoblasts (24); enhances natural killer (NK) cell adhesion to tumor endothelium (25); and recruits monocyte and endothelial cell progenitors to the vasculature (26). Furthermore, VEGF is an important autocrine/paracrine inducer of MM cell growth, migration, and survival *via* VEGFR-1 (27,28). Binding of MM cells to BMSCs also enhances production and secretion of IGF-1. IGF-1 induces MM cell growth, survival, and migration, as well as confers drug resistance (29–34). Moreover IGF-1 induces HIF-1α, which triggers VEGF expression; consequently, inhibition of IGFR-1 activity markedly decreases VEGF secretion in MM/BMSC co-cultures. Importantly, IL-6 is active specifically in early-stage disease, whereas IGF-1 is also implicated in late stages of MM (35). Although SDF-1α and TNF-α have only minor direct effects on MM cell proliferation and survival, they regulate the initial recruitment of MM cells to a conductive microenvironment niche. Specifically, they increase adhesion of MM cells to BMSCs by upregulation of adhesion proteins on tumor as well as stromal cells (LFA-1, VLA-4, ICAM-1, VCAM-1, CD49d, CD54), thereby inducing MM cell proliferation, drug-resistance, as well as IL-6, IGF-1, and VEGF secretion (14,36). In addition to IL-6, VEGF, IGF-1, SDF-1α, and TNFα, other factors which modestly control growth and survival of MM cells include the growth factors IGF-2, HGF, bFGF, G-CSF, SCF; the cytokines IL-1, IL-10, IL-11, IL-15, and IL-21; ciliary neutropic factor, LIF, oncostatin M, and TGF-β; as well as MIP-1α and IFN-α (37,38). Furthermore, some MM cell lines and patient cells express the heparin-binding epidermal growth factor-like growth factor (HB-EGF) and its receptors encoded by ErbB1 or ErbB4 genes. In the presence of IL-6, HB-EGF stimulates the proliferation of ErbB1 and ErbB2 postitive cells through a PI3-kinase/Akt dependent pathway. Conversely, a pan-ErbB inhibitor blocked HB-EGF-induced signaling and MM cell growth (39).

THE VASCULAR NICHE OF THE BM AND TUMOR-ANGIOGENESIS

The BM vasculature represents the anatomic barrier between the hemato-poietic compartment, which is well protected by the surrounding bone, and the peripheral circulation. It thereby allows blood cell production, differ-entiation, as well as mobilization into the blood stream and homing to selective sites. Anatomically, the "vascular niche" of the BM consists of a network of sinusoidal vessels which are formed by a single layer of endo-thelial cells and directly supported by the surrounding hematopoietic marrow. Indeed, the intimate anatomical and functional association of hematopoietic and endothelial cells led to the concept of a common pre-cursor cell, the hemangioblast (40,41). For example, it is now clear that the vascular niche is not only a transfer system for mature blood cells to the peripheral circulation, but also a site required for the differentiation and maturation of hematopoietic progenitors due both to production and secretion of various cytokines and growth factors as well as direct contact (42–44). Moreover, hematopoietic cells including megakaryocytes can in turn prolong survival of BM endothelial cells by secreting endothelial cell survival factors such as VEGF (45,46). The interdependent pathophysio-logic role of the vascular niche in MM remains under active investigation.

The role of tumor-angiogenesis in solid tumors is well established and correlates with tumor growth and metastatic potential. Specifically, blood vessels are required for tumor growth and progression, as well as for pro-vision of vital oxygen and nutrients. An increasing number of studies also demonstrates a role for angiogenesis in hematologic malignancies, including MM. Increased MVD within the BM of MM patients correlates with disease progression and poor prognosis. Indeed, BM MVD at the time of initial diagnosis is an important prognostic factor for median overall survival and median progression-free survival in patients undergoing autologous trans-plantation as frontline therapy for MM. These data, coupled with the anti-angiogenic properties of thalidomide, provided the rationale for the therapeutic use of thalidomide in MM. Clinical responses to thalidomide were observed in 30% of MM patients whose disease is refractory to conventional and high-dose therapy. One of the main factors of angiogenesis, VEGF, is secreted by several MM cell lines and is present in patient MM BM aspirates. MM endothelial cells typically express high levels of several vascular markers including Tie2, VEGFR2, FGFR2, CD105-endoglin, and VE-cadherin, as well as CXC chemokines (47,48). Our own and other studies demonstrate that

VEGFR-1 is highly expressed by MM cells (49) providing the preclinical rationale to test several antiangiogenic compounds including the VEGFR tyrosine kinase inhibitor PTK787/ZK222584 and the pan-VEGFR inhibitor pazopanib for their therapeutic potential in MM (90,91).

Importantly, the discrepancy between marked antitumor activity of antiangiogenic inhibitors (e.g., VEGF receptor inhibitors) in animal models versus the disappointing clinical results when these inhibitors were used as single agents has resulted in their clinical use combined with chemotherapy. Besides increasing the efficacy of chemotherapeutics, this strategy will (1) allow the use of doses significantly below the maximum tolerated dose (MTD), thereby decreasing adverse side effects; and (2) permit drug administration for prolonged uninterrupted periods, thereby preventing development of overcoming drug resistance. Therefore administration of VEGF-receptor inhibitors in combination with other drugs may be required to achieve maximal efficacy. The clinical success of antiangiogenic agents will also likely depend on tumor stage and prior treatment. For example, one approach to decrease toxic side-effects and improve antitumor effects is metronomic chemotherapy, which is characterized by the use of frequent uninterrupted administration of conventional chemotherapeutics in doses significantly below MTD for prolonged periods. The advantage of metronomic therapy is the possibility to combine antiangiogenic therapies with either other antiangiogenic therapies or novel and conventional low-dose therapies.

MYELOMA BONE DISEASE AND THE OSTEOBLASTIC NICHE

Osteolytic bone ("punch-out") lesions are a typical clinical feature in almost all MM patients, most prominently located in the central skeleton, the skull, and the long bones and associated with bone pain, pathologic fractures, and diffuse osteoporosis. Both increased osteoclast formation and activity in the vicinity of MM cells as well as lower numbers of osteoblasts and decreased bone formation, mediate these effects (50).

Specifically, increased osteoclast (OC) activity is triggered by a variety of osteoclast-activating factors (OAFs) produced by both tumor as well as stromal cells. These factors include macrophage inflammatory protein-1α (MIP-1α) and receptor of NFκB ligand (RANKL; also named tumor necrosis factor-related activation induced cytokine, TRANCE; or osteoprotegerin ligand, OPGL), VEGF, TNFα, IL-1β, parathyroid hormone-related protein (PTHrP), HGF, and IL-6. In turn, osteoclast activity modulates MM cell growth and survival (51,52). Consequently, inhibitors of bone resorption, e.g., pamidronate, also have anti-MM activity (53,54). MIP-1α belongs to the Regulated on Activation Normal T cell Expressed and Secreted (RANTES) family of chemokines and binds CCR1, CCR5, and CCR9. It directly acts on human OCL progenitors and at later stages of osteoclast differentiation. In MM, MIP-1α is expressed and secreted by MM cells and enhances OCL formation induced by PTHrP, RANKL, and IL-6 (55). Interestingly, FGFR3 overexpression in t(4;14) MM cells is closely linked with MIP-1α upregulation, thereby providing the first association between an initiating IgH translocation in MM and associated bone disease (56). Conversely, antibodies against MIP-1α and MIP-1β or their receptor CCR5, as well as an antisense construct to MIP-1α, reduce enhanced bone resorption (57–59). RANKL, which is expressed by osteoblasts, endothelial cells, and stromal cells, induces differentiation, formation, fusion, and survival of preosteoclasts, as well as activates mature osteoclasts to resorb bone *via* RANK, on osteoclast precursors and mature osteoclasts (60,61). For physiologic bone homeostasis a balanced ratio of RANKL and OPG, a decoy receptor antagonist for RANKL secreted by osteoblasts and stromal cells, is required (62,63). In MM, this ratio is disrupted. Although the expression of RANKL in MM cells remains controversial, several studies demonstrate that RANKL expression is strongly upregulated in coculture systems of MM cells with BMSCs or preosteoblasts, whereas OPG production is downregulated (64–69). Moreover, heparan sulfates within the proteoglycan syndecan-1 (CD138) sequestrate OPG due to its binding to MM cells, internalization, and degradation (70). In vivo studies have demonstrated both a decrease in osteolysis, as well as an indirect anti-MM effect, using RANKL:Fc or OPG:Fc (68,71). A phase I study with recombinant OPG construct AMGN-0007 showed rapid, sustained, and profound suppression of bone resorption and was well tolerated (72).

In addition to increased osteoclast formation and activity, MM patients with lytic lesions have lower numbers of osteoblasts and decreased bone formation. Dysregulation of several molecules contribute to this effect, including Runx2/Cbfa1, Wnt, and IL-3. Specifically, MM cells block activity and function of the transcription factor Runx2/Cbfa1 in human BM osteoblast progenitors through direct VLA-4/VCAM-1-mediated contact or IL-7 secretion (73–75), and increase osteoclastogenesis *via* enhanced secretion of OPG in osteoprogenitor cells (76). Moreover, recent studies also suggest the importance of the canonical Wingless-type (Wnt) signaling pathway in MM bone disease. Specifically, the Wnt-signaling antagonist dickkopf-1 (DKK1), an inhibitor of osteoblast differentiation, is significantly overexpressed in patients with MM presenting with lytic bone lesions. Inhibition of osteoblast precursors by DKK1 shifts the balance towards osteoclasts and blocks establishment of the BM microenvironment required for hematopoietic stem cell differentiation, thereby contributing to immunosuppression and anemia in MM patients. Consequently, administration of a polyclonal DKK1 antibody ameliorated the bone-specific morbidity of MM (77). Moreover, immuno depletion of secreted frizzled-related protein (sFRP)-2, which prevents the binding of Wnt proteins to their receptors and thereby inhibits osteoblast function, significantly restored mineralized nodule formation in vitro (78). Finally, IL-3 is increased in the BM plasma from MM patients and triggers increased OCL formation, as well as blocks differentiation of preosteoblasts to mature osteoblasts. Importantly, CD3+ T cells, another cellular component within the BM microenvironment, have recently been identified as the main source of IL-3 in MM patients (79–81). A potential critical role of CD3+ T cells in MM bone disease is supported both by their increased production of RANKL; as well as their support of osteoclastogenesis involving OPG/TRAIL interaction (69,82). Another molecule that may contribute to MM bone disease is the proteoglycan serglycin, which is increased in some MM cell lines and patient MM cells, and inhibits bone mineralization by inhibiting crystal growth rate of hydroxyapatite (83).

The BM microenvironment, and osteoblasts in particular, are required for HSC development (84,85). Specifically, HSCs reside either next to osteoblasts within the osteoblastic/endosteal niche (trabecular bone surface), which provides a quiescent microenvironment for HSC maintenance; or adjacent to endothelial cells of the sinusoids within the vascular niche, which favors HSC differentiation and mobilization into the periphery. Therefore the stem cell niche regulates the balance between cellular self-renewal and blood cell-lineage-dependent differentiation, specifically by asymmetric division (generating another stem cell and a progenitor cell) or symmetric division (generating two stem cells). This process occurs in a discrete topological and chronological pattern dependent on different physiologic conditions (86,87). Ongoing studies are now directed to identify the specific MM stem cell, and to define a likely role for the osteoblastic/endosteal niche in its development, proliferation, and survival.

FUTURE ASPECTS: STROMAL THERAPY AS A NEW THERAPEUTIC STRATEGY

The similarities in gene expression profiles in monoclonal gammopathy of undetermined significance (MGUS) and MM cells versus normal plasma cells strongly support the hypothesis that the MM BM microenvironment plays a pivotal role in malignant transformation (88). Indeed, the development of MM can be seen as a complex multistep process involving both genetic changes in the tumor cell, as well as the selective supportive conditions of the BM niche to stimulate MM cell growth, survival, migration, and drug resistance (89). Importantly, bortezomib (Millenium Pharmaceuticals, Cambridge, MA) and lenalidomide (Celgene Corporation, Warren, NJ) are two novel agents recently approved by the US Food and Drug Administration (FDA) for treatment of relapsed/refractory MM. Besides their direct activity against MM cells, the therapeutic success of bortezomib and lenalidomide is also based on their activity against the BM microenvironment. Specifically, bortezomib inhibits MM cell growth triggered by

BMSC adhesion, as well as production and secretion of cytokines that mediate MM cell growth and survival. Moreover, bortezomib down-regulates caveolin-1 expression and phosphorylation required for VEGF-mediated MM cell migration on fibronectin. The antiangiogenic effect of bortezomib is another potential mechanism of its anti-MM activity. Similar to bortezomib, lenalidomide overcomes growth and survival advantage conferred by the BM milieu and also downregulates VEGF. In addition, lenalidomide costimulates T cells, enhances antitumor immunity mediated by IFNγ and IL-2, and augments NK cell cytotoxicity.

Our understanding of the BM microenvironment structure and its impact on hematopoietic cell homing, seeding, proliferation and survival is increasing. Within MM, ongoing and future studies are directed to develop in vitro MM BM model systems that simulate the complex interactions of the cellular and liquid compartments within the BM. These model systems will not only further delineate molecular processes of MM pathogenesis, but also provide the preclinical framework for clinical evaluation of novel targeted therapies to improve patient outcome in MM.

REFERENCES

1. Jensen GS, Belch AR, Mant MJ, Ruether BA, Yacyshyn BR, Pilarski LM. Expression of multiple beta 1 integrins on circulating monoclonal B cells in patients with multiple myeloma. Am J Hematol 1993; 43:29–36.
2. Damiano JS, Cress AE, Hazlehurst LA, Shtil AA, Dalton WS. Cell adhesion mediated drug resistance (CAM-DR): role of integrins and resistance to apoptosis in human myeloma cell lines. Blood 1999; 93:1658–67.
3. Vacca A, Ria R, Presta M, et al. Alpha(v)beta(3) integrin engagement modulates cell adhesion, proliferation, and protease secretion in human lymphoid tumor cells. Exp Hematol 2001; 29:993–1003.
4. Ria R, Vacca A, Ribatti D, Di Raimondo F, Merchionne F, Dammacco F. Alpha(v)beta(3) integrin engagement enhances cell invasiveness in human multiple myeloma. Haematologica 2002; 87:836–45.
5. Uchiyama H, Barut BA, Chauhan D, Cannistra SA, Anderson KC. Characterization of adhesion molecules on human myeloma cell lines. Blood 1992; 80:2306–14.
6. Uchiyama H, Barut BA, Mohrbacher AF, Chauhan D, Anderson KC. Adhesion of human myeloma-derived cell lines to bone marrow stromal cells stimulates interleukin-6 secretion. Blood 1993; 82:3712–20.
7. Hazlehurst LA, Damiano JS, Buyuksal I, Pledger WJ, Dalton WS. Adhesion to fibronectin via beta1 integrins regulates p27kip1 levels and contributes to cell adhesion mediated drug resistance (CAM-DR). Oncogene 2000; 19: 4319–27.
8. Tai YT, Li XF, Breitkreutz I, et al. Role of B-cell-activating factor in adhesion and growth of human multiple myeloma cells in the bone marrow microenvironment. Cancer Res 2006; 66:6675–82.

9. Podar K, Hideshima T, Chauhan D, Anderson KC. Targeting signalling pathways for the treatment of multiple myeloma. Expert Opin Ther Targets 2005; 9:359–81.

10. Gupta D, Treon SP, Shima Y, et al. Adherence of multiple myeloma cells to bone marrow stromal cells upregulates vascular endothelial growth factor secretion: therapeutic applications. Leukemia 2001; 15:1950–61.

11. Gado K, Domjan G, Hegyesi H, Falus A. Role of Interleukin-6 in the pathogenesis of multiple myeloma. Cell Biol Int 2000; 24:195–209.

12. Urashima M, Chauhan D, Uchiyama H, Freeman GJ, Anderson KC. CD40 ligand triggered interleukin-6 secretion in multiple myeloma. Blood 1995; 85: 1903–12.

13. Tai YT, Podar K, Gupta D, et al. CD40 activation induces p53-dependent vascular endothelial growth factor secretion in human multiple myeloma cells. Blood 2002; 99:1419–27.

14. Hideshima T, Chauhan D, Schlossman R, Richardson P, Anderson KC. The role of tumor necrosis factor alpha in the pathophysiology of human multiple myeloma: therapeutic applications. Oncogene 2001; 20:4519–27.

15. Costes V, Portier M, Lu ZY, Rossi JF, Bataille R, Klein B. Interleukin-1 in multiple myeloma: producer cells and their role in the control of IL-6 production. Br J Haematol 1998; 103:1152–60.

16. Lust JA, Donovan KA. The role of interleukin-1 beta in the pathogenesis of multiple myeloma. Hematol Oncol Clin North Am 1999; 13:1117–25.

17. Hurt EM, Wiestner A, Rosenwald A, et al. Overexpression of c-maf is a frequent oncogenic event in multiple myeloma that promotes proliferation and pathological interactions with bone marrow stroma. Cancer Cell 2004; 5: 191–9.

18. Ferrara N, Carver-Moore K, Chen H, et al. Heterozygous embryonic lethality induced by targeted inactivation of the VEGF gene. Nature 1996; 380:439–42.

19. Carmeliet P, Ferreira V, Breier G, et al. Abnormal blood vessel development and lethality in embryos lacking a single VEGF allele. Nature 1996; 380:435–9.

20. Shalaby F, Rossant J, Yamaguchi TP, et al. Failure of blood-island formation and vasculogenesis in Flk-1-deficient mice. Nature 1995; 376:62–6.

21. Gerber HP, Malik AK, Solar GP, et al. VEGF regulates haematopoietic stem cell survival by an internal autocrine loop mechanism. Nature 2002; 417:954–8.

22. Gabrilovich DI, Chen HL, Girgis KR, et al. Production of vascular endothelial growth factor by human tumors inhibits the functional maturation of dendritic cells. Nat Med 1996; 2:1096–103.

23. Henriksen K, Karsdal M, Delaisse JM, Engsig MT. RANKL and vascular endothelial growth factor (VEGF) induce osteoclast chemotaxis through an ERK1/2-dependent mechanism. J Biol Chem 2003; 278:48745–53.

24. Midy V, Plouet J. Vasculotropin/vascular endothelial growth factor induces differentiation in cultured osteoblasts. Biochem Biophys Res Commun 1994; 199:380–6.

25. Melder RJ, Koenig GC, Witwer BP, Safabakhsh N, Munn LL, Jain RK. During angiogenesis, vascular endothelial growth factor and basic fibroblast growth factor regulate natural killer cell adhesion to tumor endothelium. Nat Med 1996; 2:992–7.

26. Lyden D, Hattori K, Dias S, et al. Impaired recruitment of bone-marrow-derived endothelial and hematopoietic precursor cells blocks tumor angiogenesis and growth. Nat Med 2001; 7:1194–201.

27. Podar K, Tai YT, Davies FE, et al. Vascular endothelial growth factor triggers signaling cascades mediating multiple myeloma cell growth and migration. Blood 2001; 98:428–35.

28. Vincent L, Jin DK, Karajannis MA, et al. Fetal stromal-dependent paracrine and intracrine vascular endothelial growth factor-a/vascular endothelial growth factor receptor-1 signaling promotes proliferation and motility of human primary myeloma cells. Cancer Res 2005; 65:3185–92.

29. Ferlin M, Noraz N, Hertogh C, Brochier J, Taylor N, Klein B. Insulin-like growth factor induces the survival and proliferation of myeloma cells through an interleukin-6-independent transduction pathway. Br J Haematol 2000; 111: 626–34.

30. Tu Y, Gardner A, Lichtenstein A. The phosphatidylinositol 3-kinase/AKT kinase pathway in multiple myeloma plasma cells: roles in cytokine-dependent survival and proliferative responses. Cancer Res 2000; 60:6763–70.

31. Qiang YW, Kopantzev E, Rudikoff S. Insulinlike growth factor-I signaling in multiple myeloma: downstream elements, functional correlates, and pathway cross-talk. Blood 2002; 99:4138–46.

32. Qiang YW, Yao L, Tosato G, Rudikoff S. Insulin-like growth factor I induces migration and invasion of human multiple myeloma cells. Blood 2004; 103:301–8.

33. Ge NL, Rudikoff S. Insulin-like growth factor I is a dual effector of multiple myeloma cell growth. Blood 2000; 96:2856–61.

34. Tai YT, Podar K, Catley L, et al. Insulin-like growth factor-1 induces adhesion and migration in human multiple myeloma cells via activation of beta1-integrin and phosphatidylinositol 3'-kinase/AKT signaling. Cancer Res 2003; 63: 5850–8.

35. Mitsiades CS, Mitsiades NS, McMullan CJ, et al. Inhibition of the insulin-like growth factor receptor-1 tyrosine kinase activity as a therapeutic strategy for multiple myeloma, other hematologic malignancies, and solid tumors. Cancer Cell 2004; 5:221–30.

36. Hideshima T, Chauhan D, Hayashi T, et al. The biological sequelae of stromal cell-derived factor-1alpha in multiple myeloma. Mol Cancer Ther 2002; 1:539–44.

37. Lentzsch S, Gries M, Janz M, Bargou R, Dorken B, Mapara MY. Macrophage inflammatory protein 1-alpha (MIP-1 alpha) triggers migration and signaling cascades mediating survival and proliferation in multiple myeloma (MM) cells. Blood 2003; 101:3568–73.

38. Lentzsch S, Chatterjee M, Gries M, et al. PI3-K/AKT/FKHR and MAPK signaling cascades are redundantly stimulated by a variety of cytokines and contribute independently to proliferation and survival of multiple myeloma cells. Leukemia 2004.

39. Mahtouk K, Jourdan M, De Vos J, et al. An inhibitor of the EGF receptor family blocks myeloma cell growth factor activity of HB-EGF and potentiates dexamethasone or anti-IL-6 antibody-induced apoptosis. Blood 2004; 103: 1829–37.

40. Choi K, Kennedy M, Kazarov A, Papadimitriou JC, Keller G. A common precursor for hematopoietic and endothelial cells. Development 1998; 125:725–32.

41. Nishikawa SI. A complex linkage in the developmental pathway of endothelial and hematopoietic cells. Curr Opin Cell Biol 2001; 13:673–8.
42. Tavassoli M. Structure and function of sinusoidal endothelium of bone marrow. Prog Clin Biol Res 1981; 59B:249–56.
43. Rafii S, Mohle R, Shapiro F, Frey BM, Moore MA. Regulation of hematopoiesis by microvascular endothelium. Leuk Lymphoma 1997; 27: 375–86.
44. Rafii S, Shapiro F, Rimarachin J, et al. Isolation and characterization of human bone marrow microvascular endothelial cells: hematopoietic progenitor cell adhesion. Blood 1994; 84:10–19.
45. Mohle R, Green D, Moore MA, Nachman RL, Rafii S. Constitutive production and thrombin-induced release of vascular endothelial growth factor by human megakaryocytes and platelets. Proc Natl Acad Sci USA 1997; 94: 663–8.
46. Avecilla ST, Hattori K, Heissig B, et al. Chemokine-mediated interaction of hematopoietic progenitors with the bone marrow vascular niche is required for thrombopoiesis. Nat Med 2004; 10:64–71.
47. Vacca A, Ria R, Semeraro F, et al. Endothelial cells in the bone marrow of patients with multiple myeloma. Blood 2003; 102:3340–8.
48. Pellegrino A, Ria R, Pietro GD, et al. Bone marrow endothelial cells in multiple myeloma secrete CXC-chemokines that mediate interactions with plasma cells. Br J Haematol 2005; 129:248–56.
49. Podar K, Anderson KC. The pathophysiological role of VEGF in hematological malignancies: therapeutic implications. Blood 2005; 105:1383–95.
50. Giuliani N, Rizzoli V, Roodman GD. Multiple myeloma bone disease: pathophysiology of osteoblast inhibition. Blood 2006; 108(13):3992–6.
51. Yaccoby S, Pearse RN, Johnson CL, Barlogie B, Choi Y, Epstein J. Myeloma interacts with the bone marrow microenvironment to induce osteoclastogenesis and is dependent on osteoclast activity. Br J Haematol 2002; 116: 278–90.
52. Vanderkerken K, De Leenheer E, Shipman C, et al. Recombinant osteoprotegerin decreases tumor burden and increases survival in a murine model of multiple myeloma. Cancer Res 2003; 63:287–9.
53. Berenson JR, Lichtenstein A, Porter L, et al. Efficacy of pamidronate in reducing skeletal events in patients with advanced multiple myeloma. Myeloma Aredia Study Group. N Engl J Med 1996; 334:488–93.
54. Dhodapkar MV, Singh J, Mehta J, et al. Anti-myeloma activity of pamidronate in vivo. Br J Haematol 1998; 103:530–2.
55. Han JH, Choi SJ, Kurihara N, Koide M, Oba Y, Roodman GD. Macrophage inflammatory protein-1alpha is an osteoclastogenic factor in myeloma that is independent of receptor activator of nuclear factor kappaB ligand. Blood 2001; 97:3349–53.
56. Masih-Khan E, Trudel S, Heise C, et al. MIP-1{α} (CCL3) is a downstream target of FGFR3 and RAS/MAPK signaling in multiple myeloma. Blood 2006; 108(10):3465–71.
57. Choi SJ, Cruz JC, Craig F, et al. Macrophage inflammatory protein 1-alpha is a potential osteoclast stimulatory factor in multiple myeloma. Blood 2000; 96: 671–5.

58. Choi SJ, Oba Y, Gazitt Y, et al. Antisense inhibition of macrophage inflammatory protein 1-alpha blocks bone destruction in a model of myeloma bone disease. J Clin Invest 2001; 108:1833–41.

59. Oyajobi BO, Franchin G, Williams PJ, et al. Dual effects of macrophage inflammatory protein-1alpha on osteolysis and tumor burden in the murine 5TGM1 model of myeloma bone disease. Blood 2003; 102:311–9.

60. Lacey DL, Timms E, Tan HL, et al. Osteoprotegerin ligand is a cytokine that regulates osteoclast differentiation and activation. Cell 1998; 93:165–76.

61. Hsu H, Lacey DL, Dunstan CR, et al. Tumor necrosis factor receptor family member RANK mediates osteoclast differentiation and activation induced by osteoprotegerin ligand. Proc Natl Acad Sci USA 1999; 96:3540–5.

62. Bucay N, Sarosi I, Dunstan CR, et al. Osteoprotegerin-deficient mice develop early onset osteoporosis and arterial calcification. Genes Dev 1998; 12:1260–8.

63. Kong YY, Yoshida H, Sarosi I, et al. OPGL is a key regulator of osteoclastogenesis, lymphocyte development and lymph-node organogenesis. Nature 1999; 397:315–23.

64. Farrugia AN, Atkins GJ, To LB, et al. Receptor activator of nuclear factor-kappaB ligand expression by human myeloma cells mediates osteoclast formation in vitro and correlates with bone destruction in vivo. Cancer Res 2003; 63:5438–45.

65. Heider U, Langelotz C, Jakob C, et al. Expression of receptor activator of nuclear factor kappaB ligand on bone marrow plasma cells correlates with osteolytic bone disease in patients with multiple myeloma. Clin Cancer Res 2003; 9:1436–40.

66. Roux S, Meignin V, Quillard J, et al. RANK (receptor activator of nuclear factor-kappaB) and RANKL expression in multiple myeloma. Br J Haematol 2002; 117:86–92.

67. Giuliani N, Bataille R, Mancini C, Lazzaretti M, Barille S. Myeloma cells induce imbalance in the osteoprotegerin/osteoprotegerin ligand system in the human bone marrow environment. Blood 2001; 98:3527–33.

68. Pearse RN, Sordillo EM, Yaccoby S, et al. Multiple myeloma disrupts the TRANCE/osteoprotegerin cytokine axis to trigger bone destruction and promote tumor progression. Proc Natl Acad Sci USA 2001; 98:11581–6.

69. Giuliani N, Colla S, Sala R, et al. Human myeloma cells stimulate the receptor activator of nuclear factor-kappa B ligand (RANKL) in T lymphocytes: a potential role in multiple myeloma bone disease. Blood 2002; 100:4615–21.

70. Standal T, Seidel C, Hjertner O, et al. Osteoprotegerin is bound, internalized, and degraded by multiple myeloma cells. Blood 2002; 100:3002–7.

71. Croucher PI, Shipman CM, Lippitt J, et al. Osteoprotegerin inhibits the development of osteolytic bone disease in multiple myeloma. Blood 2001; 98:3534–40.

72. Body JJ, Greipp P, Coleman RE, et al. A phase I study of AMGN-0007, a recombinant osteoprotegerin construct, in patients with multiple myeloma or breast carcinoma related bone metastases. Cancer 2003; 97:887–92.

73. Komori T. Regulation of skeletal development by the Runx family of transcription factors. J Cell Biochem 2005; 95:445–53.

74. Komori T, Yagi H, Nomura S, et al. Targeted disruption of Cbfa1 results in a complete lack of bone formation owing to maturational arrest of osteoblasts. Cell 1997; 89:755–64.

75. Giuliani N, Colla S, Morandi F, et al. Myeloma cells block RUNX2/CBFA1 activity in human bone marrow osteoblast progenitors and inhibit osteoblast formation and differentiation. Blood 2005; 106:2472–83.

76. Thirunavukkarasu K, Halladay DL, Miles RR, et al. The osteoblast-specific transcription factor Cbfa1 contributes to the expression of osteoprotegerin, a potent inhibitor of osteoclast differentiation and function. J Biol Chem 2000; 275:25163–72.

77. Tian E, Zhan F, Walker R, et al. The role of the Wnt-signaling antagonist DKK1 in the development of osteolytic lesions in multiple myeloma. N Engl J Med 2003; 349:2483–94.

78. Oshima T, Abe M, Asano J, et al. Myeloma cells suppress bone formation by secreting a soluble Wnt inhibitor, sFRP-2. Blood 2005; 106:3160–5.

79. Lee JW, Chung HY, Ehrlich LA, et al. IL-3 expression by myeloma cells increases both osteoclast formation and growth of myeloma cells. Blood 2004; 103:2308–15.

80. Ehrlich LA, Chung HY, Ghobrial I, et al. IL-3 is a potential inhibitor of osteoblast differentiation in multiple myeloma. Blood 2005; 106:1407–14.

81. Giuliani N, Morandi F, Tagliaferri S, et al. Interleukin-3 (IL-3) is over-expressed by T lymphocytes in multiple myeloma patients. Blood 2006; 107: 841–2.

82. Colucci S, Brunetti G, Rizzi R, et al. T cells support osteoclastogenesis in an in vitro model derived from human multiple myeloma bone disease: the role of the OPG/TRAIL interaction. Blood 2004; 104:3722–30.

83. Theocharis AD, Seidel C, Borset M, et al. Serglycin constitutively secreted by myeloma plasma cells is a potent inhibitor of bone mineralization in vitro. J Biol Chem 2006; 281(46):35116–28.

84. Zhang J, Niu C, Ye L, et al. Identification of the haematopoietic stem cell niche and control of the niche size. Nature 2003; 425:836–41.

85. Calvi LM, Adams GB, Weibrecht KW, et al. Osteoblastic cells regulate the haematopoietic stem cell niche. Nature 2003; 425:841–6.

86. Fuchs E, Tumbar T, Guasch G. Socializing with the neighbors: stem cells and their niche. Cell 2004; 116:769–78.

87. Watt FM, Hogan BL. Out of Eden: stem cells and their niches. Science 2000; 287:1427–30.

88. Davies FE, Dring AM, Li C, et al. Insights into the multistep transformation of MGUS to myeloma using microarray expression analysis. Blood 2003; 102(13): 4504–11.

89. Kuehl WM, Bergsagel PL. Multiple myeloma: evolving genetic events and host interactions. Nat Rev Cancer 2002; 2:175–87.

90. Lin B, Podar K, Gupta D, et al. The vascular endothelial growth factor receptor tyrosine kinase inhibitor PTK787/ZK222584 inhibits growth and migration of multiple myeloma cells in the bone marrow micro environment. Cancer Res 2002; 62(17):5019–26.

91. Podar K, Tonon G, Sattler M, et al. The small-molecule VEGF receptor inhibitor pazopanib (GW786034B) targets both tumor and endothelial cells in multiple myeloma. Proc Acad Sci USA 2006; 103(51):19478–83.

5

Novel Therapeutic Targets in Multiple Myeloma

Giovanni Tonon

*Department of Medical Oncology, Dana-Farber Cancer Institute,
Harvard Medical School, Boston, Massachusetts, U.S.A.*

INTRODUCTION

Among cancers of different origin, multiple myeloma (MM) has carved out a position of prominence, as an effective model system to test and validate leading therapeutic compounds. Indeed, several drugs now in clinical practice were first successfully tested in MM, and then their use extended to other hematological and epithelial tumors.

Many recent developments in identifying drugs targeting MM have been the result of fruitful collaborations between academia and industry, where academia has tested in MM cell line and in vivo models compounds developed by industry and targeting cancer-specific pathways. On a parallel track, two highly effective drugs against MM have been identified somewhat serendipitously: Thalidomide, which has helped to reveal the importance of angiogenesis in the initiation and maintenance of MM, and bortezomib, which has brought to light the concept of protein metabolism as a critical therapeutic target in MM cells.

The future challenge will be to exploit the data coming from comprehensive expression and genomic profiling, as well as sequencing and proteomic approaches, to identify novel targets not linked to previously known cancer-relevant pathways and not yet developed as potentially fruitful therapeutic targets.

As stressed in previous chapters, the interactions of MM cells with surrounding cells and environment are of critical importance both for understanding MM biology and its response (or resistance) to drugs. Indeed, it has been proven again and again how extensively MM cells rely on signals and interactions from their surroundings for their growth and survival (Fig. 1) (1). Moreover, it has been consistently shown how most, if not all, the compounds used or tested in MM target the MM cells and surrounding cells at the same time and disrupt their intricate and continuous cross-talk (See Chapters 2–6) (2).

THALIDOMIDE AND THE IMMUNOMODULATORY DERIVATIVES

The stunning revival of the immunomodulatory drug (ImID) Thalidomide as an anticancer drug started in 1999, when its use was proposed for the treatment of MM based on its antiangiogenic activity (3). In this landmark study, thalidomide was proposed as an effective treatment of advanced MM, with a clinical response evident in 30–40% of patients with advanced and refractory MM, with 10% of patients showing near-complete remissions.

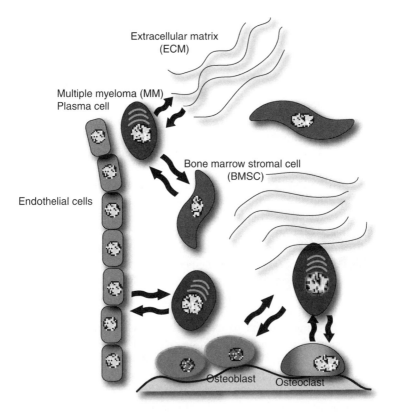

Figure 1   MM cell survival and proliferation depends and relies on the mutual interactions with endothelial, bone, and bone marrow cells and stroma.

In the following years, the multifaceted mechanism of action of thalidomide was extensively explored, and unexpected twists were discovered (Fig. 2) (4). In the context of MM, thalidomide is able to induce growth arrest associated with apoptosis in MM cells and inhibit adhesion of MM cells to bone marrow stromal cells (BMSCs). Stromal-cell expression of vascular endothelial growth factor (VEGF) and basic fibroblast growth factor

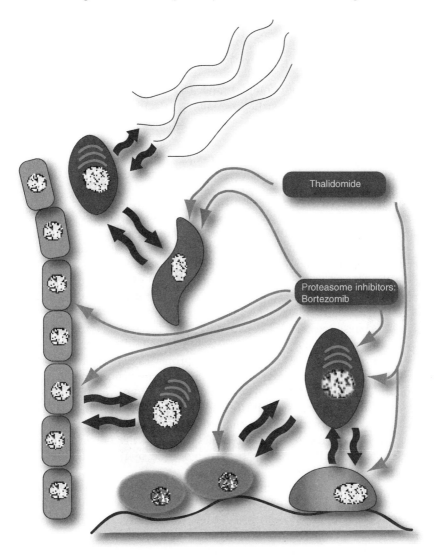

Figure 2 Multifaceted mechanism of action of thalidomide and bortezomib. In addition to multiple myeloma (MM) cells, these compounds also target other compartments in the bone marrow.

(bFGF) is reduced, thereby decreasing angiogenesis. Expression of interleukin-6 (IL-6) and tumor necrosis factor-α (TNF-α) by BMSC was also reduced. Thalidomide was also able to induce T-cell stimulation and proliferation, with release of IL-2 and interferon-γ (IFN-γ), followed by the activation of natural killer (NK) cells and subsequent MM-cell death. Given the teratogenic effects of thalidomide, major efforts have been directed on identifying other related compounds devoid of side effects. Using thalidomide as the lead compound, other immunomodulatory derivatives (ImiDs) in particular 4-amino analogues in which an amino group is added to the fourth carbon of the pthaloyl ring of thalidomide, were found to be up to 50,000 times more potent than the parent compound in vitro. In particular, CC-5013 (lenalidomide) and CC-4047 (actimid) have been introduced in the clinical practice as equally effective but with far fewer side effects than thalidomide (4).

BORTEZOMIB AND THE RELEVANCE OF PROTEIN METABOLISM IN THE TREATMENT OF MM

MM cells present a high protein turnover. Protein metabolism is therefore finely tuned to prevent overloading that could lead to apoptosis. Compounds targeting different phases of this metabolic process have become the cornerstone of the treatment of this disease, prominent among them bortezomib, a major breakthrough in the treatment of MM (5,6). Among the targets of the proteasome inhibitors are the IL-6 pathway (7) and the nuclear factor-κ B (NF-κB) pathway (8), but it should be noted that bortezomib acts also on other cascades, not immediately linked to the proteasome physiology (6,9). Lee et al. (10) have, for example, reported that bortezomib targets a signaling pathway called the unfolded protein response (UPR) that allows MM cells to handle the proper folding of the increased load of proteins. Additionally, bortezomib exerts its action on other cells residing in the bone marrow milieu (Fig. 2). For example, bortezomib disrupts the interaction between BMSC and MM cells, through the down-regulation of adhesion molecules and reduced NF-κB-dependent secretion of cytokines from BMSC. An additional effect is through inhibition of angiogenesis and cell migration, due to blockade of the VEGF-caveolin 1 axis (11–13).

Latterly, other proteasome inhibitors have been proposed for the treatment of MM. Among the most promising ones are two orally-available compounds, NPI-0052 (14) and PR-171 (6). Interestingly, their mechanism of action is not completely overlapping with bortezomib, and they induce a response even in bortezomib-resistant cells.

A recent development in the treatment of MM in the context of protein metabolism has been the identification of the aggresome as a potential target. Recent work has suggested that this pathway is critical for the survival of MM cells as well, since inhibition of HDAC6 with tubacin-induced apoptosis in MM cells (11,15) and was synergistic with bortezomib. LBH589, another histone deacetylase inhibitor, was recently reported to induce MM cell apoptosis (16).

Drugs inhibiting Hsp90, which contributes to the folding and activation of several cancer-relevant proteins, are also effective in targeting MM cells (17). It has been recently shown that the geldanamycin analog 17-AAG induces apoptosis of MM cells acting at several levels, simultaneously suppressing the insulin-like growth factor receptor (IGF1R) and the interleukin-6 receptor (IL-6R) signaling (including the NF-KB, PI3K/AKT, and MAPK pathways) (18). Moreover, NZ28, an inhibitor of heat shock proteins strongly sensitized myeloma cells to proteasome and Hsp90 inhibitors (19).

COMPOUNDS TARGETING CANCER-SPECIFIC PATHWAYS

Recent advances in the understanding of cancer biology have allowed us to gain a more detailed view of the " molecular circuitry of cancer" (Fig. 3) (20). A few essential "hubs," including the mitogen activated protein kinase (MAPK) and phosphatidylinositol-3 kinase/AKT (PI3K/AKT) pathway, in most tumors, associated with NF-KB and STAT3, more specifically in hematological tumors, are consistently dysregulated in cancers and provide

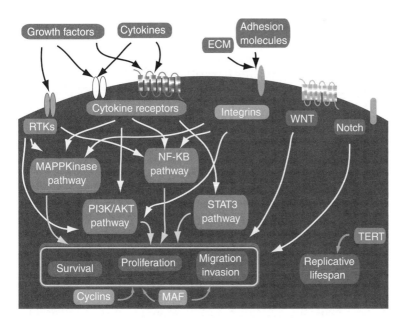

Figure 3   Major signaling pathways involved in MM tumorigenesis.

potent survival, proliferation, and migration signals to the cells. The activation of these " hubs" is induced by dysregulation of various receptors and/or receptor ligands that act upstream and whose activity is tightly controlled in physiological conditions; however, after mutations or genomic rearrangements, they become constitutively active. These receptors include receptor tyrosine kinases and tyrosine-associated receptors (including cytokine receptors and integrins) and their ligands. Other pathways, whose dysregulation have been shown to be critical in several cancers including MM, are WNT and NOTCH. No specific compounds targeting these cascades have been tested as yet in MM, with the exception of neutralizing antibodies blocking the activity of Dickkopf-1 (DKK1), a soluble inhibitor of WNT signaling, which has shown a reduction of osteolytic bone resorption, increased bone formation, and reduced MM growth (21).

LIGANDS AND RECEPTORS

Receptor Tyrosine Kinases

IGF1R

It has been known for a long time that MM cells express insulin-like growth factor (IGF) as well as its receptor IGF1R (22,23). Stimulation of MM cell lines with IGF induced cell proliferation and had an anti-apoptotic effect, mostly through activation of the MAPK, PI3/AKT (24), and NF-κ B (25) pathways. In addition to an autocrine effect based on the production of IGF by MM cells, activation of the IGF1R receptor results from the interaction between MM cells and BMSC (26). Recently, a role for this receptor has also been shown in cell adhesion and migration (27).

Several compounds specific for this pathway have been proposed and seem to have dramatic effect on the survival of MM cell lines [see (28) for a recent review] , including, e.g., the selective kinase inhibitor NVP-ADW742 (29), in both in vitro and in vivo MM models. More recently, both small molecules and monoclonal antibodies against IGF1R have been tested in MM cell lines and provided encouraging results (30– 33).

VEGF

The role of vascular endothelial growth factor (VEGF) and its receptor in tumor neovascularization in the context of solid tumors has been known for many years. More recently, the relevance of fibroblast growth factor and the fibroblast growth factor receptor 1, FLT1 (VEGFR1) [but not KDR (VEGFR2)] has been also proposed for MM. VEGF is expressed and secreted by MM tumor cells as well as by BMSCs (34,35). More recently, it has been shown that VEGF is directly linked to proliferation and migration of human MM cells, suggesting an autocrine VEGF loop in MM through the activation of at least two signaling pathways: The Raf-1-MEK-extracellular signal-regulated protein kinase (ERK) pathway that mediates proliferation, and PI3K-dependent PKC alpha activation cascade, inducing migration (36,37). As mentioned above, both thalidomide and bortezomib inhibit this pathway. Additionally, other, more specific, VEGFR-inhibitors have been proposed and tested in MM. Among them are PTK787/ZK 222584 (PTK787), designed to bind specifically to the tyrosine kinase domain of VEGFR (38); GW654652, a pan-inhibitor of VEGF receptors (39); indolinone derivative BIBF 1000, which competitively binds to the ATP binding sites within the kinase domains of VEGFR1 through VEGFR3; FGFR1 and FGFR3, as well as PDGFRα (40) and, most recently, GW786034B (41), which act directly on and MM cells to inhibit proliferation, as well as on the bone marrow microenvironment. Several clinical trials evaluating bevacizumab, a monoclonal antibody directed at vascular endothelial growth factor, are ongoing or just completed. While preliminary clinical studies with first-generation VEGF inhibitor have shown little or no benefits (42,43), several additional clinical trials are ongoing to determine whether the promising results seen in in vitro studies could bear fruit in the clinical setting.

FGFR3

The receptor tyrosine kinase FGFR3 is dysregulated in approximately 15% of MM, as a result of a chromosomal translocation t(4;14) which dysregulates the gene *MMSET* as well (44). Patients presenting with this translocation have a poor prognosis. While it is not yet clear whether the dysregulation of FGFR3 expression by itself has a prominent role in MM pathogenesis (45), several compounds targeting mutated FGFR3 and specifically tested on cell lines harboring the t(4;14) have demonstrated encouraging results. SU5402, SU10991, and PD173074 (46–48), Chir-258 (49), PKC412 (50) are all kinase inhibitors with proven activity against MM cell lines with mutated FGFR3 expression.

Other Receptor-Tyrosine Receptors

c-Met is expressed on germinal center B cells and on terminally differentiated plasma cells. Moreover, c-Met is expressed in MM cells, and high levels of its ligand HGF were found in the serum of MM patients and correlated with a poor prognosis (51,52). A clear role for the MET/HGF pathway has been established in MM (53), and a connection between overexpression of HGF and reduced bone synthesis and HGF-stimulated adhesion of myeloma cells to fibronectin (54,55) have been demonstrated. Recently, a novel selective small molecule tyrosine kinase inhibitor PHA-665752 directed against the receptor has been shown to reduce proliferation, migration, and adhesion of myeloma cells (56).

Recent findings have suggested that various ErbB receptors are expressed in MM cells and activated by heparin-binding epidermal growth factor-like growth factor (HB-EGF) and amphiregulin (AREG). The exposure of MM cells to PD169540 (a pan-ErbB inhibitor) and IRESSA (an ErbB1-specific inhibitor) was able to induce apoptosis in MM cells. Additionally, crosstalk occurs between ErbB3 and the interferon-α (IFN-α) signaling complex in the myeloma cell line KAS-6/1 which contributes to the regulation of cell proliferation (57,58).

CD117 (c-Kit) has been identified on the surface of MM but its functional relevance has not been determined (59–61). Also, overexpression of Her2/Neu has been reported in a subset of MM patients, but its relevance on the prognosis and the pathogenesis of the disease has not been established (61).

Tyrosine-Kinase-Associated Receptors: Cytokine Receptors and Integrins

Cytokines are subdivided, based on their structure and mechanism of action, in several subgroups including hematopoietins, interferons, and tumor-necrosis factors.

While several members of the hematopoietin family have been implicated in MM cell proliferation (62), the cytokine interleukin-6 (IL-6) cascade and several members belonging to the TNF receptor pathways have been studied more extensively.

IL-6

The role of IL-6 and its receptors in MM has been uncovered almost 20 years ago (63). Further studies have confirmed the central role of this pathway in the context of normal plasma cell physiology as well as MM pathogenesis. Through interaction with gp130 and IL-6R, IL-6 activates the Janus kinase/signal transducer and activator of transcription (JAK/STAT) pathway promoting survival, the proliferation-associated MAPK cascade, and often the PI3K/AKT pathway (64). Moreover, IL-6 represents one of the first examples of a cytokine produced by both MM cell lines (autocrine effect) (63,65) and BMSC (paracrine action) (65,66). In particular, interaction of MM cells with BMSC induces the secretion of IL-6 from BMSC (1), mostly through the activation of NF-κB (67). Given its central role in MM pathogenesis, IL-6 has been one of the most sought-after targets in MM (68). While several compounds effective against MM indirectly affect the IL-6 pathway, targeted biological therapies including mAbs directed against IL-6 and IL-6R and IL-6-conjugated toxins have provided mixed results. While phase II clinical trials using mABs have shown responses in MM patients and a pilot study has shown encouraging results with the murine anti-interleukin-6 (anti-IL-6) monoclonal antibody BE-8 (69), a recent multicenter prospective randomized trial did not show any advantage on adding BE-8 to high dose melphalan as part of the second conditioning regimen for autologous stem cell transplantation (IFM 99-04 protocol) (70). A recent study by Tassone et al. has provided encouraging results through the use of the IL-6 superantagonist Sant7, both in vitro and in vivo (71). Further clinical studies will be needed to conclusively define the utility of targeted IL-6 therapies in MM patients.

TNF

Several members of the TNF family are critical for MM proliferation and survival and many promising drugs targeting these compounds have been proposed (72,73). Among the subgroup of TNF receptors that induce cell death upon activation, the tumor necrosis factor (TNF)-related apoptosis-inducing ligand/Apo2 ligand (TRAIL/Apo2L) induces apoptosis in MM cells (74). Recently, 2 human mAbs directed against TNFRSF10A (HGS-ETR1) and TNFRSF10B (HGS-ETR2) have demonstrated an ability to induce apoptosis in MM cell lines (75), albeit recent data also suggests that recombinant TRAIL might induce apoptosis in the osteoblast compartment exacerbating the MM-induced bone disease (76). Among the TNF receptors that induce proliferation, CD40 and CD40 ligand promote proliferation mediated by IL-6 (77) as well as migration of MM cells and angiogenesis via upregulation of NF-κB, PI3K/AKT (78), and VEGF (79). SGN-14 (80), and more recently CHIR-12.12 (81) and SGN-40 (82) antibodies directed against CD40, induce MM cell death.

Another subset of TNF ligands and receptors that play a major role in inducing proliferation and preventing apoptosis in MM are the ligands APRIL and BAFF, as well as their corresponding receptors TACI, BAFF-R, and BCMA (83,84). These proteins activated NF-κB, PI3K/AKT, and MAPK pathways and induced a strong up-regulation of the Mcl-1 and Bcl-2 antiapoptotic proteins in myeloma cells (84). Several therapeutic monoclonal antibodies, receptor-Fc fusion proteins, or small molecule compounds are under study to inhibit this pathway (85).

MM cells recruit and activate osteoclasts mostly through TNF receptors. In addition to osteoclast-activating factors such as tumor necrosis factor α (TNF-α) (8), IL-1β (86), IL-6, and PTHrP, the RANK receptor and ligand, as well as the chemokine CCL3 (also known as MIP-1α) (87,88) promote osteoclast formation and ultimately bone absorption. These effects are counteracted by the decoy receptor of RANKL, osteoprotegerin (89), as well as by other compounds, such as AMGN-0007, a recombinant osteoprotegerin construct (90) and Denosumab (AMG 162), a fully human monoclonal antibody to RANKL (91). Another chemokine implicated in the process of osteoclast precursor recruitment and activation seen in MM is SDF-1α (92).

Integrins

The relevance of integrins in MM has been extensively studied, but not fully elucidated as yet (93). Several attempts have been made to directly target integrins, as for example, α4 integrin (94,95), NCAM1 (CD56) (96) and ICAM-1 (CD54) (97), with encouraging results.

Signaling "Hubs"—RAS and the MAPKinases, PI3K/AKT, NF-κ B, and STAT3

Within cancer cells in general and MM specifically, there are few pathways that seem to exert a major role in driving proliferation and preventing the tumor cells from undergoing apoptosis. These pathways are activated by signals from receptors, as for example receptor tyrosine kinases or cytokine receptors. While some of these pathways are altered in almost all cancers, as for example the MAPK and the PI3KCA/AKT, others seem to be more specifically dysregulated in hematological tumors, including MM, as for example the NF-κB and the STAT3 pathway (Fig. 3).

Given its central role in cancer and MM, the RAS pathway represents an attractive and obvious candidate for targeted therapy. Among the drugs that have received more interest are the farnesyltransferase inhibitors. Several groups have reported that compounds belonging to this family are able to induce apoptosis in MM cell lines, alone or in combination (98– 103). However, compounds of this family effective in vitro (and even in vivo) often have demonstrated modest therapeutic activity (104). The root of the problem lies in the fact that, although HRAS is exclusively modified by farnesyltransferase, KRAS and, to a lesser extent, NRAS can also be modified by geranylgeranyltransferase (GGT). Concomitant targeting of the two enzymes is not feasible, given the high toxicity of the combined therapy. Indeed clinical trials with these compounds in MM patients have not provided solid results, and so far these compounds have not been introduced in the current clinical practice for the treatment of MM patients (101,105). Compounds targeting the RAS downstream signaling cascade has been tested and proven effective on MM models (104,106).

Another pathway that is frequently altered in human cancers, the PI3K/AKT pathway, is also often dysregulated in MM (107,108). Recently, several compounds specifically targeting the PI3K/AKT axis have been tested in MM cell lines and patients, with encouraging results. In particular, the mTOR inhibitor rapamycin and analogues of this compound are highly effective in vitro against MM cell lines, both alone (109–113), and in combination (114).

Among the pathways more specifically altered in hematological cancers, the NF-κB pathway exerts a central role in MM. While the genetic causes of NF-κB dysregulation in MM are largely unknown (115,116), the involvement of NF-κB in MM tumorigenesis and the interaction of this pathway with other genes critically relevant for MM pathogenesis, as for example IL-6 (67), has been recognized for a long time. Several drugs highly effective for the treatment of MM inhibit, as part of their mechanism of action, the NF-κB pathway, including dexamethasone, thalidomide and IMiDs, proteasome inhibitor PS-341, and As(2) O(3) (117).

Finally, another central signaling "hub" that has recently gained in relevance is STAT3 (116), not only in the context of IL-6 activation, but more generally after stimulation by other mechanisms, such as FGFR3 overexpression (118).

TARGETS RELATED TO PROLIFERATION, SURVIVAL, AND REPLICATIVE LIFESPAN

Among the compounds targeting genes and pathways more directly involved in cell proliferation, there is the class of inhibitors of cyclin-dependent kinases (CDK) that drive the progression of the cell cycle through the G1 phase in cooperation with cyclins. Several members of this family have shown a significant ability to reduce proliferation in MM cells, including the CDK4/6 inhibitors flavopiridol (119), R-roscovitine (CYC202 or Seliciclib) (120), and PD 0332991 (121), albeit the specific activity of the different compounds against CDK4/6 has not always been firmly demonstrated.

Telomeres, the repetitive DNA sequences at the ends of eukaryotic chromosomes, both protect the chromosome ends from degradation and regulate the life span of human cell lineages. Instead of progressively losing telomeric DNA sequences during successive cell cycles, cancer cells, usually through the reactivation of the reverse transcriptase that extends telomeric DNA telomerase, or alternative mechanisms, maintain a constant length on the telomeres, thereby conferring replicative immortality to cancer cells. MM cells do frequently present high telomerase activity, which are directly correlated with poor survival (122). Targeting telomerase is therefore an attractive therapeutic strategy in MM, and several compounds targeting telomerase have been proposed, including GRN163 (123,124), TMPyP4 (125), and telomestatin (126). As for the prosurvival mechanisms, recent work has demonstrated that small-molecule Bcl-2 inhibitor HA14-1, as well as a low molecular weight Smac mimetic LBW242 (127), directly induce apoptosis of MM cells (128).

FUTURE CHALLENGES AND OPPORTUNITIES

Recent surveys of expression profiling (129–131) as well as of DNA copy number changes in MM cell lines and patient samples (132) have provided a wealth of information that will profoundly change the whole approach to target discovery and validation. Ongoing sequencing efforts will also provide information on targets against which monoclonal antibodies or small molecules could be devised. These new technologies will likely introduce the new era of tailored treatments based on specific genetic lesions in individual patients, therefore allowing for more targeted, effective, and less toxic treatments.

REFERENCES

1. Uchiyama H, Barut BA, Mohrbacher AF, et al. Adhesion of human myeloma-derived cell lines to bone marrow stromal cells stimulates interleukin-6 secretion. Blood 1993; 82(12):3712–20.
2. Yasui H, Hideshima T, Richardson PG, et al. Novel therapeutic strategies targeting growth factor signalling cascades in multiple myeloma. Br J Haematol 2006; 132(4):385–97.
3. Singhal S, Mehta J, Desikan R, et al. Antitumor activity of thalidomide in refractory multiple myeloma. N Engl J Med 1999; 341(21):1565–71.
4. Bartlett JB, Dredge K, Dalgleish AG. The evolution of thalidomide and its IMiD derivatives as anticancer agents. Nat Rev Cancer 2004; 4(4): 314–22.
5. Adams J. The development of proteasome inhibitors as anticancer drugs. Cancer Cell 2004; 5(5):417–21.
6. Joazeiro CAP, Anderson KC, Hunter T. Proteasome inhibitor drugs on the rise. Cancer Res 2006; 66(16):7840–2.
7. Hideshima T, Chauhan D, Hayashi T, et al. Proteasome inhibitor PS-341 abrogates IL-6 triggered signaling cascades via caspase-dependent down-regulation of gp130 in multiple myeloma. Oncogene 2003; 22(52):8386–93.
8. Hideshima T, Chauhan D, Schlossman R, et al. The role of tumor necrosis factor alpha in the pathophysiology of human multiple myeloma: therapeutic applications. Oncogene 2001; 20(33):4519–27.
9. Lipford JR, Smith GT, Chi Y, et al. A putative stimulatory role for activator turnover in gene expression. Nature 2005; 438(7064):113–16.
10. Lee AH, Iwakoshi NN, Anderson KC, et al. Proteasome inhibitors disrupt the unfolded protein response in myeloma cells. Proc Natl Acad Sci USA 2003; 100(17):9946–51.
11. Hideshima T, Bradner JE, Chauhan D, et al. Intracellular protein degradation and its therapeutic implications. Clin Cancer Res 2005; 11(24 Pt 1): 8530–3.
12. Podar K, Shringarpure R, Tai YT, et al. Caveolin-1 is required for vascular endothelial growth factor-triggered multiple myeloma cell migration and is targeted by bortezomib. Cancer Res 2004; 64(20):7500–6.
13. Roccaro AM, Hideshima T, Raje N, et al. bortezomib mediates antiangiogenesis in multiple myeloma via direct and indirect effects on endothelial cells. Cancer Res 2006; 66(1):184–91.
14. Chauhan D, Catley L, Li G, et al. A novel orally active proteasome inhibitor induces apoptosis in multiple myeloma cells with mechanisms distinct from bortezomib. Cancer Cell 2005; 8(5):407–19.
15. Hideshima T, Bradner JE, Wong J, et al. Small-molecule inhibition of proteasome and aggresome function induces synergistic antitumor activity in multiple myeloma. Proc Natl Acad Sci USA 2005; 102(24):8567–72.
16. Catley L, Weisberg E, Kiziltepe T, et al. Aggresome induction by proteasome inhibitor bortezomib and alpha-tubulin hyperacetylation by tubulin

deacetylase (TDAC) inhibitor LBH589 are synergistic in myeloma cells. Blood 2006; 108(10):3441–9.

17. Whitesell L, Lindquist SL. HSP90 and the chaperoning of cancer. Nat Rev Cancer 2005; 5(10):761–72.

18. Mitsiades CS, Mitsiades NS, McMullan CJ, et al. Antimyeloma activity of heat shock protein-90 inhibition. Blood 2006; 107(3):1092–100.

19. Zaarur N, Gabai VL, Porco JA, Jr, et al. Targeting heat shock response to sensitize cancer cells to proteasome and Hsp90 inhibitors. Cancer Res 2006; 66(3):1783–91.

20. Hahn WC, Weinberg RA. Modelling the molecular circuitry of cancer. Nat Rev Cancer 2002; 2(5):331–41.

21. Yaccoby S, Ling W, Zhan F, et al. Antibody-based inhibition of DKK1 suppresses tumor- induced bone resorption and multiple myeloma growth in-vivo. Blood 2006; 109(5):2106–11.

22. Freund GG, Kulas DT, Mooney RA. Insulin and IGF-1 increase mitogenesis and glucose metabolism in the multiple myeloma cell line, RPMI 8226. J Immunol 1993; 151(4):1811–20.

23. Georgii-Hemming P, Wiklund HJ, Ljunggren O, et al. Insulin-like growth factor I is a growth and survival factor in human multiple myeloma cell lines. Blood 1996; 88(6):2250–8.

24. Ge NL, Rudikoff S. Insulin-like growth factor I is a dual effector of multiple myeloma cell growth. Blood 2000; 96(8):2856–61.

25. Mitsiades CS, Mitsiades N, Poulaki V, et al. Activation of NF-kappaB and upregulation of intracellular anti-apoptotic proteins via the IGF-1/Akt signaling in human multiple myeloma cells: therapeutic implications. Oncogene 2002; 21(37):5673–83.

26. Asosingh K, Gunthert U, Bakkus MH, et al. In vivo induction of insulin-like growth factor-I receptor and CD44v6 confers homing and adhesion to murine multiple myeloma cells. Cancer Res 2000; 60(11):3096–104.

27. Tai YT, Podar K, Catley L, et al. Insulin-like growth factor-1 induces adhesion and migration in human multiple myeloma cells via activation of beta1-integrin and phosphatidylinositol 3' -kinase/AKT signaling. Cancer Res 2003; 63(18):5850–8.

28. Mitsiades CS, Mitsiades N. Treatment of hematologic malignancies and solid tumors by inhibiting IGF receptor signaling. Expert Rev Anticancer Ther 2005; 5(3):487–9.

29. Mitsiades CS, Mitsiades NS, McMullan CJ, et al. Inhibition of the insulin-like growth factor receptor-1 tyrosine kinase activity as a therapeutic strategy for multiple myeloma, other hematologic malignancies, and solid tumors. Cancer Cell 2004; 5(3):221–30.

30. Descamps G, Wuilleme-Toumi S, Trichet V, et al. CD45neg but not CD45pos human myeloma cells are sensitive to the inhibition of IGF-1 signaling by a murine anti-IGF-1R monoclonal antibody, mAVE1642. J Immunol 2006; 177 (6):4218–23.

31. Wu KD, Zhou L, Burtrum D, et al. Antibody targeting of the insulin-like growth factor I receptor enhances the anti-tumor response of multiple myeloma to chemotherapy through inhibition of tumor proliferation and angiogenesis. Cancer Immunol Immunother 2006; 56(3):343–57.

32. Stromberg T, Ekman S, Girnita L, et al. IGF-1 receptor tyrosine kinase inhibition by the cyclolignan PPP induces G2/M-phase accumulation and apoptosis in multiple myeloma cells. Blood 2006; 107(2):669–78.

33. Menu E, Jernberg-Wiklund H, Stromberg T, et al. Inhibiting the IGF-1 receptor tyrosine kinase with the cyclolignan PPP: an in vitro and in vivo study in the 5T33MM mouse model. Blood 2006; 107(2):655–60.

34. Bellamy WT, Richter L, Frutiger Y, et al. Expression of vascular endothelial growth factor and its receptors in hematopoietic malignancies. Cancer Res 1999; 59(3):728–33.

35. Dankbar B, Padro T, Leo R, et al. Vascular endothelial growth factor and interleukin-6 in paracrine tumor-stromal cell interactions in multiple myeloma. Blood 2000; 95(8):2630–6.

36. Podar K, Tai YT, Davies FE, et al. Vascular endothelial growth factor triggers signaling cascades mediating multiple myeloma cell growth and migration. Blood 2001; 98(2):428–35.

37. Podar K, Tai YT, Lin BK, et al. Vascular endothelial growth factor-induced migration of multiple myeloma cells is associated with beta 1 integrin- and phosphatidylinositol 3-kinase-dependent PKC alpha activation. J Biol Chem 2002; 277(10):7875–81.

38. Lin B, Podar K, Gupta D, et al. The vascular endothelial growth factor receptor tyrosine kinase inhibitor PTK787/ZK222584 inhibits growth and migration of multiple myeloma cells in the bone marrow microenvironment. Cancer Res 2002; 62(17):5019–26.

39. Podar K, Catley LP, Tai YT, et al. GW654652, the pan-inhibitor of VEGF receptors, blocks the growth and migration of multiple myeloma cells in the bone marrow microenvironment. Blood 2004; 103(9):3474–9.

40. Bisping G, Kropff M, Wenning D, et al. Targeting receptor kinases by a novel indolinone derivative in multiple myeloma: abrogation of stroma-derived interleukin-6 secretion and induction of apoptosis in cytogenetically defined subgroups. Blood 2006; 107(5):2079–89.

41. Podar K, Tonon G, Sattler M, et al. The small-molecule VEGF receptor inhibitor pazopanib (GW786034B) targets both tumor and endothelial cells in multiple myeloma. Proc Natl Acad Sci USA 2006; 103(51):19478–83.

42. Zangari M, Anaissie E, Stopeck A, et al. Phase II study of SU5416, a small molecule vascular endothelial growth factor tyrosine kinase receptor inhibitor, in patients with refractory multiple myeloma. Clin Cancer Res 2004; 10(1 Pt 1): 88–95.

43. Kovacs MJ, Reece DE, Marcellus D, et al. A phase II study of ZD6474 (Zactima, a selective inhibitor of VEGFR and EGFR tyrosine kinase in patients with relapsed multiple myeloma—NCIC CTG IND.145. Invest New Drugs 2006; 24(6):529–35.

44. Kuehl WM, Bergsagel PL. Multiple myeloma: evolving genetic events and host interactions. Nat Rev Cancer 2002; 2(3):175–87.

45. Chesi M, Bergsagel PL, Kuehl WM. The enigma of ectopic expression of FGFR3 in multiple myeloma: a critical initiating event or just a target for mutational activation during tumor progression. Curr Opin Hematol 2002; 9(4):288–93.

46. Trudel S, Ely S, Farooqi Y, et al. Inhibition of fibroblast growth factor receptor 3 induces differentiation and apoptosis in t(4;14) myeloma. Blood 2004; 103(9):3521–28.
47. Grand EK, Chase AJ, Heath C, et al. Targeting FGFR3 in multiple myeloma: inhibition of t(4; 14) -positive cells by SU5402 and PD173074. Leukemia 2004; 18(5):962–6.
48. Paterson JL, Li Z, Wen XY, et al. Preclinical studies of fibroblast growth factor receptor 3 as a therapeutic target in multiple myeloma. Br J Haematol 2004; 124(5):595–603.
49. Trudel S, Li ZH, Wei E, et al. CHIR-258, a novel, multitargeted tyrosine kinase inhibitor for the potential treatment of t(4; 14) multiple myeloma. Blood 2005; 105(7):2941–8.
50. Chen J, Lee BH, Williams IR, et al. FGFR3 as a therapeutic target of the small molecule inhibitor PKC412 in hematopoietic malignancies. Oncogene 2005; 24(56):8259–67.
51. Borset M, Hjorth-Hansen H, Seidel C, et al. Hepatocyte growth factor and its receptor c-met in multiple myeloma. Blood 1996; 88(10):3998–4004.
52. Seidel C, Borset M, Turesson I, et al. Elevated serum concentrations of hepatocyte growth factor in patients with multiple myeloma. The Nordic Myeloma Study Group. Blood 1998; 91(3):806–12.
53. Derksen PW, de Gorter DJ, Meijer HP, et al. The hepatocyte growth factor/ Met pathway controls proliferation and apoptosis in multiple myeloma. Leukemia 2003; 17(4):764–74.
54. Standal T, Abildgaard N, Fagerli UM, et al. HGF inhibits BMP-induced osteoblastogenesis: possible implications for the bone disease of multiple myeloma. Blood 2006; 109(7):3024–30.
55. Holt RU, Baykov V, Ro TB, et al. Human myeloma cells adhere to fibronectin in response to hepatocyte growth factor. Haematologica 2005; 90(4):479–88.
56. Hov H, Holt RU, Ro TB, et al. A selective c-met inhibitor blocks an autocrine hepatocyte growth factor growth loop in ANBL-6 cells and prevents migration and adhesion of myeloma cells. Clin Cancer Res 2004; 10(19): 6686–94.
57. Walters DK, Jelinek DF. A role for Janus kinases in crosstalk between ErbB3 and the interferon-alpha signaling complex in myeloma cells. Oncogene 2004; 23(6):1197–205.
58. Walters DK, French JD, Arendt BK, et al. Atypical expression of ErbB3 in myeloma cells: cross-talk between ErbB3 and the interferon-alpha signaling complex. Oncogene 2003; 22(23):3598–607.
59. Kraj M, Poglod R, Kopec-Szlezak J, et al. C-kit receptor (CD117) expression on plasma cells in monoclonal gammopathies. Leuk Lymphoma 2004; 45(11): 2281–9.
60. Lugli A, Went P, Khanlari B, et al. Rare KIT (CD117) expression in multiple myeloma abrogates the usefulness of imatinib mesylate treatment. Virchows Arch 2004; 444(3):264–8.
61. Potti A, Ganti AK, Koch M, et al. Immunohistochemical identification of HER-2/neu overexpression and CD117 (c-kit) expression in multiple myeloma. Leuk Lymphoma 2002; 43(12):2427–30.

62. Lauta VM. A review of the cytokine network in multiple myeloma: diagnostic, prognostic, and therapeutic implications. Cancer 2003; 97(10): 2440–52.
63. Kawano M, Hirano T, Matsuda T, et al. Autocrine generation and requirement of BSF-2/IL-6 for human multiple myelomas. Nature 1988; 332(6159):83–5.
64. Heinrich PC, Behrmann I, Haan S, et al. Principles of interleukin (IL) -6-type cytokine signalling and its regulation. Biochem J 2003; 374(Pt 1):1–20.
65. Klein B, Zhang XG, Jourdan M, et al. Paracrine rather than autocrine regulation of myeloma-cell growth and differentiation by interleukin-6. Blood 1989; 73(2):517–26.
66. Caligaris-Cappio F, Bergui L, Gregoretti MG, et al. Role of bone marrow stromal cells in the growth of human multiple myeloma. Blood 1991; 77(12): 2688–93.
67. Chauhan D, Uchiyama H, Akbarali Y, et al. Multiple myeloma cell adhesion-induced interleukin-6 expression in bone marrow stromal cells involves activation of NF-kappa B. Blood 1996; 87(3):1104–12.
68. Trikha M, Corringham R, Klein B, et al. Targeted anti-interleukin-6 monoclonal antibody therapy for cancer: a review of the rationale and clinical evidence. Clin Cancer Res 2003; 9(13):4653–65.
69. Rossi JF, Fegueux N, Lu ZY, et al. Optimizing the use of anti-interleukin-6 monoclonal antibody with dexamethasone and 140 mg/m2 of melphalan in multiple myeloma: results of a pilot study including biological aspects. Bone Marrow Transplant 2005; 36(9):771–9.
70. Moreau P, Hullin C, Garban F, et al. Tandem autologous stem cell transplantation in high-risk de novo multiple myeloma: final results of the prospective and randomized IFM 99-04 protocol. Blood 2006; 107(1): 397–403.
71. Tassone P, Neri P, Burger R, et al. Combination therapy with interleukin-6 receptor superantagonist Sant7 and dexamethasone induces antitumor effects in a novel SCID-hu In vivo model of human multiple myeloma. Clin Cancer Res 2005; 11(11):4251–8.
72. Bodmer JL, Schneider P, Tschopp J. The molecular architecture of the TNF superfamily. Trends Biochem Sci 2002; 27(1):19–26.
73. Aggarwal BB. Signalling pathways of the TNF superfamily: a double-edged sword. Nat Rev Immunol 2003; 3(9):745–56.
74. Mitsiades CS, Treon SP, Mitsiades N, et al. TRAIL/Apo2L ligand selectively induces apoptosis and overcomes drug resistance in multiple myeloma: therapeutic applications. Blood 2001; 98(3):795–804.
75. Menoret E, Gomez-Bougie P, Geffroy-Luseau A, et al. Mcl-1L cleavage is involved in TRAIL-R1- and TRAIL-R2-mediated apoptosis induced by HGS-ETR1 and HGS-ETR2 human mAbs in myeloma cells. Blood 2006; 108(4): 1346–52.
76. Tinhofer I, Biedermann R, Krismer M, et al. A role of TRAIL in killing osteoblasts by myeloma cells. FASEB J 2006; 20(6):759–61.
77. Urashima M, Chauhan D, Uchiyama H, et al. CD40 ligand triggered interleukin-6 secretion in multiple myeloma. Blood 1995; 85(7):1903–12.

78. Tai YT, Podar K, Mitsiades N, et al. CD40 induces human multiple myeloma cell migration via phosphatidylinositol 3-kinase/AKT/NF-kappaB signaling. Blood 2003; 101(7):2762–9.
79. Tai YT, Podar K, Gupta D, et al. CD40 activation induces p53-dependent vascular endothelial growth factor secretion in human multiple myeloma cells. Blood 2002; 99(4):1419–27.
80. Francisco JA, Donaldson KL, Chace D, et al. Agonistic properties and in vivo antitumor activity of the anti-CD40 antibody SGN-14. Cancer Res 2000; 60(12):3225–31.
81. Tai YT, Li X, Tong X, et al. Human anti-CD40 antagonist antibody triggers significant antitumor activity against human multiple myeloma. Cancer Res 2005; 65(13):5898–906.
82. Tai YT, Catley LP, Mitsiades CS, et al. Mechanisms by which SGN-40, a humanized anti-CD40 antibody, induces cytotoxicity in human multiple myeloma cells: clinical implications. Cancer Res 2004; 64(8):2846–52.
83. Novak AJ, Darce JR, Arendt BK, et al. Expression of BCMA, TACI, and BAFF-R in multiple myeloma: a mechanism for growth and survival. Blood 2004; 103(2):689–94.
84. Moreaux J, Legouffe E, Jourdan E, et al. BAFF and APRIL protect myeloma cells from apoptosis induced by interleukin 6 deprivation and dexamethasone. Blood 2004; 103(8):3148–57.
85. Dillon SR, Gross JA, Ansell SM, et al. An APRIL to remember: novel TNF ligands as therapeutic targets. Nat Rev Drug Discov 2006; 5(3):235–46.
86. Costes V, Portier M, Lu ZY, et al. Interleukin-1 in multiple myeloma: producer cells and their role in the control of IL-6 production. Br J Haematol 1998; 103(4):1152–60.
87. Han JH, Choi SJ, Kurihara N, et al. Macrophage inflammatory protein-1alpha is an osteoclastogenic factor in myeloma that is independent of receptor activator of nuclear factor kappaB ligand. Blood 2001; 97(11): 3349–53.
88. Choi SJ, Oba Y, Gazitt Y, et al. Antisense inhibition of macrophage inflammatory protein 1-alpha blocks bone destruction in a model of myeloma bone disease. J Clin Invest 2001; 108(12):1833–41.
89. Croucher PI, Shipman CM, Lippitt J, et al. Osteoprotegerin inhibits the development of osteolytic bone disease in multiple myeloma. Blood 2001; 98(13):3534–40.
90. Body JJ, Greipp P, Coleman RE, et al. A phase I study of AMGN-0007, a recombinant osteoprotegerin construct, in patients with multiple myeloma or breast carcinoma related bone metastases. Cancer 2003; 97(3 Suppl):887–92.
91. Body JJ, Facon T, Coleman RE, et al. A study of the biological receptor activator of nuclear factor-kappaB ligand inhibitor, denosumab, in patients with multiple myeloma or bone metastases from breast cancer. Clin Cancer Res 2006; 12(4):1221–8.
92. Zannettino AC, Farrugia AN, Kortesidis A, et al. Elevated serum levels of stromal-derived factor-1alpha are associated with increased osteoclast activity and osteolytic bone disease in multiple myeloma patients. Cancer Res 2005; 65(5):1700–9.

93. Cook G, Dumbar M, Franklin IM. The role of adhesion molecules in multiple myeloma. Acta Haematol 1997; 97(1–2):81–9.
94. Mori Y, Shimizu N, Dallas M, et al. Anti-alpha4 integrin antibody suppresses the development of multiple myeloma and associated osteoclastic osteolysis. Blood 2004; 104(7):2149–54.
95. Olson DL, Burkly LC, Leone DR, et al. Anti-alpha4 integrin monoclonal antibody inhibits multiple myeloma growth in a murine model. Mol Cancer Ther 2005; 4(1):91–9.
96. Tassone P, Gozzini A, Goldmacher V, et al. In vitro and in vivo activity of the maytansinoid immunoconjugate huN901-N2' -deacetyl-N2' -(3-mercapto-1-oxopropyl) -maytansine against CD56+ multiple myeloma cells. Cancer Res 2004; 64(13):4629–36.
97. Smallshaw JE, Coleman E, Spiridon C, et al. The generation and anti-myeloma activity of a chimeric anti-CD54 antibody, cUV3. J Immunother 2004; 27(6):419–24.
98. David E, Sun SY, Waller EK, et al. The combination of the farnesyl transferase inhibitor lonafarnib and the proteasome inhibitor bortezomib induces synergistic apoptosis in human myeloma cells that is associated with down-regulation of p-AKT. Blood 2005; 106(13):4322–9.
99. Pei XY, Dai Y, Rahmani M, et al. The farnesyltransferase inhibitor L744832 potentiates UCN-01-induced apoptosis in human multiple myeloma cells. Clin Cancer Res 2005; 11(12):4589–600.
100. Beaupre DM, McCafferty-Grad J, Bahlis NJ, et al. Farnesyl transferase inhibitors enhance death receptor signals and induce apoptosis in multiple myeloma cells. Leuk Lymphoma 2003; 44(12):2123–34.
101. Alsina M, Fonseca R, Wilson EF, et al. Farnesyltransferase inhibitor tipifarnib is well tolerated, induces stabilization of disease, and inhibits farnesylation and oncogenic/tumor survival pathways in patients with advanced multiple myeloma. Blood 2004; 103(9):3271–7.
102. Ochiai N, Uchida R, Fuchida S, et al. Effect of farnesyl transferase inhibitor R115777 on the growth of fresh and cloned myeloma cells in vitro. Blood 2003; 102(9):3349–53.
103. Le Gouill S, Pellat-Deceunynck C, Harousseau JL, et al. Farnesyl transferase inhibitor R115777 induces apoptosis of human myeloma cells. Leukemia 2002; 16(9):1664–7.
104. Downward J. Targeting RAS signalling pathways in cancer therapy. Nat Rev Cancer 2003; 3(1):11–22.
105. Cortes J, Albitar M, Thomas D, et al. Efficacy of the farnesyl transferase inhibitor R115777 in chronic myeloid leukemia and other hematologic malignancies. Blood 2003; 101(5):1692–7.
106. Dai Y, Landowski TH, Rosen ST, et al. Combined treatment with the checkpoint abrogator UCN-01 and MEK1/2 inhibitors potently induces apoptosis in drug-sensitive and -resistant myeloma cells through an IL-6-independent mechanism. Blood 2002; 100(9):3333–43.
107. Tu Y, Gardner A, Lichtenstein A. The phosphatidylinositol 3-kinase/AKT kinase pathway in multiple myeloma plasma cells: roles in cytokine-dependent survival and proliferative responses. Cancer Res 2000; 60(23):6763–70.

108. Hsu J, Shi Y, Krajewski S, et al. The AKT kinase is activated in multiple myeloma tumor cells. Blood 2001; 98(9):2853–5.

109. Shi Y, Gera J, Hu L, et al. Enhanced sensitivity of multiple myeloma cells containing PTEN mutations to CCI-779. Cancer Res 2002; 62(17): 5027–34.

110. Stromberg T, Dimberg A, Hammarberg A, et al. Rapamycin sensitizes multiple myeloma cells to apoptosis induced by dexamethasone. Blood 2004; 103(8):3138–47.

111. Zhang J, Choi Y, Mavromatis B, et al. Preferential killing of PTEN-null myelomas by PI3K inhibitors through Akt pathway. Oncogene 2003; 22(40): 6289–95.

112. Raje N, Kumar S, Hideshima T, et al. Combination of the mTOR inhibitor rapamycin and CC-5013 has synergistic activity in multiple myeloma. Blood 2004; 104(13):4188–93.

113. Hideshima T, Catley L, Yasui H, et al. Perifosine, an oral bioactive novel alkylphospholipid, inhibits Akt and induces in vitro and in vivo cytotoxicity in human multiple myeloma cells. Blood 2006; 107(10):4053–62.

114. Francis LK, Alsayed Y, Leleu X, et al. Combination mammalian target of rapamycin inhibitor rapamycin and HSP90 inhibitor 17-allylamino-17-demethoxygeldanamycin has synergistic activity in multiple myeloma. Clin Cancer Res 2006; 12(22):6826–35.

115. Fracchiolla NS, Lombardi L, Salina M, et al. Structural alterations of the NF-kappaB transcription factor lyt-10 in lymphoid malignancies. Oncogene 1993; 8(10):2839–45.

116. Bharti AC, Shishodia S, Reuben JM, et al. Nuclear factor-kappaB and STAT3 are constitutively active in CD138+ cells derived from multiple myeloma patients, and suppression of these transcription factors leads to apoptosis. Blood 2004; 103(8):3175–84.

117. Hideshima T, Chauhan D, Richardson P, et al. NF-kappaB as a therapeutic target in multiple myeloma. J Biol Chem 2002; 277(19):16639–47.

118. Plowright EE, Li Z, Bergsagel PL, et al. Ectopic expression of fibroblast growth factor receptor 3 promotes myeloma cell proliferation and prevents apoptosis. Blood 2000; 95(3):992–8.

119. Gojo I, Zhang B, Fenton RG. The cyclin-dependent kinase inhibitor flavopiridol induces apoptosis in multiple myeloma cells through transcriptional repression and down-regulation of Mcl-1. Clin Cancer Res 2002; 8(11): 3527–38.

120. Raje N, Kumar S, Hideshima T, et al. Seliciclib (CYC202 or R-roscovitine), a small-molecule cyclin-dependent kinase inhibitor, mediates activity via down-regulation of Mcl-1 in multiple myeloma. Blood 2005; 106(3):1042–7.

121. Baughn LB, Di Liberto M, Wu K, et al. A novel orally active small molecule potently induces G1 arrest in primary myeloma cells and prevents tumor growth by specific inhibition of cyclin-dependent kinase 4/6. Cancer Res 2006; 66(15):7661–7.

122. Wu KD, Orme LM, Shaughnessy J, Jr, et al. Telomerase and telomere length in multiple myeloma: correlations with disease heterogeneity, cytogenetic status, and overall survival. Blood 2003; 101(12):4982–9.

123. Akiyama M, Hideshima T, Shammas MA, et al. Effects of oligonucleotide N3'→P5' thio-phosphoramidate (GRN163) targeting telomerase RNA in human multiple myeloma cells. Cancer Res 2003; 63(19):6187–94.

124. Wang ES, Wu K, Chin AC, et al. Telomerase inhibition with an oligonucleotide telomerase template antagonist: in vitro and in vivo studies in multiple myeloma and lymphoma. Blood 2004; 103(1):258–66.

125. Shammas MA, Shmookler Reis RJ, Akiyama M, et al. Telomerase inhibition and cell growth arrest by G-quadruplex interactive agent in multiple myeloma. Mol Cancer Ther 2003; 2(9):825–33.

126. Shammas MA, Shmookler Reis RJ, Li C, et al. Telomerase inhibition and cell growth arrest after telomestatin treatment in multiple myeloma. Clin Cancer Res 2004; 10(2):770–6.

127. Chauhan D, Neri P, Velankar M, et al. Targeting mitochondrial factor Smac/ DIABLO as therapy for multiple myeloma (MM). Blood 2006; 109(3):1220–7.

128. Pei XY, Dai Y, Grant S. The small-molecule Bcl-2 inhibitor HA14-1 interacts synergistically with flavopiridol to induce mitochondrial injury and apoptosis in human myeloma cells through a free radical-dependent and Jun NH2-terminal kinase-dependent mechanism. Mol Cancer Ther 2004; 3(12):1513–24.

129. Zhan F, Hardin J, Kordsmeier B, et al. Global gene expression profiling of multiple myeloma, monoclonal gammopathy of undetermined significance, and normal bone marrow plasma cells. Blood 2002; 99(5):1745–57.

130. Zhan F, Huang Y, Colla S, et al. The molecular classification of multiple myeloma. Blood 2006; 108(6):2020–8.

131. Davies FE, Dring AM, Li C, et al. Insights into the multistep transformation of MGUS to myeloma using microarray expression analysis. Blood 2003; 102(13):4504–11.

132. Carrasco DR, Tonon G, Huang Y, et al. High-resolution genomic profiles define distinct clinico-pathogenetic subgroups of multiple myeloma patients. Cancer Cell 2006; 9(4):313–25.

6

Monoclonal Gammopathy of Undetermined Significance

Robert A. Kyle and S. Vincent Rajkumar

*Division of Hematology, Mayo Clinic College of Medicine,
Rochester, Minnesota, U.S.A.*

INTRODUCTION

Monoclonal gammopathy of undetermined significance (MGUS) is defined by a monoclonal immunoglobulin in serum of <3 g/dL, fewer than 10% plasma cells in the bone marrow and no evidence of lytic bone lesions, anemia, hypercalcemia, or renal insufficiency related to the plasma cell proliferative process. More than 50% of patients with a monoclonal gammopathy at Mayo Clinic have MGUS. IgG is the most common type of M protein.

RECOGNITION OF MONOCLONAL GAMMOPATHIES

Testing for monoclonal gammopathies is performed when multiple myeloma (MM), primary amyloidosis (AL), Waldenström's macroglobulinemia (WM), or a related disorder is suspected in any given patient. Agarose gel serum protein electrophoresis is the preferred method of detection of monoclonal proteins and also allows for the quantification of the size of the M protein. In addition, immunofixation is performed in order to detect smaller monoclonal proteins that are not apparent on Agarose gel electrophoresis to confirm the presence of an M protein that has been detected on electrophoresis and to determine the immunoglobulin heavy- and light-chain types. Traditionally, both serum and urine are tested with electrophoresis and immunofixation when a monoclonal plasma cell disorder is suspected clinically. Recently, it has been shown that such screening can be performed using the combination of serum protein electrophoresis, serum immunofixation, and the serum-free light-chain (FLC) assay, eliminating the need for urine studies. In a series of 428 patients with an M protein in the urine, the presence of a monoclonal protein was detected in all but two patients utilizing examination of the serum with protein electrophoresis, immunofixation, and the FLC ratio. These two patients had a small MGUS. Thus, incorporation of the FLC assay as described above eliminated the need for electrophoresis and immunofixation of an aliquot from a 24-hour urine specimen (1). However, if a monoclonal gammopathy is found on such screening, a 24-hour urine specimen must be collected and examined by electrophoresis and immunofixation.

In patients diagnosed with monoclonal gammopathies, quantification of serum immunoglobulins should be performed with a rate nephelometer because it is not influenced by molecular size and therefore measures 7S IgM, polymers of IgA, and aggregates of IgG accurately. Levels of IgM obtained with nephelometry may be 1 to 2 g/dL higher than that expected on the basis of the serum protein electrophoretic tracing. The IgG and IgA values may also be increased with nephelometric studies.

Measurement of the FLC has been utilized in clinical practice (2). This is an automated nephelometric assay that measures the level of free kappa and free light-chains in the serum (normal ratio for FLC kappa/lambda is 0.26 to 1.65). Eighty-eight percent of 1020 patients at Mayo Clinic in whom an FLC assay was requested had a monoclonal plasma cell disorder. All 121 patients who did not have a monoclonal gammopathy had a normal FLC-kappa/lambda ratio. The FLC-kappa/lambda ratio was abnormal in 91% of 110 untreated patients with AL. The combination of immunofixation of serum and urine and the serum FLC assay detected an abnormal result in 99% of patients with AL (3).

A search for a monoclonal protein with immunofixation of serum and urine and the FLC assay should be seriously considered in any patient who has unexplained weakness or fatigue, anemia, back pain of unknown cause, osteoporosis, osteolytic lesions or fractures, hypercalcemia, renal insufficiency, Bence Jones proteinuria, or an increased erythrocyte sedimentation rate. The tests should also be performed in adults with unexplained sensorimotor peripheral neuropathy, carpal tunnel syndrome, refractory congestive heart failure, nephrotic syndrome, orthostatic hypotension, or malabsorption, because a monoclonal protein may indicate AL. In addition, these tests should be done in patients with macroglossia or change in their voice, increased bruising or bleeding, or steatorrhea. Immunofixation should be performed whenever MM, WM, AL, or a related disorder is suspected clinically, even when the electrophoretic pattern appears normal. Patients older than 40 years with a nephrotic syndrome of an unknown cause should also have immunofixation because the presence of a monoclonal light chain is a strong indication of AL or light-chain deposition disease. The FLC assay is beneficial for the diagnosis of nonsecretory multiple myeloma, light-chain deposition disease, and AL, as well as screening for the presence of a monoclonal gammopathy. It is also useful in determining prognosis of MGUS, solitary plasmacytoma of bone, and AL amyloidosis following stem cell transplantation.

PREVALENCE OF MGUS

Monoclonal proteins have been detected without evidence of MM, WM, AL, or related disorders in approximately 1.5% of persons >50 years of age and 3% of persons >70 years of age (4–6).

The first population-based study using sensitive laboratory techniques to detect monoclonal gammopathies was recently reported (7). Serum samples were obtained from 21,463 (77%) of the 28,038 enumerated residents of Olmsted County, Minnesota who were ≥50 years of age or older; 694 (3.2%) of these patients had MGUS. The age-adjusted rates were 4% in men and 2.7% in women. MGUS was found in 5.3% of persons ≥70 years of age, while 7.5% of those ≥85 years had MGUS (Fig. 1). In fact, 8.9% of men greater than ≥85 years of age had MGUS (Fig. 1). The size of the M protein was ≥2 g/dL in only 4.5% of the 694 patients. The median size of the M protein was 0.5 g/dL, while 13% had a nonmeasurable M protein. One or both uninvolved immunoglobulins were reduced in 28% of 447 patients tested. Of 79 patients tested, 21% had a monoclonal light chain in the urine.

The prevalence of MGUS is higher in black patients than in white patients. In one study, an M protein was found in 8.6% of 916 black patients compared with 3.2% in white patients (8). In a large study of

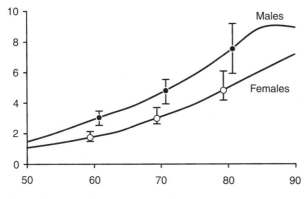

Figure 1 Prevalence of monoclonal gammopathy of undertermined significance according to age. Six hundred and ninety four of 21,463 residents ≥ 50 years of age had M protein. The I bars represent 95% confidence intervals. Years of age > 90 have been condensed to 90 years of age. *Source*: Adapted from Ref. 7.

inpatients from the US Veteran Affairs Hospitals, the age-adjusted prevalence rate for MGUS was 3.0-fold higher in African-Americans than in Caucasians (9).

LONG-TERM OUTCOME OF MGUS

MGUS is a common finding in the medical practice of all physicians. It is important for both the patient and physician to determine whether MGUS will remain stable or progress to MM or a related disorder.

Between 1956 and 1970, the outcome of patients with MGUS who were evaluated at Mayo Clinic were described (10,11). Two hundred and forty one patients were followed for 3,579 person-years (median: 13.7 years; range: 0–39 years). At last follow-up, only 14 (6%) were alive and had no substantial increase in M protein during a median follow-up of 33 years. The serum M protein value increased to ≥3 g/dL in 25 patients (10%) but did not require chemotherapy for symptomatic MM, WM, or AL. One hundred and thirty eight patients (57%) died without evidence of symptomatic MM, WM, AL, lymphoma, or a related disorder. Cardiac disease, cerebrovascular disease, or a nonplasma cell malignancy accounted for the majority of deaths. MM, WM, AL, or a lymphoproliferative disorder developed in 64 patients (27%). The actuarial risk of progression was 17% at 10 years, 34% at 20 years, and 39% at 25 years, a rate of approximately 1.5% per year (69% of the 64 patients who progressed developed MM). The interval from diagnosis of MGUS to the diagnosis of MM ranged from 1 to 32 years (median, 10.6 years). AL was found in eight patients 6 to 19 years (median, 9 years) after the serum M protein was recognized. WM developed in seven patients 4 to 16 years (median, 10.3 years) after the M protein was detected, while a lymphoproliferative disorder developed in five other patients (malignant lymphoma, 3; chronic lymphocytic leukemia, 1; and atypical lymphoproliferative disorder, 1).

Because the 241 Mayo Clinic patients from all parts of the US and other countries may be subject to referral bias, we conducted a study of 1384 patients with MGUS from the 11 counties of southeastern Minnesota evaluated at Mayo Clinic from 1960 to 1994, in an effort to confirm the findings of the original study (12). The median age at diagnosis was 72 years, in contrast to 64 years for the 241 cohort. Fifty-four percent were male. Only 2% were younger than 40 years at diagnosis and 59% were 70 years of age or older. The size of the M protein ranged from unmeasurable to 3 g/dL. An IgG was found in 70%, IgM in 15%, IgA in 12%, and biclonal gammopathies in 3%. The uninvolved (normal or background) immunoglobulins were reduced in 38% of 840 patients who were studied. Thirty-one percent of the 418 patients who had immunofixation of urine had a monoclonal light chain. The bone marrow contained 0–10% plasma cells (median, 3%) in the 160 patients who underwent the procedure.

A follow-up of 11,009 person-years (median, 15.4 years; range, 0–35 years) was done. Nine hundred and sixty three (70%) died, indicating a robust follow-up. MM, AL, lymphoma with an IgM serum protein, WM, plasmacytoma, or chronic lymphocytic leukemia developed in 115 patients (8%) during follow-up. Progression to one of these disorders occurred in 1% of patients each year. At 10 years, 10% progressed; at 20 years, 21%, and at 25 years, 26% had progressed (Fig. 2). Patients were at risk for progression of MGUS even after more than 25 years of observation. Thirty-two additional patients were identified in whom the serum M protein increased to ≥3 g/dL, or the percentage of bone marrow plasma cells exceeded 10% but in whom symptomatic MM or WM did not develop. Thus, these findings confirm the results of the initial Mayo Clinic study of 241 patients.

The number of patients with progression to a plasma cell disorder (115 patients) was 7.3 times the number expected. The risk of developing MM was increased 25-fold, WM 46-fold, and AL 8.4-fold. The risk of lymphoma was increased 2.4-fold, but this risk is underestimated because only lymphoma associated with an M protein was counted in the observed number, while the incidence rates for lymphoma associated with IgG, IgA, and IgM proteins were used to calculate the expected number. Sixty-five percent

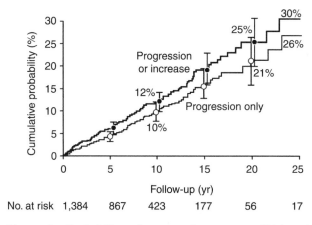

Figure 2 Probability of progression among 1384 residents of southeastern Minnesota in whom monoclonal gammopathy of undetermined significance (MGUS) was diagnosed from 1960 through 1994. The top curve shows the probability of a progression to a plasma-cell cancer (115 patients) or of an increase in the monoclonal protein concentration to more than 3 g/dL or the proportion of plasma cells in bone marrow to more than 10% (32 patients). The bottom curve shows only the probability of progression of MGUS to multiple myeloma, IgM lymphoma, primary amyloidosis, macroglobulinemia, chronic lymphocytic leukemia, or plasmacytoma (115 patients). The bars show 95% confidence intervals. *Source*: Adapted from Ref. 12.

(n=75) of the 115 patients who progressed developed MM. The characteristics of these 75 patients were comparable with those of 1027 patients with newly-diagnosed myeloma who were referred to Mayo Clinic between 1985 and 1998 (13).

Other Series

Similar findings have been reported in several other series. In one group, 13 of 128 patients with MGUS developed a malignant disease during a median follow-up of 56 months (14). In another study, 6.6% of 334 patients with MGUS had progression after a median follow-up of 8.4 years (15). During a median follow-up of 70 months, 6.8% of 335 persons with MGUS progressed (16). The actuarial probability of development of malignancy was 31% at 20 years in a series of 263 patients with MGUS (17). Malignant transformation was the cause of death in 97 of 1324 patients with MGUS in North Jutland, Denmark (only 4.9 deaths were expected) (18). Sixty-four new cases of malignancy (5 expected; relative risk, 12.9) were found among 1229 patients with MGUS (19). The risk of developing MM, WM, or lymphoma was 34.3-fold, 63.8-fold, and 5.9-fold, respectively. In a series of, 504 patients with MGUS from Iceland, malignancy developed in 10% after a median follow-up of six years (20). Thus, these series confirm a risk of progression from MGUS to MM or a related disorder of approximately 1% per year. It must be emphasized that this risk does not disappear even after long-term follow-up.

PATHOGENESIS OF PROGRESSION OF MGUS

Genetic changes, bone marrow angiogenesis, cytokines related to myeloma bone disease, and possibly infectious agents may all play a role in the progression of MGUS to MM or a related disorder.

Cytogenetic changes are common in MGUS. IgH (14q32) translocations were reported in 46% of patients with MGUS (21). In another study, 27 of 59 patients (46%) with MGUS had IgH translocations consisting of t(11;14)(q13;q32) in 25%, t(4;14)(p16.3;q32) in 9%, and t(14;16)(q32;q23) in 5% (22). These translocations lead to the dysregulation of oncogenes such as cyclin D1 (11q13), C-MAF (16q23), FGF-R3/MMSET (fibroblast growth factor receptor 3/MM SET domain), (4p16.3) and cyclin D3 (6p21) and may be involved with the initiation of the MGUS clone rather than progression of MGUS to MM. Recently, Chng et al. (23) reported that 40% (11 of 28) patients with smoldering MM (SMM) or MGUS had hyperdiploidy. This is similar to that found in MM. It appears that genomic instability is common in MGUS (about one-half of patients with MGUS have an IgH translocation), while hyperdiploidy (IgH nontranslocated MGUS) is present in most of the remaining patients.

Avet-Loiseau et al. (24) found that deletions of chromosome 13, which have an adverse prognostic effect in MM, are found in similar frequencies in both MM and MGUS. Detection of monosomal chromosome 13 by conventional cytogenetics is associated with an adverse effect in MM, but it is not clear whether the rate of progression from MGUS to MM is altered because the frequency of deletion of chromosome 13 is similar in both MGUS and MM.

Angiogenesis

Bone marrow angiogenesis is increased in MM and has prognostic value (25,26). Four hundred patients with MGUS, SMM, newly-diagnosed MM, relapsed MM, and AL were studied at Mayo Clinic. The median microvessel density (in vessels per high-power field) was 1.3 in the 42 normal controls, 1.7 in AL, 3 in MGUS, 4 in SMM, 11 in MM, and 20 in relapsed MM (27). Bone marrow angiogenesis increased progressively from MGUS to advanced MM, but it is not known if angiogenesis plays an etiological role. Sixty-three percent of MGUS serum samples inhibited angiogenesis, while 43% of SMM and 4% of MM serum samples did so. This inhibitory activity was heat stable and was not overcome by the addition of VEGF (28). Thus, the increased angiogenesis that occurs with disease progression may be due to the loss of an endogenous angiogenesis inhibitor.

The most important feature that differentiates MGUS from MM is the occurrence of lytic bone lesions, pathological fractures, osteopenia, and hypercalcemia in MM. Osteoclast activation and inhibition of osteoblast differentiation is responsible for the development of bone lesions. Various cytokines activate osteoclasts in myeloma (29). Myeloma bone disease can occur from excess receptor activator of nuclear factor kappa β ligand (RANK-L) or reduced levels of osteoprotegerin (OPG) (30). Interleukin-1-beta, tumor necrosis factor-alpha and interleukin-6 (IL-6) have also been implicated in myeloma bone disease.

PREDICTORS OF PROGRESSION OF MGUS TO MM OR RELATED DISORDERS

One cannot distinguish a patient whose condition will remain stable from one in whom MGUS progresses to a plasma cell malignancy. However, certain parameters are useful for prediction of progression from MGUS to MM.

The size of the M protein at diagnosis was the most important predictor of progression to a plasma cell disorder in a series of 1384 patients with MGUS from southeastern Minnesota. The risk of progression to MM or a related disorder 20 years after diagnosis of MGUS was 49% for those presenting with an M spike of 2.5 g/dL, but was 14% for patients with an initial M-protein value less than 0.5 g/dL. The risk of progression with 2.5 g/dL was 4.6 times the risk of a value of 0.5 g/dL. The reduction of uninvolved immunoglobulins; presence, type, and amount of urinary light chain; number of bone marrow plasma cells; age; gender; presence of hepatosplenomegaly; and levels of hemoglobin, creatinine, and serum albumin were not predictors for progression (12).

Patients with an IgM or an IgA M protein have an increased risk of progression compared to those who have an IgG M protein. In one series, the transformation rate was 6.8% when the bone marrow plasma cell level was less than 10%, but was 37% in the patients who had a bone marrow plasma cell level between 10% and 30% (16). In another study, Cesana et al. (31) noted that the presence of more than 5% bone marrow plasma cells was an independent risk factor for progression. In a large study, serum samples obtained within 30 days of diagnosis were available in 1148 of 1384 patients with MGUS from southeastern Minnesota. At a median follow-up of 15 years, malignant progression occurred in 87 patients (7.6%). An abnormal FLC ratio was detected in 379 of the 1148 patients (33%). The risk of progression in patients with an abnormal FLC ratio was significantly higher than in patients with a normal ratio (hazard ratio, 3.5) and was independent of the size and type of serum M protein.

RISK STRATIFICATION MODEL FOR MGUS

A new risk stratification model for determining the risk of progression of MGUS was developed using the data discussed above. Patients with an elevated serum M protein ($\geq$1.5 g/dL), abnormal serum FLC ratio, and IgA or IgM MGUS, had a risk of progression at 20 years of 58% (high-risk MGUS), compared with 37% with any two risk factors (high intermediate-risk MGUS), 21% with one risk factor (low intermediate-risk MGUS), and 5% with none of the risk factors with present (low-risk MGUS) (32).

In the management of patients with MGUS, one must be aware that death from other causes (cardiovascular or cerebrovascular diseases or nonplasma cell malignancies) is far greater than that from MGUS. In the 1,384 MGUS patients from southeastern Minnesota, plasma cell disorders had developed in 10%, whereas 72% had died of other causes after 20 years of follow-up (Fig. 3).

DIFFERENTIATION OF MGUS FROM MM

To differentiate MGUS from MM or a related disorder, one must take a complete clinical history and perform a physical examination. Laboratory tests include a complete blood count (CBC), serum calcium and creatinine levels, and a radiographic bone survey including the long bones. A bone marrow aspirate and biopsy is indicated in all patients with an M protein $\geq$1.5 g/dL, patients with an IgA or an IgM MGUS, those with an abnormal FLC ratio, and all patients who have an abnormality of the CBC, calcium or

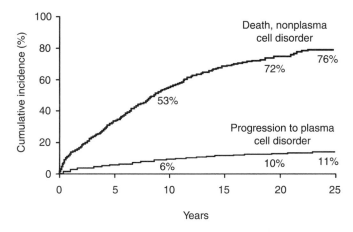

Figure 3 Rate of death from nonplasma cell disorders compared with progression to plasma cell disorders in 1384 patients with monoclonal gammopathy of undertermined significance from southeastern Minnesota. *Source*: Adapted from Ref. 33.

creatinine levels, or the radiographic bone survey. The size of the serum and urine M protein, hemoglobin level, percentage of bone marrow plasma cells, presence of hypercalcemia or renal insufficiency, and the presence of lytic bone lesions are helpful in the differential diagnosis.

Patients with a serum M protein level ≥3 g/L and/or bone marrow plasma cells ≥10% in the absence of anemia, renal insufficiency, hypercalcemia, lytic bone lesions or other clinical manifestations related to a malignant plasma cell proliferative disorder are considered to have SMM (34). Although SMM is associated with a higher risk of malignant transformation than MGUS, these patients must not be treated with chemotherapy until progression occurs because they remain stable for many years.

A reduction of uninvolved (polyclonal or background) immunoglobulins cannot be used to differentiate MM from MGUS, even though 90% of patients with MM have a reduction of 1 or more immunoglobulins (13). Thirty to forty percent of patients with MGUS also have a decrease in uninvolved immunoglobulins (11, 12, 14, 16). The presence of an M protein in the urine (Bence Jones proteinuria) cannot be used to distinguish MGUS and MM because monoclonal light chains are often found in patients with MGUS. Thirty-one percent of the 418 tested patients with MGUS from southeastern Minnesota had a monoclonal light chain in the urine (12).

An elevated plasma cell labeling index strongly suggests that the patient has or will soon have symptomatic MM and should be followed more closely (35). However, more than one-third of patients with symptomatic MM requiring therapy have a normal plasma cell labeling index. Furthermore, the test is not widely available. The presence of circulating plasma cells in the peripheral blood is also an indicator of active disease. The presence of osteolytic lesions suggests the diagnosis of MM, but metastatic carcinoma must be excluded.

Conventional cytogenetic studies or interphase fluorescence in situ hybridization (FISH) are not useful in differential diagnosis because abnormalities are found in both MGUS and MM. Increased levels of beta-2-microglobulin, expression of CD56, or increased serum levels of IL-6 fail to differentiate MM from MGUS.

MANAGEMENT OF MGUS

Patients with MGUS require indefinite follow-up. Generally, serum protein electrophoresis should be repeated in six months and, if stable, annually thereafter. Patients who have a low risk of progression characterized by a serum M protein <1.5 g/dL, IgG type and normal FLC ratio (low-risk MGUS) can be followed less often (32). In these patients, routine skeletal radiography and bone marrow examination are usually unnecessary. A roentgenographic metastatic bone survey and a bone marrow examination should be performed initially in patients with a serum M spike ≥1.5 g/dL, IgA or IgM MGUS, or an abnormal FLC ratio. These studies are also indicated in patients who have unexplained anemia, renal insufficiency, hypercalcemia, or bone lesions. Performance of interphase FISH, determination of the plasma cell labeling index, and search for circulating for plasma cells in the peripheral blood should be done if possible. Computed tomography or ultrasound examination of the abdomen may be helpful in patients with an IgM monoclonal gammopathy. Patients should always be advised to contact their physicians if there is any change in their clinical condition.

VARIANTS OF MGUS

IgM MGUS

IgM MGUS was found in 56% of 430 patients with a monoclonal IgM serum protein seen at Mayo Clinic between 1956 and 1978 (36). Currently at Mayo Clinic, about one-half of patients with a monoclonal gammopathy have MGUS. Approximately 20% of MGUS patients have an IgM monoclonal protein.

IgM MGUS was recognized in 213 Mayo Clinic patients who resided in the 11 counties of southeastern Minnesota (37). During follow-up, non-Hodgkin's lymphoma ($n=17$), WM ($n=6$), CLL ($n=3$), or AL ($n=3$) developed in 29 (14%) of the 213 IgM patients with a relative risk of 15-, 262-, 6-, and 16-fold, respectively. Progression occurred at a rate of 1.5%

per year. Independent predictors of progression included the size of the serum M protein at recognition and the serum albumin value (37).

Biclonal Gammopathies

Biclonal gammopathies are characterized by the presence of two different M proteins and occur in 2–6% of patients with monoclonal gammopathies. In a series of 57 patients with a biclonal gammopathy, 65% had biclonal gammopathy of undetermined significance (38). The clinical findings in biclonal gammopathies were similar to those in monoclonal gammopathies.

Triclonal Gammopathies

Grosbois et al. (39) described a patient with triclonal gammopathy (IgM kappa, IgG kappa, and IgA kappa) and then reviewed 24 cases from the literature. Sixteen cases were associated with a malignant lymphoproliferative disorder, five occurred in nonhematologic diseases, and three were of undetermined significance.

Idiopathic Bence Jones (Light Chain) Proteinuria

Bence Jones proteinuria may be a major feature in MM, AL, WM, or other malignant lymphoplasma cell disorders, but occasional patients may produce large amounts of Bence Jones protein in the absence of end-organ damage. Seven patients with Bence Jones protein (>1.0 g/24h) in whom no serum M protein was found and who had no evidence of MM or a related disorder were described (40). Two of the seven patients developed MM, SMM occurred in one, and AL in another, while two patients died of unrelated causes. One of these patients excreted up to 1.8 g/24h of kappa light chain for 37 years without developing evidence of renal insufficiency or amyloidosis. Although idiopathic Bence Jones proteinuria may remain stable for years, MM or AL often occurs and, consequently, these patients must be followed up indefinitely.

IgD MGUS

Almost all patients with an IgD M protein have MM, AL, or plasma cell leukemia. However, MGUS of the IgD type has been reported (41).

ASSOCIATION OF MGUS WITH OTHER DISEASES

In an older population, one might expect certain diseases to be associated with MGUS. The association of two diseases depends on the frequency with which each occurs independently. Furthermore, an apparent association may occur because of the difference in the referral practice or in other selected patient groups. Appropriate statistical and epidemiologic methods must be used to evaluate these associations. The necessity of an appropriate control population cannot be overemphasized. More detailed reviews of the association of an M protein with nonplasma cell disorders have been published (42,43).

Lymphoproliferative Disorders

In 1957, Azar et al. (44) reported that malignant lymphoma and lymphatic leukemia may be associated with a myeloma-type serum protein. Kyle et al. (45) described six patients with lymphoma who had serum protein electrophoretic patterns consistent with those of MM. Alexanian (46) reported that only 4 of 292 patients (1%) with a nodular lymphoma had an M protein, while 44 of 640 patients (7%) with diffuse non-Hodgkin's lymphoma or CLL had an M protein. We reviewed the medical records of 430 patients in whom an IgM monoclonal gammopathy had been identified between 1956 and 1978 at Mayo Clinic. Patients were classified as having WM, lymphoma, CLL, AL, MGUS, or malignant lymphoproliferative disease. Patients with a malignant lymphoproliferative process were characterized by an IgM protein value <3 g/dL, but bone marrow infiltration with lymphocytes or plasmacytoid lymphocytes and need for therapy because of anemia or constitutional symptoms was absent. Interestingly, the median survival of the patients with a malignant lymphoproliferative disorder requiring therapy was similar to that of patients with WM (5.5 and five years, respectively) (36).

Fifty-nine percent of 382 patients with a lymphoid neoplasm and an associated IgM monoclonal protein consisted of lymphoplasmacytic/lymphoma WM. The remainder represented CLL/small lymphocytic lymphoma (20%), marginal zone lymphoma (7%), follicular lymphoma (5%), mantle cell lymphoma (3%), diffuse large B-cell lymphoma (2%), and miscellaneous (4%) (47). An M protein was detected in seven of 26 patients (27%) with extranodal marginal-zone lymphoma (48).

Leukemia

In a series of 100 patients with CLL and an M protein in the serum or urine, the type of serum M protein was IgG in 51%, IgM in 38%, IgA in 1%, and only monoclonal light chains in 10% (49). Twenty-six patients with CLL/SLL with an IgM M protein were compared with 52 patients with CLL/SLL without an IgM M protein. The authors reported that the survival was not different between the two groups (50). Monoclonal gammopathies have also been reported in acute leukemia, hairy-cell leukemia, T-cell leukemia, and chronic myelocytic leukemia.

Other Hematological Diseases

Acquired von Willebrand's disease may be associated with a monoclonal gammopathy (51). Monoclonal gammopathies have also been reported with lupus anticoagulant activity, pernicious anemia, refractory anemia, pure red cell aplasia, polycythemia vera, idiopathic myelofibrosis, Gaucher's disease, and congenital dyserythropoietic anemia III. Macrocytosis has also been noted in patients with MGUS (52).

Connective Tissue Disorders

Rheumatoid arthritis has been reported in patients with monoclonal gammopathies. MGUS has also been described in lupus erythematosis, discoid lupus erythematosis, polymyositis, inclusion body myositis, scleroderma, and ankylosing spondylitis. Polymyalgia rheumatica has also been described with MGUS, but because both conditions occur more commonly, in an older population, the relationship is questionable.

Neurologic Disorders

In 279 patients who had a sensorimotor peripheral neuropathy of unknown cause, 16 (6%) had MGUS (53). In another series, 16 of 56 patients with MGUS had a peripheral neuropathy. The incidence of MGUS in peripheral neuropathy is variable and depends on patient selection, the vigor with which the presence of the M protein is sought, and whether peripheral neuropathy is diagnosed on the basis of clinical features or electrophysiologic examination. The association of neuropathy and monoclonal gammopathies has been the subject of an excellent review (54).

The most common M protein found in peripheral neuropathy is IgM followed by IgG and IgA. In approximately one-half of patients with IgM MGUS and peripheral neuropathy, the M protein binds to myelin-associated glycoprotein (MAG). The IgM protein may also bind to gangliosides, glycolipids, or chrondroitin sulphate. The clinical significance of the binding of the M protein to these components is not clear. Quarles and Weiss (55) published an extensive review of antibodies associated with peripheral neuropathy. We reported 65 patients with MGUS and sensorimotor peripheral neuropathy at Mayo Clinic; 31 had IgM, 24 had IgG, and 10 had IgA. We found no difference in the type and severity of neuropathy in patients who did and those who did not have anti-MAG activity. The level of the M-protein did not correlate with the severity of the neuropathy (56).

The differential diagnosis of MGUS-associated neuropathy includes AL and POEMS syndrome. Postural hypotension, anhidrosis, sphincter dysfunction, and heart or kidney failure often occur in AL but not in MGUS-associated neuropathy. Clinical neuropathy was found in 74% and electrodiagnostic findings in 89% of 29 patients with hepatitis C-related mixed cryoglobulinemia. In general, peripheral neuropathy progressed despite treatment with alpha-2 interferon or corticosteroids (57).

Therapy of peripheral neuropathy and MGUS is challenging. Plasmapheresis has been of benefit for some patients. Rituximab, intravenous gamma globulin, fludarabine, and alkylating agents have all produced some benefit, but the overall results are disappointing.

Motor Neuron and Other Neurologic Diseases

Eleven of 120 patients (9%) with motor neuron disease had an associated M protein. Ten of the 11 patients had amyotrophic lateral sclerosis. Nemaline (rod) myopathy has been reported with an IgG monoclonal gammopathy. Ataxia-telangectasia has also been described with MGUS.

Dermatologic Diseases

Lichen myxedematosus (papular mucinosis or scleromyxedema) is a rare dermatologic condition usually associated with a cathodal IgG lambda monoclonal protein. MGUS has been associated with pyoderma gangrenosum (58). An IgG monoclonal protein was recognized in 16 of 22 patients (73%) with necrobiotic xanthogranuloma (59). Subcorneal pustular dermatosis has been reported with monoclonal gammopathy. Schnitzler syndrome, which is characterized by chronic urticaria and an IgM monoclonal protein, has been reported in 36 patients. A detailed review of monoclonal gammopathies and skin disorders has been published (60).

Liver Disease

There is an association between hepatitis C virus (HCV) and monoclonal gammopathy. An M protein was found in 11% of 239 HCV-positive patients with chronic liver disease, but in only 1% of 98 HCV-negative patients (61). Although polyclonal increases in immunoglobulins are characteristic of chronic liver disease, an M protein was reported in 11 of 31 patients with chronic active hepatitis.

Endocrine Disorders

Monoclonal gammopathies have been reported in patients with hyperparathyroidism. We reviewed the records of 911 patients at Mayo Clinic who had hyperparathyroidism, were ≥50 years of age, and in whom immunoelectrophoresis had been performed. Nine of these 911 patients (1%) had MGUS; the prevalence was similar to that in a normal population (62). In another report, 20 of 101 patients with hyperparathyroidism had an M protein, compared with only 2 of 127 controls (63). Thus, the association of hyperparathyroidism and MGUS is unresolved.

Immunosuppression

Monoclonal gammopathies are frequently found after liver (64), kidney, or heart (65) transplantation. Autologous (66) and allogenic bone marrow transplantations have also been reported with monoclonal gammopathies. The effect of transplantation on patients with MGUS is not clear, but in one report, SMM developed in two and the M protein increased in another one of the five patients with MGUS undergoing transplantation (67).

Monoclonal proteins may also be associated with antibody activity: von Willebrand factor, thyroglobulin, riboflavin, dextran, actin, insulin, antistreptolysin O, double-stranded DNA, thyroxine, antinuclear activity, apolipoprotein, cephalin, and lactate dehydrogenase, as well as several antibiotics (68).

Binding of calcium by an M protein may produce hypercalcemia without pathologic consequences because the ionized calcium level remains normal (69). Transferrin, phosphorus, or copper may also bind to M proteins.

Miscellaneous Conditions

A wide variety of other diseases have been reported to have an association with MGUS. Angioedema and acquired deficiency of C-1 esterase inhibitor may be associated with an M protein (70,71). Systemic capillary leak syndrome is also associated with an M protein, usually of IgG type (72), as well as focal and segmental glomerulosclerosis (73).

The association of MGUS with silicone breast implants is controversial. In one report, five of 288 women with silicone breast implants had MGUS, while an M protein was found in 4 of 288 patients without implants (74). Corneal crystal deposits have been recognized in patients with MGUS (75). Monoclonal gammopathies have been reported in a wide variety of patients, including purpura fulminans, septic arthritis, Hashimoto's thyroiditis, idiopathic pulmonary fibrosis, Henoch–Schönlein purpura, pulmonary alveolar proteinosis, idiopathic pulmonary hemosiderosis, sarcoidosis, hereditary spherocytosis, hyperlipoproteinemia, and thymoma. However, the relationship of MGUS to these conditions is not clear and may simply be coincidental.

ACKNOWLEDGMENT

This work was supported in part by Grant CA-62242 and CA-107476 from the National Cancer Institute.

REFERENCES

1. Katzmann JA, Dispenzieri A, Kyle RA, et al. Elimination of the need for urine studies in the screening algorithm for monoclonal gammopathies by using serum immunofixation and free light chain assays. Mayo Clinic Proc 2006; 81 (12):1575–8.

2. Katzmann JA, Clark RJ, Abraham RS, et al. Serum reference intervals and diagnostic ranges for free kappa and free lambda immunoglobulin light chains: relative sensitivity for detection of monoclonal light chains. Clin Chem 2002; 48 (9):1437–44.

3. Katzmann JA, Abraham RS, Dispenzieri A, Lust JA, Kyle RA. Diagnostic performance of quantitative κ and λ free light chain assays in clinical practice. Clin Chem 2005; 51(5):878–81.

4. Axelsson U, Bachmann R, Hallen J. Frequency of pathological proteins (M-components) on 6,995 sera from an adult population. Acta Medica Scand 1966; 179(2):235–47.

5. Kyle RA, Finkelstein S, Elveback LR, Kurland LT. Incidence of monoclonal proteins in a Minnesota community with a cluster of multiple myeloma. Blood 1972; 40(5):719–24.

6. Saleun JP, Vicariot M, Deroff P, Morin JF. Monoclonal gammopathies in the adult population of Finistere, France. J Clin Pathol 1982; 35(1):63–8.

7. Kyle RA, Therneau TM, Rajkumar SV, et al. Prevalence of monoclonal gammopathy of undetermined significance. N Engl J Med 2006; 354(13): 1362–9.

8. Cohen HJ, Crawford J, Rao MK, Pieper CF, Currie MS. Racial differences in the prevalence of monoclonal gammopathy in a community-based sample of the elderly [erratum appears in Am J Med 1998; 105(4):362]. Am J Med 1998; 104(5):439–44.

9. Landgren O, Gridley G, Turesson I, et al. Risk of monoclonal gammopathy of undetermined significance (MGUS) and subsequent multiple myeloma among African American and white veterans in the United States. Blood 2006; 107(3): 904–6.

10. Kyle RA. Monoclonal gammopathy of undetermined significance: natural history in 241 cases. Am J Med 1978; 64(5):814–26.

11. Kyle RA, Therneau TM, Rajkumar SV, Larson DR, Plevak MF, Melton LJ, III. Long-term follow-up of 241 patients with monoclonal gammopathy of undetermined significance: the original Mayo Clinic series 25 years later. Mayo Clinic Proc 2004; 79(7):859–66.

12. Kyle RA, Therneau TM, Rajkumar SV, et al. A long-term study of prognosis in monoclonal gammopathy of undetermined significance. N Engl J Med 2002; 346(8):564–9.

13. Kyle RA, Gertz MA, Witzig TE, et al. Review of 1027 patients with newly diagnosed multiple myeloma. Mayo Clinic Proc 2003; 78(1):21–33.

14. Blade J, Lopez-Guillermo A, Rozman C, et al. Malignant transformation and life expectancy in monoclonal gammopathy of undetermined significance. Br J Haematol 1992; 81(3):391–4.

15. van de Poel MH, Coebergh JW, Hillen HF. Malignant transformation of monoclonal gammopathy of undetermined significance among out-patients of a community hospital in southeastern Netherlands. Br J Haematol 1995; 91(1): 121–5.

16. Baldini L, Guffanti A, Cesana BM, et al. Role of different hematologic variables in defining the risk of malignant transformation in monoclonal gammopathy. Blood 1996; 87(3):912–8.

17. Pasqualetti P, Festuccia V, Collacciani A, Casale R. The natural history of monoclonal gammopathy of undetermined significance: a 5- to 20-year follow-up of 263 cases. Acta Haematol 1997; 97(3):174–9.

18. Gregersen H, Ibsen J, Mellemkjoer L, Dahlerup J, Olsen J, Sorensen H. Mortality and causes of death in patients with monoclonal gammopathy of undetermined significance. Br J Haematol 2001; 112(2):353–7.

19. Gregersen H, Mellemkjoer L, Salling Ibsen J, et al. Cancer risk in patients with monoclonal gammopathy of undetermined significance. Am J Hematol 2000; 63(1):1–6.

20. Ogmundsdottir HM, Haraldsdottir V, Jóhannesson GM, et al. Monoclonal gammopathy in Iceland: a population-based registry and follow-up. Br J Haematol 2002; 118(1):166–73.

21. Avet-Loiseau H, Facon T, Daviet A, et al. 14q32 translocations and monosomy 13 observed in monoclonal gammopathy of undetermined significance delineate a multistep process for the oncogenesis of multiple myeloma. Intergroupe Francophone du Myelome. Cancer Res 1999; 59(18):4546–50.

22. Fonseca R, Bailey RJ, Ahmann GJ, et al. Genomic abnormalities in monoclonal gammopathy of undetermined significance. Blood 2002; 100(4): 1417–24.

23. Chng WJ, Van Wier SA, Ahmann GJ, et al. A validated FISH trisomy index demonstrates the hyperdiploid and nonhyperdiploid dichotomy in MGUS. Blood 2005; 106(6):2156–61.

24. Avet-Loiseau H, Li JY, Morineau N, et al. Monosomy 13 is associated with the transition of monoclonal gammopathy of undetermined significance to multiple myeloma. Intergroupe Francophone du Myelome. Blood 1999; 94(8): 2583–9.

25. Vacca A, Ribatti D, Roncali L, et al. Bone marrow angiogenesis and progression in multiple myeloma. Br J Haematol 1994; 87(3):503–8.

26. Rajkumar SV, Leong T, Roche PC, et al. Prognostic value of bone marrow angiogenesis in multiple myeloma. Clin Cancer Res 2000; 6(8):3111–6.

27. Rajkumar SV, Mesa RA, Fonseca R, et al. Bone marrow angiogenesis in 400 patients with monoclonal gammopathy of undetermined significance, multiple myeloma, and primary amyloidosis. Clin Cancer Res 2002; 8(7): 2210–6.

28. Kumar S, Witzig TE, Timm M, et al. Bone marrow angiogenic ability and expression of angiogenic cytokines in myeloma: evidence favoring loss of marrow angiogenesis inhibitory activity with disease progression. Blood 2004; 104(4):1159–65.

29. Roodman GD, III. Biology of myeloma bone disease. In: Broudy VC, Abkowitz JL, Vose JM, eds. Hematology 2002: American Society of Hematology Education Program Book. Washington, DC; 2002: 227–32.

30. Croucher PI, Shipman CM, Lippitt J, et al. Osteoprotegerin inhibits the development of osteolytic bone disease in multiple myeloma. Blood 2001; 98 (13):3534–40.

31. Cesana C, Klersy C, Barbarano L, et al. Prognostic factors for malignant transformation in monoclonal gammopathy of undetermined significance and smoldering multiple myeloma. J Clin Oncol 2002; 20(6):1625–34.

32. Rajkumar SV, Kyle RA, Therneau TM, et al. Serum free light chain ratio is an independent risk factor for progression in monoclonal gammopathy of undetermined significance. Blood 2005; 106(3):812–7. Epub 2005 Apr 26.

33. Monoclonal gammopathies of undetermined significance: a review. Immunolog Rev 2003; 194:(24):112–39.

34. Kyle RA, Greipp PR. Smoldering multiple myeloma. N Engl J Med 1980; 302 (24):1347–9.

35. Greipp PR, Witzig TE, Gonchoroff NJ, et al. Immunofluorescence labeling indices in myeloma and related monoclonal gammopathies. Mayo Clinic Proc 1987; 62(11):969–77.

36. Kyle RA, Garton JP. The spectrum of IgM monoclonal gammopathy in 430 cases. Mayo Clinic Proc 1987; 62(8):719–31.

37. Kyle RA, Therneau TM, Rajkumar SV, et al. Long-term follow-up of IgM monoclonal gammopathy of undetermined significance. Blood 2003; 102(10): 3759–64.

38. Kyle RA, Robinson RA, Katzmann JA. The clinical aspects of biclonal gammopathies: review of 57 cases. Am J Med 1981; 71(6):999–1008.

39. Grosbois B, Jego P, de Rosa H, et al. Triclonal gammopathy and malignant immunoproliferative syndrome. (French). Revue de Medecine Interne 1997; 18(6):470–3.

40. Kyle RA, Greipp PR. "Idiopathic" Bence Jones proteinuria: long-term follow-up in seven patients. N Engl J Med 1982; 306(10):564–7.

41. Blade J, Kyle RA. IgD monoclonal gammopathy with long-term follow-up. Br J Haematol 1994; 88(2):395–6.

42. Kyle RA, Blade J, Rajkumar SV. Monoclonal gammopathies of undetermined significance. In: Malpas J, et al., eds., Myeloma: Biology and Management. 3rd ed. Philadelphia, PS: Saunders, 2004:315–52.

43. Kyle RA, Rajkumar SV. Monoclonal gammopathy of undetermined significance. Br J Haematol 2006; 134(6):573–89.

44. Azar HA, Hill WT, Osserman EF. Malignant lymphoma and lymphatic leukemia. Am J Med 1957; 23:239–49.

45. Kyle RA, Bayrd ED, McKenzie BF, Heck FJ. Diagnostic criteria for electrophoretic patterns of serum and urinary proteins in multiple myeloma: study of one hundred and sixty-five multiple myeloma patients with similar electrophoretic patterns. J Am Med Assoc 1960; 174:245–51.

46. Alexanian R. Monoclonal gammopathy in lymphoma. Arch Int Med 1975; 135(1):62–6.

47. Lin P, Hao S, Handy BC, Bueso-Ramos CE, Medeiros LJ. Lymphoid neoplasms associated with IgM paraprotein: a study of 382 patients. Am J Clin Pathol 2005; 123(2):200–5.

48. Asatiani E, Cohen P, Ozdemirli M, Kessler CM, Mavromatis B, Cheson BD. Monoclonal gammopathy in extranodal marginal zone lymphoma (ENMZL) correlates with advanced disease and bone marrow involvement. Am J Hematol 2004; 77(2):144–6.

49. Noel P, Kyle RA. Monoclonal proteins in chronic lymphocytic leukemia. Am J Clin Pathol 1987; 87(3):385–8.

50. Yin CC, Lin P, Carney DA, et al. Chronic lymphocytic leukemia/small lymphocytic lymphoma associated with IgM paraprotein. Am J Clin Pathol 2005; 123(4):594–602.
51. Lamboley V, Zabraniecki L, Sie P, Pourrat J, Fournie B. Myeloma and monoclonal gammopathy of uncertain significance associated with acquired von Willebrand's syndrome: seven new cases with a literature review. Joint, Bone, Spine: Revue du Rhumatisme 2002; 69(1):62–7.
52. Horstman AL, Serck SL, Go RS. Macrocytosis associated with monoclonal gammopathy. Eur J Haematol 2005; 75(2):146–9.
53. Kelly JJ, Jr, Kyle RA, Miles JM, O'Brien PC, Dyck PJ. The spectrum of peripheral neuropathy in myeloma. Neurology 1981; 31(1):24–31.
54. Ropper AH, Gorson KC. Neuropathies associated with paraproteinemia. N Engl J Med 1998; 338(22):1601–7.
55. Quarles RH, Weiss MD. Autoantibodies associated with peripheral neuropathy. Muscle Nerve 1999; 22(7):800–22.
56. Gosselin S, Kyle RA, Dyck PJ. Neuropathy associated with monoclonal gammopathies of undetermined significance. Ann Neurol 1991; 30(1):54–61.
57. Ammendola A, Sampaolo S, Ambrosone L, et al. Peripheral neuropathy in hepatitis-related mixed cryoglobulinemia: electrophysiologic follow-up study. Muscle Nerve 2005; 31(3):382–5.
58. Powell FC, Schroeter AL, Su WP, Perry HO. Pyoderma gangrenosum and monoclonal gammopathy. Arch Dermatol 1983; 119(6):468–72.
59. Finan MC, Winkelmann RK. Necrobiotic xanthogranuloma with paraproteinemia. A review of 22 cases. Medicine 1986; 65(6):376–88.
60. Daoud MS, Lust JA, Kyle RA, Pittelkow MR. Monoclonal gammopathies and associated skin disorders. J Am Acad Dermatol 1999; 40(4):507–35.
61. Andreone P, Zignego AL, Cursaro C, et al. Prevalence of monoclonal gammopathies in patients with hepatitis C virus infection. Ann Int Med 1998; 129(4):294–8.
62. Mundis RJ, Kyle RA. Primary hyperparathyroidism and monoclonal gammopathy of undetermined significance. Am J Clin Pathol 1982; 77(5):619–21.
63. Arnulf B, Bengoufa D, Sarfati E, et al. Prevalence of monoclonal gammopathy in patients with primary hyperparathyroidism: a prospective study. Arch Int Med 2002; 162(4):464–7.
64. Badley AD, Portela DF, Patel R, et al. Development of monoclonal gammopathy precedes the development of Epstein-Barr virus-induced posttransplant lymphoproliferative disorder. Liver Transplant Surg 1996; 2(5):375–82.
65. Caforio AL, Gambino A, Belloni Fortina A, et al. Monoclonal gammopathy in heart transplantation: risk factor analysis and relevance of immunosuppressive load. Transplant Proc 2001; 33(1–2):1583–4.
66. Zent CS, Wilson CS, Tricot G, et al. Oligoclonal protein bands and Ig isotype switching in multiple myeloma treated with high-dose therapy and hematopoietic cell transplantation. Blood 1998; 91(9):3518–23.
67. Rostaing L, Modesto A, Abbal M, Durand D. Long-term follow-up of monoclonal gammopathy of undetermined significance in transplant patients. Am J Nephrol 1994; 14(3):187–91.

68. Merlini G, Farhangi M, Osserman EF. Monoclonal immunoglobulins with antibody activity in myeloma, macroglobulinemia and related plasma cell dyscrasias. Seminars Oncol 1986; 13(3):350–65.

69. Annesley TM, Burritt MF, Kyle RA. Artifactual hypercalcemia in multiple myeloma. Mayo Clin Proc 1982; 57(9):572–5.

70. Gelfand JA, Boss GR, Conley CL, Reinhart R, Frank MM. Acquired C1 esterase inhibitor deficiency and angioedema: a review. Medicine 1979; 58(4): 321–8.

71. Fremeaux-Bacchi V, Guinnepain MT, Cacoub P, et al. Prevalence of monoclonal gammopathy in patients presenting with acquired angioedema type 2. Am J Med 2002; 113(3):194–9.

72. Droder RM, Kyle RA, Greipp PR. Control of systemic capillary leak syndrome with aminophylline and terbutaline. Am J Med 1992; 92(5):523–6.

73. Dingli D, Larson DR, Plevak MF, Grande JP, Kyle RA. Focal and segmental glomerulosclerosis and plasma cell proliferative disorders. Am J Kidney Dis 2005; 46(2):278–82.

74. Karlson EW, Tanasijevic M, Hankinson SE, et al. Monoclonal gammopathy of undetermined significance and exposure to breast implants. Arch Int Med 2001; 161(6):864–7.

75. Bourne WM, Kyle RA, Brubaker RF, Greipp PR. Incidence of corneal crystals in the monoclonal gammopathies. Am J Ophthalmol 1989; 107(2):192–3.

7

Prognostic Factors and Classification in Multiple Myeloma

Jesús F. San Miguel, Ramón García-Sanz, and Norma C. Gutiérrez

Department of Hematology, University Hospital of Salamanca and Center for Cancer Research of Salamanca, Salamanca, Spain

INTRODUCTION

Multiple myeloma (MM) is a clonal B-cell disorder in which malignant plasma cells (PCs) accumulate in the bone marrow (BM) and produce lytic bone lesions and excessive amounts of monoclonal protein. The survival duration of patients with MM ranges from a few months to more than 10 years. In the main, this heterogeneity relates to specific characteristics of the tumor itself and the host. The identification of those characteristics associated with either a good or poor prognosis are most important not only for doctors but also for patients, in order to obtain more individualized information about disease outcome, instead of simply offering a general median survival rate. For the last 30 years many groups have reported on their investigations into the clinical and biological disease characteristics influencing survival. In fact, there is a disassociation between the large body of information generated in this field and its translation into clinical practice.

Three main reasons justify investigation of prognostic factors in multiple myeloma: (*i*) to provide a direct individualized information on the disease outcome, something very appreciated by patients and relatives, (*ii*) to identify risk groups in order to explore new treatment strategies in uniform cohort of patients and to allow the subsequent comparison of the results obtained by different investigators, and (*iii*) to reveal the clinical implications of certain biological features of the tumor cell, which could help to better understand the pathogenesis of the disease. However, the current availability of highly efficient new drugs is changing the myeloma panorama and this will also affect the investigation of prognostic factors with the new challenge of the identification of factors influencing the response to these novel therapies.

Traditionally, three main categories of prognostic factors have been considered in oncology: (*i*) factors related to the host, (*ii*) factors reflecting characteristics of the malignant clone, and (*iii*) factors resulting from the interaction between the tumor clone and the host, which mainly reflect the tumor burden and disease complications. However, this view could be slightly modified, since the availability of massive gene expression profiling (GEP) will allow the simultaneous evaluation of thousands of genes with potential prognostic influence. Thus, some groups consider that the prognosis and classification of myeloma should be mainly based on the genetic abnormalities present in the tumor cell clone (1,2). However, it should be kept in mind that there are some other parameters that may also have a relevant influence on the outcome of MM patients.

FACTORS RELATED TO THE TUMOR CELL CLONE

This group of prognostic factors reflects the intrinsic characteristics of the myelomatous plasma cells, including morphology, immunophenotyping and multidrug resistance, cytogenetics, gene expression profiling, and the proliferative activity of PC.

Morphology

In contrast to other hematological malignancies where the morphological features of the malignant cells are quite significant for classification and prognosis, little attention has yet been paid to the morphology of tumor PC. Nevertheless, an immature or plasmablastic morphology is associated with a poor outcome and has independent prognostic significance (3–6).

Immunophenotype

Several groups have explored the prognostic implications of the antigenic profile of PC (7–15). However, these studies are usually based on small series of patients and not uniformly treated, which may account, at least in part, to the existence of discrepant results. Some studies suggest that markers associated to an early PC phenotype (CD20, CD45, sIg) correlate with a poor outcome (10,11,16). Downregulation of CD56 and a greater expression of CD44 has been associated with an extramedullary spreading of malignant PC (8,9). The expression of CD28 has been related to disease activity, probably confined to highly proliferative accelerated phases of the disease (9,14,15). An additional observation is that certain cancer testis antigens (17) are frequently expressed in myelomatous PC as tumor-specific antigens, providing the basis for immunotherapeutic approaches (18–22). Moreover, expression of some of these CTAs, such as SSX1, SSX4, SSX5 and, especially, SSX2, is associated with reduced survival (23).

In recent years, CD45 expression has been extensively studied but the French group, and lack of CD45 expression was associated with adverse prognosis (16,24). Nevertheless, interestingly, the proliferating myeloma compartment was restricted to the CD45 bright minor subset in BM (25). This could be explained because this compartment is directly dependent on interleukin-6 (IL-6), and CD45 is a phosphatase required for IL-6-mediated growth (26–28). The Mayo Clinic group have obtained similar results in terms of relationship between a high percentage of CD45+ cells and indolent forms of the disease or better prognosis in symptomatic MM (29). By contrast, in our series, CD45 antigen did not emerge as a relevant prognostic marker (unpublished data).

We have recently analyzed in a series of 587 uniformly treated transplanted patients, the prognostic influence of the antigenic expression (30). Although the results should still be considered as preliminary due to short follow-up, it was observed that the lack of CD56 or the overexpression of CD19 and CD28 antigens confers an adverse prognosis. By contrast, acquisition of CD117 was associated with a favorable outcome. Moreover, patients with a CD28–CD117- or CD56–CD28+ phenotypic profile had adverse prognosis.

Upon analyzing prognostic factors, it is also important to consider the ability of tumor cells to overcome the toxic effect of chemotherapeutic drugs. Several approaches have been used to assess it, such as the expression of p-glycoprotein (MDR-1) which is usually observed in patients who have been exposed to anthracyclines and Vinca Alkaloids (31,32), although its prognostic is not very clear (33,34). A more interesting approach seem to be the assessment of LRP (lung resistant protein), since according to the Dutch group this protein is expressed in 50% of MM patients and it identifies a subgroup of patients with low probability to respond to conventional chemotherapy that can be resolved with high-dose chemotherapy and ASCT (35).

In any case, the prognostic impact of most of these antigens has not been confirmed in multivariate analysis, so routine immunophenotyping should not be used as a tool for prognostic evaluation purposes. In contrast, these studies can be of help for differential diagnosis between MGUS and MM (36–38) as well as for monitoring changes in the PC compartment after treatment (39,40).

Genetic Abnormalities

As in other hematological malignancies, cytogenetics has become one of the most important prognostic factor for MM. Therefore, cytogenetic evaluation is now mandatory in all patients with newly diagnosed MM, and should include interphase FISH in purified PC or in combination with immuno-fluorescent detection of light-chain restricted PC (cIg-FISH). In fact, molecular cytogenetic investigations of myeloma cells have demonstrated that almost all cases of MM are cytogenetically abnormal. Nowadays, translocations involving immunoglobulin heavy chain (IgH) gene, which are detectable in 40–60% of the patients, are considered an early event in PC disorders with significant prognostic implications. Thus, several groups have demonstrated that t(4;14)(p16;q32) and t(14;16)(q32;q23) are associated with poor survival (41–43). In contrast, the presence of t(11;14)(q13;q32) was shown to have either a favorable or irrelevant influence on the prog-nosis (44–46). Monosomy 13/13q deletions (present in about 50% of cases) have been associated with short survival in almost all large series of patients treated with both conventional or high dose therapy (43,47–54). However, the independent prognostic influence of monosomy 13 is currently under review, since its adverse prognosis can be, at least in part, influenced by the association with other cytogenetic aberrancies such as 14q32 translocations or p53 deletions (45,46). Thus, recent data suggests that the adverse prog-nostic value of 13q deletion would disappear in the absence of t(4;14) (45,46).

Other potential adverse cytogenetic features are 17p13 deletion (p53), gains on 1q (55–59). In addition, the presence of complex as well as hypo-diploid karyotypes is also associated with treatment failure (47,54).

Tumor clone development is believed to be a consequence of a multi-step process that accumulates sequential genetic changes (60). Oncogenic events associated with disease progression include several genetic changes such as translocations, mutations, deletions, and epigenetic abnormalities. Some of these genetic abnormalities were found to have an impact on the aggressiveness and prognosis of the disease. P53 mutations (61) or deletions (46,56–58) are associated with progressive disease and relapse, and patients who display K-ras mutations have significantly shorter survival as compared to those who do not (62,63). Methylation of *p16* is a frequent event in MM that inhibits *p16* gene expression (64,65), which has been described to be associated with high proliferative activity of PC and poor prognosis (66–71). However, the prognostic influence of *p16* methylation has not been repro-duced by other groups (72,73) and in our hands is not an independent prognostic factor due to its relationship with the proliferative activity of PC cells in S-phase, which is a more powerful prognostic indicator (71). It is possible that p16 methylation represent an epigenetic change inserted within the overall epigenetic changes that occur with disease progression (74–77). However, we have recently found that a low transcription of the p16 gene measured by RQ-PCR is associated with short survival (78), which suggests a real impact of this gene in the MM pathogenesis. The inactivation of other tumor suppressor genes such as p14, p15, p18, p21, and p27[kip1] have also been associated with poor prognosis in different series (1,77–80), which is in line with the view that D cyclins are the central key of myeloma pathogenesis, since their main targets, the CDK4/6, result inhibited by these suppressors (77,81).

Gene Expression Profiling

Massive GEP has allowed the recognition of new biological findings with prognostic impact in MM (82–85). Initially, MM patients were classified into different types based on different gene expression profiles (86), or its relationship with chromosomal translocations (87). These results have been refined more recently and thus, MM has been subsequently subclassified in up to seven MM types with the aim of developing a prognostically relevant molecular classification (1). The first group is characterized by the overexpression of numerous cell cycle- and proliferation-related genes and cancer–testis antigen genes. Accordingly, it was designed as proliferation (PR) subgroup. The second group is characterized by the elevated expression of endothelin 1 (*EDN1*), a positive osteoblastic stimulus, and reduced expression of *DKK1*, an osteoblastic inhibitor. Consistent with these genetic changes, this group of patients has a less extensive bone disease than the remaining groups which justify the term of low bone disease (LB) group. Another well-defined group is the MS group (group 3), which is characterized by an *MMSET* spike in the gene expression profiling, as well as by an overexpression of the *FGFR3* gene in 75% of these cases, which are the two genes hyperactivated in the reciprocal t(4;14)(p16;q32) translocation. The fourth subgroup is mainly characterized by the presence of hyperdiploidy, most often associated with trisomies of chromosomes 3, 5, 7, 9, 11, 15, 19, and 21. This group, named HY, is characterized by the overexpression of several genes related to bone metabolism (*TRAIL, FRZB, DKK1, CCR5*) and several interferon-induced genes. Groups 5 and 6 are mainly defined by the expression of cyclins D1 and D3, that are activated by the t(11;14)(q13;q32) and t(6;14)(p21;q32), respectively. Although cases with *CCND1* and *CCND3* spikes are clustered together, they split into two distinct groups (termed CD-1 and CD-2) because there are at least 123 genes differentially expressed between them. Finally, the last group (group 7) is characterized by the overexpression of MAF or MAFB genes, justifying the MF denomination. The expression of these two genes is mutually exclusive, but they are selected in the same group by the analysis. Probably, one of the most important contributions of this classification is its prognostic implication, since groups HY, CD1, CD2, and LB have a very good prognosis in opposition to PR, MF, and MS (1).

In addition, all this information has contributed to establish a new hypothesis for MM pathogenesis that presumes the existence of a universal unifying event: the cyclin D overexpression. In this hypothesis, the earliest oncogenic changes would involve three overlapping pathways: IgH translocations, multiple trisomies, and monosomy 13 or 13q14 deletion, which could be partially overlapped. The final fact would be the essentially invariant deregulation of a cyclin D (88,89).

DNA Ploidy Studies and Proliferative Activity of Plasma Cells

Measurement of cell DNA contents by flow cytometry (FCM) provides rapid and objective information about the quantitative abnormalities in the total DNA content per cell.

Hypodiploidy is associated with a poor response to treatment and short survival (90). However, the incidence of DNA hypodiploid cases by FCM is very low. Interestingly, a high incidence of hypodiploid cases has been reported in plasma cell leukemia (91,92), which supports the hypothesis of a worse prognosis for DNA hypodiploid MM. As for hyperdiploidy, although some studies have suggested that it could be associated with a worse prognosis, especially when the DNA index is higher than 1.15 (93), in our experience, DNA hyperdiploid MM patients show a significantly better outcome as compared to the nonhyperdiploid cases (94,95), which has been recently confirmed with other approaches (1,88,96).

The proliferative activity of PC, also named PC labeling index (LI) correlated with the percentage of plasma cells in S-phase of the cell cycle. Initially, LI was assessed by the incorporation of [H3]thymidine and it proved to be an excellent independent prognostic factor in MM. Accordingly, it has been shown that patients with a high tumor cell mass and more than 3% of myeloma cells incorporating [H3]thymidine had a median survival of only 5 months (97). Interestingly, Joshua et al. (98) have shown that the proliferative activity is almost entirely attributable to an increase of the LI of the immature PC. However, this technique uses in vitro radioactive labeling and therefore it is difficult to be applied in routine laboratories. Due to these limitations, nonradioactive approaches, such as the use of bromodeoxyuridine, another thymidine analogue, have been developed showing a similar prognostic impact (99). The use of propidium iodide (PI) stainings for PC, and its subsequent analysis at FCM, permits the discrimination of PC distribution along the different cell cycle phases, upon using appropriate mathematical models (7). However, due to the fact that in the BM of MM patients, many other cells apart from myelomatous PC exist, the first requisite for an accurate analysis of the S-phase PC in MM, based on the measurement of cell DNA contents, is the simultaneous identification of the neoplastic cells present in the sample so that their cell cycle distribution can be analyzed separately from that of the normal hematopoietic residual cells. In this sense, we have reported that the combined assessment of PC-related antigens (CD38+++ and CD138+) and propidium iodide can be used to assess the cell cycle distribution of MM PC separately from that of normal residual hamopoietic cells, by FCM (100).

With this method, we have found a clear correlation between a high percentage of S-phase plasma cells (>3%) and poor outcome (101,102).

Very recently, the availability of GEP has allowed the use of a new concept for plasma cell labeling index, since the proliferative activity of PC can be estimated using the normalized value of 11 genes associated with proliferation (*TOP2A, BIRC5, CCNB2, NEK2, ANAPC7, STK6, BUB1, CDC2, C10orf3, ASPM,* and *CDCA1*) (1,88). This system has been validated by comparing PC from healthy donors, MM patients and MM cells lines, but it has not yet been tested for survival analysis.

HOST FACTORS AND THEIR INTERACTIONS

Prognostic Factors Depending on the Host

Among host factors, the favorable influence of a good performance status and young age are well established. An age lower than 60–70 years is associated with prolonged survival (103–108). Moreover, it has been reported that patients under 40 years with normal renal function and low B2M have a median survival of over eight years (109). By contrast, very advanced age is a poor prognostic factor; thus, we have observed that patients over 80 years of age have a much worse prognosis than patients between 65 and 80 years of age, independently of other prognostic factors (102). Nevertheless, several groups support that age is not an independent prognostic factor (110) and in fact they recommend transplants to MM patients over the age of 70 years (111). However, in any case, age is so important that in most centers the decision making processes, such as the exclusion for transplantation (112), are mainly based on the age of the patients.

A poor performance status (ECOG scale of 2 to 4) clearly confer a poor prognosis to the patient (108), but this parameter is rather subjective and, in consequence, it is usually excluded from prognostic factor analysis. However, recent data have reinforced its importance, since albumin, an objective measurable parameter closely related to performance status, together with beta-2-microglobulin, are considered as the two most relevant independent parameters for predicting survival in the ISS classification (Table 1) (113).

There are some other important factors related with the host, such as the genetics of normal cells, which may have an important influence on disease outcome. As far as race is concerned, the initial information from a SWOG study showed that black and white patients have similar survival rates (114), but another more recent USA study suggests a better response and longer survival for African American patients compared to non-African Americans (115). In any case, the influence of constitutional genomics will be reinvestigated, since the study of genetic polymorphisms has recognized

Table 1 International Staging System for Multiple Myeloma

Stage	Parameters	Median survival (months)
1	β2M < 3.5 mg/L and albumin > 3.5 g/dL	62
2	β2M < 3.5 mg/L and albumin < 3.5 g/dL, or β2M 3.5–5.5	44
3	β2M > 5.5 mg/L	29

several conditions that can be related not only with a predisposition to develop myeloma (116–121) but also with the tolerance to the therapy, and the probability to develop complications, etc. (122,123). The possibility to evaluate thousands of polymorphisms through the SNIP technology opens a new area for analyses of genomic polymorphisms and MM outcome.

The immune status in cancer patients plays an important role in the control of the tumor growth and survival. The number of peripheral blood CD4+ cells is significantly reduced in MM patients, particularly in those with advanced clinical stages. The reduction mainly affects to memory and not naive CD4+ cells. Moreover, patients with low CD4+ levels (< 700 10^6 cells/L) display a short survival, although this is not an independent prognostic factor (7). Similar results have been reproduced by the ECOG (124). In addition, this group observed that high levels of peripheral blood CD19+ cells are positively associated with prolonged survival (125). Within NK cells there are several NK cell subpopulations with antigenic and functional differences, which have generated discrepant results along the literature (126,127). In our experience, the overall number of NK cells is significantly increased in patients with MM, but their distribution according to clinical stages differs depending on the type of NK subpopulation. Thus, the number of mature NK cells increases in the early stages of the disease (probably in an attempt to control the tumor growth), while in advanced stages, the number of PB mature NK cells decreases, while the relative number of immature NK cells increases (127). Another important finding concerning the prognostic influence of immune surveillance is that MM patients might develop T-cell clones which can recognize autologous idiotypic Ig structures as tumor specific antigens. The occurrence of expanded T cell cytotoxic clones within the CD8+CD57+CD28– compartment is associated with an improved prognosis (128,129).

Prognostic Factors Associated with Tumor Burden and Disease Complications

Tumor Burden and Disease Activity

The Durie & Salmon classification was the first attempt to measure tumor burden. The system was obtained with mathematical models that established a relationship between the tumor mass and M-component size. However, the amount of M-component is not usually recognized as a prognostic factor. Regarding the isotype of the monoclonal immunoglobulin, the British group has reviewed 2,592 patients, and they observed that light chain only (LCO) patients had the worst median survival (1.9 years) compared to 2.3 and 2.5 year in patients with IgA and IgG paraproteins. However, IgA and IgG patients with levels of LC excretion similar to those of LCO patients also had poor survival times because of renal failure, resulting in worse survival during induction therapy and at relapse. We have to keep in mind that patients included in series were treated long time ago, this justifying the short survival that these patients exhibit (130). The proportion of PC in BM may also reflect the tumor burden, as well as the pattern of bone marrow infiltration, and the presence of circulating PC. A high number of PC in BM as well as a diffuse pattern of infiltration are generally associated with a poor prognosis. However, they are not consistent prognostic factors, probably due to the heterogeneous distribution of PC in BM. The detection of circulating PC, identified either by morphology or immunophenotyping, is associated with advanced disease, and it has been reported that the presence of high levels of circulating PC (>4% PC) is an independent adverse prognostic factor (102,131).

There is a wide array of biochemical markers that reflect tumor burden and/or disease activity. Uncorrected β2M levels increases as a result of both tumor burden growth and renal function deterioration. Actually, β2M is a very sensitive indicator of renal function and this parameter is related to any variable that affects renal function such as the MM impact on kidney, age, infections and other kidney problems. This is the reason why β2M abrogates the independent prognostic value of other renal indicators (creatinine, urea, etc.) in multivariate analyses. Several threshold values for β2M (3–6 mg/dL) have been used to discriminate prognostic subgroups (99,101,132–135) but β2M can also be used as a continuous variable since the higher the β2M value, the shorter the survival. This finding makes the assessment of serum β2M levels at diagnosis in MM, as well as the albumin mandatory, since they are the two parameters that define the three stages of the new International Staging System (ISS). This system is derived from more than 11,000 patients, and it has shown been that β2M and albumin are the best combination of easily available markers to discriminate prognostic subgroups: Stage I (β2M< 3.5 & albumin >3.5 mg/dL), Stage III (β2M >5.5) and Stage II (the rest) (56,113). In contrast, β2M is not helpful for monitoring the course of the disease since there are patients that relapse without a previous increase in β2M level (false negative), while others show increased levels without any evidence of disease progression (135,136).

Other markers of disease activity, such as thymidin-kinase, neopterin and lactate dehydrogenase, do not usually remain as independent prognostic factors in multivariate analyses (137). Interleukin-6 (IL6) is a major PC growth factor, and elevated serum levels have been described to be associated with short survival (138,139). Similarly, high levels of its soluble receptor (sIL-6R) correlate with poor prognosis (140). Nevertheless, discrepant results have also been reported (141), so these two markers are not extensively used in clinical practice to asses the prognosis in MM patients. Moreover, IL-6 influences the hepatic synthesis of several acute phase reactant proteins such as C-reactive protein (CRP), α1-antitrypsin (α1-AT) and orosomucoid that could be used in its place. Actually, serum CRP levels represent a surrogate marker for IL-6 concentration (142), and the same could be applied for α1-AT (143). The use of CRP together with β2M constitute a very useful combination to predict survival in MM patients allowing to stratify MM patients into three groups according to CRP and β2M serum levels (142). Finally, the Nordic Myeloma Study Group reported that patients with high serum soluble syndecan-1 or CD138 ($\geq$ 1170 units/mL) display a short survival (20 vs. 44 months) (144), data that have been recently confirmed by the group from Birmingham in an extensive series of 324 cases (145).

Disease Complications

Disease complications such as anemia, thrombocytopenia, and renal insufficiency have a relevant influence on disease outcome (108). Skeletal lesions also have an adverse impact on survival. They have usually been evaluated by X ray, but more recently they have been also studied by magnetic resonance imaging (MRI) showing utility as a prognostic factor. Thus, the Greek group has evaluated 142 symptomatic MM patients with MRI. Focal marrow lesions were identified in 50% of patients, diffuse marrow replacement in 28%, a variegated pattern in 14%, and normal pattern in 8%. These patterns were of prognostic value, since median survival was only 24 months for patients with the diffuse pattern, while it was longer than 50 months for the remaining patterns ($p=0.001$) (146). In addition, this information was capable to add prognostic information to the ISS stages. Other groups have found a close relationship between the MRI and duration of response, since those patients with signs of bone marrow infiltration quickly relapse (147). Similar results have also been reported by using whole-body PET with (18) F-FDG (148,149). Bone resorption markers, such as urinary levels of pyridinoline and deoxy-pyridinoline, are augmented in patients with advanced clinical stages and progressive disease, and they are correlated with CRP, creatinine, and albumin levels, but the relationship with survival is not very close (150,151). In addition, cytokines influence bone lesions and can be related with the prognosis. High levels of IL-6 or metaloprotease-9 are associated with advanced bone disease (152,153). Elevated serum levels of stromal-derived factor-1α have been described to be associated with increased osteoclast activity and osteolytic bone disease in MM patients (154). In addition, soluble receptor activator of nuclear κB (sRANKL) is elevated in patients with advanced bone disease and the ratio between sRANKL and osteroprotegerin is a very good predictor for survival (155). In the same line, proinflammatory enzymes such as cyclooxygenase-2 (156) can be produced by MM cells to support local inflammation and its high expression is associated with poor outcome (156).

RESPONSE TO THERAPY

In most hematological malignancies, response to front-line therapy is one, if not the most, important prognostic factor. In MM this statement is not so clear. The reason for this is probably because, until the introduction of high dose chemotherapy, complete remission were extremely rare and the only available comparison was between responding patients (achieving partial or minor responses) and nonresponding patients, the former category having a better outcome (157). In the Oxford meta-analysis comparing melphalan and prednisone versus combination polychemotherapy (158), improvements in response led to prolongation of event free and progression free survival, but not in overall survival. An additional difficulty on the assessment of the prognostic impact of response in MM was the definition of response. The EBMT/IBMTR introduced the criteria of negative immunofixation and <5% PC in bone marrow for definition of complete remission (CR). However, it is evident that more sensitive techniques may contribute to a better assessment of the response. These techniques include: (*i*) immuno-phenotypic evaluation of bone marrow residual disease either using a clonality k/l test or a more sensitive approach based on multiparametric FCM, which identify residual PC based on the aberrant phenotype of myelomatous PC (CD56$^+$CD19$^-$CD45$^-$ or CD28$^+$ or CD117$^+$); (*ii*) molecular analysis of BM PC by ASO-PCR or RQ-ASO-PCR; (*iii*) the serum free-light chain (FLC) test and finally, (*iv*) imaging techniques such as MRI or PET in order to detect myeloma activity outside of the BM. The expectation is that these more sensitive tests will contribute to a more precise definition of response and, similar to what occurs in other hematological malignancies, terms such as immunophenotypic or molecular remission or PET/MRI negative will be better predictors of the final outcome. In the mean time, the International Working Group has introduced the term stringent complete remission (sCR, defined as CR—negative immunofixation on the serum and urine and disappearance of any soft-tissue plasmacytomas and ≤5% plasma cells in bone marrow—plus normal FLC ratio and absence of clonal cells in bone marrow by immunohistochemistry or immunofluorescence) as a new response category, and in addition the term minor response has been deleted, these cases being now considered as stable disease. Using the EBMT/IBMTR criteria, several groups have shown that achievement of CR is a surrogate marker for survival (159–166). Thus, treatment strategies designed to improve the CR rate either using autologous stem cell transplantation (159,160) or the thalidomide-melphalan-prednisone regimen (161,162) were associated with higher CR rates and an increased overall survival. Using a landmark analysis, the ECOG has shown that newly diagnosed patients who achieve CR improved survival (163), and a similar observation was reported by the Spanish PETHEMA/GEM group in patients undergoing ASCT (164), as well as in a retrospective study conducted at the MD Anderson cancer center (166). In contrast, the SWOG has reported that time to first progression is a more important outcome predictor that respond to front-line therapy (167). In addition, the Arkansas Group using thalidomide and autologous transplantation have shown that higher CR rates are associated with prolonged EFS but not OS (168). The availability of highly efficient rescue treatments, based on novel agents, makes more and more difficult the design of appropriate analysis devoted to define the role of response to initial therapy in the final overall survival. In any case, we believe that in MM, similar to other hematological malignancies, achievement of CR should be a priority, but clearly improved criteria for definition of CR (both in and outside of the BM milieu) are clearly required. A final comment about those cases which return to a "MGUS-like status" following intensive treatment. These patients could enjoy a prolonged survival in spite of having a residual M-component: and therefore the definition of the underlying biological and genetic characteristics of these patients is a challenge for future investigations.

PREDICTING TRANSFORMATION IN ASYMPTOMATIC MYELOMAS, MGUS, AND SOLITARY PLASMACYTOMA

There is an increase in the number of patients now being diagnosed as asymptomatic MM and, among them, a relatively high proportion have a young age at presentation. Therefore, it is of interest to identify factors which may predict the risk of transformation from an indolent status to a symptomatic MM.

The French group conducted a study (169) which included 91 stage I asymptomatic MM patients. Forty-one of them experienced disease progression at a median of 48 months. The factors independently favoring a bad outcome were: Hb $< 12\,g/dL$, BM plasmacytosis $> 25\%$, and MC $> 30\,g/L$. Patients with 2 or 3 risk factors progressed in < 6 months, while those without any of them remained stable for > 50 months.

A second study, conducted at MD Anderson (170), included 101 asymptomatic patients with a normal skeletal survey. Those patients with two out of the following factors had a high risk of early progression: M-component $> 30\,g/L$, BJ protein $> 50\,g/L$, and IgA isotype. In addition, in patients with only one adverse factor, MRI proved to be a useful tool for the identification of cases at risk of progression.

Using multiparametric FCM we have evaluated bone marrow aspirate samples from 78 patients with smoldering MM. The percentage of phenotypically aberrant PC within the BMPC compartment (aPC/BMPCc) at diagnosis discriminate two groups of patients with a significantly different risk of progression (PFS at 5 years of 64% vs. 8% for patients with $\geq$ or $<95\%$ aPC/ BMPCc, $p < 0.0001$). On multivariate analysis only the percentage of aPC/ BMPCc ($p = 0.004$) and the presence of immunoparesis ($p = 0.007$) showed independent prognostic value. Using these two variables we have identified three different risk categories (PFS at 5 years of 9%: $n = 32$, 42%: $n = 27$, and 82%: $n = 27$, respectively $p < 0.0001$) (171).

For MGUS patients, the largest study was published in 2002 by RA. Kyle (172). It included 1384 patients followed from 1960 through 1994 reviewing 11,009 person-years of follow-up and 115 progressions to MM, IgM lymphoma, primary amyloidosis, macroglobulinemia, chronic lymphocytic leukemia, or plasmacytoma. The risk of progression to MM or a related cancer was only associated with the size of the M-component at diagnosis. Thus, 10 years after the diagnosis of MGUS the risk of this progression was 6% for an initial monoclonal protein value ≤ 0.5 g/dL, 7% for a value of 1 g/dL, 11% for 1.5 g/dL, 20% for 2 g/dL, 24% for 2.5 g/dL, and 34% for >3.0 g/dL ($p < 0.001$). More recently, the same group has published an interesting study using flow cytometry to evaluate MGUS patients. They observed that among 325 analyzed patients, 63 (19%) had circulating PCs. Patients with circulating PCs were twice as likely to experience progression to another plasma cell disorder, most commonly myeloma, compared with those without circulating PCs (95% CI, 1.1 to 4.3; $p = 0.03$). Thus, patients with circulating PCs had a median progression-free survival of 138 months compared with a median not reached for those without circulating PCs ($p = 0.028$) (38).

As far as the risk of progression to overt myeloma after solitary plasmacytoma (SP) is concerned, there is a recent study by Knobel et al. (173) who reviewed what parameters were associated with this event in 206 patients with bone SP. The only parameter associated with a higher risk of MM at 10 years was advanced age. In addition, favorable factors for prolonged survival were younger age and tumor size < 5 cm. Finally, a vertebral anatomic localization and the type of radiotherapy were associated with a prolonged local control (173).

Further studies based on cytogenetic/molecular parameters are needed in order to improve risk progression assessment in this cohort of patients.

SUMMARY

In the previous pages we have discussed a large number of prognostic factors, but perhaps only a few of them have real independent value. A summary of the most important would include: (*i*) two host factors that reflect the ability of the patient to tolerate chemotherapy (age and performance status) and (*ii*) two intrinsic characteristics of the malignant clone (cytogenetics and proliferative activity LI) together with two biochemical markers that reflect tumor burden/disease complications (β2M and albumin).

REFERENCES

1. Zhan F, Huang Y, Colla S, et al. The molecular classification of multiple myeloma. Blood 2006; 108:2020–8.
2. Bergsagel PL. Prognostic factors in multiple myeloma: it's in the genes. Clin Cancer Res 2003; 9:533–4.
3. Bartl R, Frisch B, Burkhardt R, et al. Bone marrow histology in myeloma: its importance in diagnosis, prognosis, classification and staging. Br J Haematol 1982; 51:361–75.
4. Greipp PR. Advances in the diagnosis and management of myeloma. Semin Hematol 1992; 29:24–45.
5. Rajkumar SV, Fonseca R, Lacy MQ, et al. Plasmablastic morphology is an independent predictor of poor survival after autologous stem-cell transplantation for multiple myeloma. J Clin Oncol 1999; 17:1551–7.
6. Greipp PR, Leong T, Bennett JM, et al. Plasmablastic morphology—an independent prognostic factor with clinical and laboratory correlates: Eastern Cooperative Oncology Group (ECOG) myeloma trial E9486 report by the ECOG Myeloma Laboratory Group. Blood 1998; 91:2501–7.
7. San Miguel JF, Garcia-Sanz R, Gonzalez M, et al. Immunophenotype and DNA cell content in multiple myeloma. Baillieres Clin Haematol 1995; 8: 735–59.
8. Pellat-Deceunynck C, Barille S, Puthier D, et al. Adhesion molecules on human myeloma cells: significant changes in expression related to malignancy, tumor spreading, and immortalization. Cancer Res 1995; 55:3647–53.
9. Pellat-Deceunynck C, Bataille R, Robillard N, et al. Expression of CD28 and CD40 in human myeloma cells: a comparative study with normal plasma cells. Blood 1994; 84:2597–603.
10. Omede P, Boccadoro M, Fusaro A, et al. Multiple myeloma: 'early' plasma cell phenotype identifies patients with aggressive biological and clinical characteristics. Br J Haematol 1993; 85:504–13.
11. San Miguel JF, Gonzalez M, Gascon A, et al. Immunophenotypic heterogeneity of multiple myeloma: influence on the biology and clinical course of the disease. Castellano-Leones (Spain) Cooperative Group for the Study of Monoclonal Gammopathies. Br J Haematol 1991; 77:185–90.
12. Sahara N, Takeshita A. Prognostic significance of surface markers expressed in multiple myeloma: CD56 and other antigens. Leuk Lymphoma 2004; 45: 61–5.
13. Mateo G, Castellanos M, Rasillo A, et al. Genetic abnormalities and patterns of antigenic expression in multiple myeloma. Clin Cancer Res 2005; 11: 3661–7.

14. Robillard N, Jego G, Pellat-Deceunynck C, et al. CD28, a marker associated with tumoral expansion in multiple myeloma. Clin Cancer Res 1998; 4:1521–6.
15. Shapiro VS, Mollenauer MN, Weiss A. Endogenous CD28 expressed on myeloma cells up-regulates interleukin-8 production: implications for multiple myeloma progression. Blood 2001; 98:187–93.
16. Moreau P, Robillard N, Avet-Loiseau H, et al. Patients with CD45 negative multiple myeloma receiving high-dose therapy have a shorter survival than those with CD45 positive multiple myeloma. Haematologica 2004; 89: 547–51.
17. Perez-Encinas M, Rabunal Martinez MJ, Bello Lopez JL. Is thalidomide effective for the treatment of gastrointestinal bleeding in hereditary hemorrhagic telangiectasia? Haematologica 2002; 87:ELT34.
18. Wang Z, Zhang Y, Mandal A, et al. The spermatozoa protein, SLLP1, is a novel cancer-testis antigen in hematologic malignancies. Clin Cancer Res 2004; 10:6544–50.
19. Dhodapkar MV, Osman K, Teruya-Feldstein J, et al. Expression of cancer/testis (CT) antigens MAGE-A1, MAGE-A3, MAGE-A4, CT-7, and NY-ESO-1 in malignant gammopathies is heterogeneous and correlates with site, stage and risk status of disease. Cancer Immun 2003; 3:9:9.
20. Lim SH, Wang Z, Chiriva-Internati M, et al. Sperm protein 17 is a novel cancer-testis antigen in multiple myeloma. Blood 2001; 97:1508–10.
21. Pellat-Deceunynck C, Mellerin MP, Labarriere N, et al. The cancer germ-line genes MAGE-1, MAGE-3 and PRAME are commonly expressed by human myeloma cells. Eur J Immunol 2000; 30:803–9.
22. van Baren N, Brasseur F, Godelaine D, et al. Genes encoding tumor-specific antigens are expressed in human myeloma cells. Blood 1999; 94:1156–64.
23. Taylor BJ, Reiman T, Pittman JA, et al. SSX cancer testis antigens are expressed in most multiple myeloma patients: co-expression of SSX1, 2, 4, and 5 correlates with adverse prognosis and high frequencies of SSX-positive PCs. J Immunother 2005; 28:564–75.
24. Bataille R, Jego G, Robillard N, et al. The phenotype of normal, reactive and malignant plasma cells. Identification of "many and multiple myelomas" and of new targets for myeloma therapy. Haematologica 2006; 91:1234–40.
25. Robillard N, Pellat-Deceunynck C, Bataille R. Phenotypic characterization of the human myeloma cell growth fraction. Blood 2005; 105:4845–8.
26. Kulas DT, Freund GG, Mooney RA. The transmembrane protein-tyrosine phosphatase CD45 is associated with decreased insulin receptor signaling. J Biol Chem 1996; 271:755–60.
27. Liu S, Ishikawa H, Tsuyama N, et al. Increased susceptibility to apoptosis in CD45(+) myeloma cells accompanied by the increased expression of VDAC1. Oncogene 2006; 25:419–29.
28. Mahmoud MS, Ishikawa H, Fujii R, et al. Induction of CD45 expression and proliferation in U-266 myeloma cell line by interleukin-6. Blood 1998; 92: 3887–97.
29. Kumar S, Rajkumar SV, Kimlinger T, et al. CD45 expression by bone marrow plasma cells in multiple myeloma: clinical and biological correlations. Leukemia 2005; 19:1466–70.

30. Mateo G, Mateos MV, Rosinol L, et al. Prognostic influence of antigenic markers in 587 multiple myeloma patients uniformly treated with high dose therapy. Haematologica 2006; 90(S1):103.

31. Grogan TM, Spier CM, Salmon SE, et al. P-glycoprotein expression in human plasma cell myeloma: correlation with prior chemotherapy. Blood 1993; 81: 490–5.

32. Sonneveld P. Multidrug resistance in haematological malignancies. J Intern Med 2000; 247:521–34.

33. Friedenberg WR, Rue M, Blood EA, et al. Phase III study of PSC-833 (valspodar) in combination with vincristine, doxorubicin, and dexamethasone (valspodar/VAD) versus VAD alone in patients with recurring or refractory multiple myeloma (E1A95): a trial of the Eastern Cooperative Oncology Group. Cancer 2006; 106:830–8.

34. Sonneveld P, Suciu S, Weijermans P, et al. Cyclosporin A combined with vincristine, doxorubicin and dexamethasone (VAD) compared with VAD alone in patients with advanced refractory multiple myeloma: an EORTC-HOVON randomized phase III study (06914). Br J Haematol 2001; 115: 895–902.

35. Raaijmakers HG, Izquierdo MA, Lokhorst HM, et al. Lung-resistance-related protein expression is a negative predictive factor for response to conventional low but not to intensified dose alkylating chemotherapy in multiple myeloma. Blood 1998; 91:1029–36.

36. Harada H, Kawano MM, Huang N, et al. Phenotypic difference of normal plasma cells from mature myeloma cells. Blood 1993; 81:2658–63.

37. Ocqueteau M, Orfao A, Almeida J, et al. Immunophenotypic characterization of plasma cells from monoclonal gammopathy of undetermined significance patients. Implications for the differential diagnosis between MGUS and multiple myeloma. Am J Pathol 1998; 152:1655–65.

38. Kumar S, Rajkumar SV, Kyle RA, et al. Prognostic value of circulating plasma cells in monoclonal gammopathy of undetermined significance. J Clin Oncol 2005; 23:5668–74.

39. San Miguel JF, Almeida J, Mateo G, et al. Immunophenotypic evaluation of the plasma cell compartment in multiple myeloma: a tool for comparing the efficacy of different treatment strategies and predicting outcome. Blood 2002; 99:1853–6.

40. Rawstron AC, Davies FE, Dasgupta R, et al. Flow cytometric disease monitoring in multiple myeloma: the relationship between normal and neoplastic plasma cells predicts outcome after transplantation. Blood 2002; 100:3095–100.

41. Stewart AK, Fonseca R. Prognostic and therapeutic significance of myeloma genetics and gene expression profiling. J Clin Oncol 2005; 23:6339–44.

42. Moreau P, Facon T, Leleu X, et al. Recurrent 14q32 translocations determine the prognosis of multiple myeloma, especially in patients receiving intensive chemotherapy. Blood 2002; 100:1579–83.

43. Fonseca R, Blood E, Rue M, et al. Clinical and biologic implications of recurrent genomic aberrations in myeloma. Blood 2003; 101:4569–75.

44. Fonseca R, Blood EA, Oken MM, et al. Myeloma and the t(11; 14)(q13; q32); evidence for a biologically defined unique subset of patients. Blood 2002; 99: 3735–41.

45. Avet-Loiseau H, Attal M, Moureau P, et al. Genetic abnormalities in myeloma: the experience of the Intergroupe Francophone du Myélome. Blood 2007; 109:3489–95.

46. Gutierrez NC, Castellanos MV, Martin ML, et al. Prognostic and biological implications of genetic abnormalities in multiple myeloma undergoing autologous stem cell transplantation: t(4;14) is the most relevant adverse prognostic factor, whereas RB deletion as a unique abnormality is not associated with adverse prognosis. Leukemia 2007; 21:143–50.

47. Tricot G, Sawyer JR, Jagannath S, et al. Unique role of cytogenetics in the prognosis of patients with myeloma receiving high-dose therapy and autotransplants. J Clin Oncol 1997; 15:2659–66.

48. Tricot G, Barlogie B, Jagannath S, et al. Poor prognosis in multiple myeloma is associated only with partial or complete deletions of chromosome 13 or abnormalities involving 11q and not with other karyotype abnormalities. Blood 1995; 86:4250–6.

49. Fonseca R, Barlogie B, Bataille R, et al. Genetics and cytogenetics of multiple myeloma: a workshop report. Cancer Res 2004; 64:1546–58.

50. Dewald GW, Therneau T, Larson D, et al. Relationship of patient survival and chromosome anomalies detected in metaphase and/or interphase cells at diagnosis of myeloma. Blood 2005; 106:3553–8.

51. Stewart AK, Fonseca R. Prognostic and therapeutic significance of myeloma genetics and gene expression profiling. J Clin Oncol 2005; 23:6339–44.

52. Zojer N, Konigsberg R, Ackermann J, et al. Deletion of 13q14 remains an independent adverse prognostic variable in multiple myeloma despite its frequent detection by interphase fluorescence in situ hybridization. Blood 2000; 95:1925–30.

53. Perez-Simon JA, Garcia-Sanz R, Tabernero MD, et al. Prognostic value of numerical chromosome aberrations in multiple myeloma: A FISH analysis of 15 different chromosomes. Blood 1998; 91:3366–71.

54. Smadja NV, Bastard S, Brigaudeau C, et al. Hypodiploidy is a major prognostic factor in multiple myeloma. Blood 2001; 98:2229–38.

55. Gutierrez NC, Garcia JL, Hernandez JM, et al. Prognostic and biologic significance of chromosomal imbalances assessed by comparative genomic hybridization in multiple myeloma. Blood 2004; 104:2661–6.

56. Drach J, Ackermann J, Fritz E, et al. Presence of a p53 gene deletion in patients with multiple myeloma predicts for short survival after conventional-dose chemotherapy. Blood 1998; 92:802–9.

57. Drach J, Ackerman J, Kaufmann H, et al. Deletions of the p53 gene in multiple myeloma. Br J Haematol 2000; 108:886.

58. Chang H, Qi C, Yi QL, et al. p53 gene deletion detected by fluorescence in situ hybridization is an adverse prognostic factor for patients with multiple myeloma following autologous stem cell transplantation. Blood 2005; 105: 358–60.

59. Hanamura I, Stewart JP, Huang Y, et al. Frequent gain of chromosome band 1q21 in plasma-cell dyscrasias detected by fluorescence in situ hybridization: incidence increases from MGUS to relapsed myeloma and is related to prognosis and disease progression following tandem stem-cell transplantation. Blood 2006; 108:1724–32.

60. Hallek M, Bergsagel PL, Anderson KC. Multiple myeloma: increasing evidence for a multistep transformation process. Blood 1998; 91:3–21.

61. Corradini P, Inghirami G, Astolfi M, et al. Inactivation of tumor suppressor genes, p53 and Rb1, in plasma cell dyscrasias. Leukemia 1994; 8: 758–67.

62. Bezieau S, Devilder MC, Avet-Loiseau H, et al. High incidence of N and K-Ras activating mutations in multiple myeloma and primary plasma cell leukemia at diagnosis. Hum Mutat 2001; 18:212–24.

63. Rowley M, Van Ness B. Activation of N-ras and K-ras induced by interleukin-6 in a myeloma cell line: implications for disease progression and therapeutic response. Oncogene 2002; 21:8769–75.

64. Urashima M, Teoh G, Ogata A, et al. Characterization of p16(INK4A) expression in multiple myeloma and plasma cell leukemia. Clin Cancer Res 1997; 3:2173–9.

65. Tasaka T, Asou H, Munker R, et al. Methylation of the p16INK4A gene in multiple myeloma. Br J Haematol 1998; 101:558–64.

66. Mateos MV, Garcia-Sanz R, Lopez-Perez R, et al. p16/INK4a gene inactivation by hypermethylation is associated with aggressive variants of monoclonal gammopathies. Hematol J 2001; 2:146–9.

67. Galm O, Wilop S, Reichelt J, et al. DNA methylation changes in multiple myeloma. Leukemia 2004; 18:1687–92.

68. Uchida T, Kinoshita T, Ohno T, et al. Hypermethylation of p16INK4A gene promoter during the progression of plasma cell dyscrasia. Leukemia 2001; 15: 157–65.

69. Guillerm G, Gyan E, Wolowiec D, et al. p16(INK4a) and p15(INK4b) gene methylations in plasma cells from monoclonal gammopathy of undetermined significance. Blood 2001; 98:244–6.

70. Chen W, Wu Y, Zhu J, et al. Methylation of p16 and p15 genes in multiple myeloma. Chin Med Sci J 2002; 17:101–5.

71. Mateos MV, Garcia-Sanz R, Lopez-Perez R, et al. Methylation is an inactivating mechanism of the p16 gene in multiple myeloma associated with high plasma cell proliferation and short survival. Br J Haematol 2002; 118: 1034–40.

72. Gonzalez-Paz N, Chng WJ, McClure RF, et al. Tumor suppressor p16 methylation in multiple myeloma: biological and clinical implications. Blood 2006.

73. Ribas C, Colleoni GW, Felix RS, et al. p16 gene methylation lacks correlation with angiogenesis and prognosis in multiple myeloma. Cancer Lett 2005; 222: 247–54.

74. Takada S, Morita K, Hayashi K, et al. Methylation status of fragile histidine triad (FHIT) gene and its clinical impact on prognosis of patients with multiple myeloma. Eur J Haematol 2005; 75:505–10.

75. Reddy J, Shivapurkar N, Takahashi T, et al. Differential methylation of genes that regulate cytokine signaling in lymphoid and hematopoietic tumors. Oncogene 2005; 24:732–6.
76. Seidl S, Ackermann J, Kaufmann H, et al. DNA-methylation analysis identifies the E-cadherin gene as a potential marker of disease progression in patients with monoclonal gammopathies. Cancer 2004; 100:2598–606.
77. Drexler HG. Review of alterations of the cyclin-dependent kinase inhibitor INK4 family genes p15, p16, p18 and p19 in human leukemia-lymphoma cells. Leukemia 1998; 12:845–59.
78. Sarasquete ME, Garcia-Sanz R, Armellini A, et al. An increased p14$^{ARF/}$ ^{p16INK4a} and p15^{INK4b} gene expression is associated with low proliferative activity in multiple myeloma and is related with an indolent clinical course and good prognosis. Haematologica 2006.
79. Ohata M, Nakamura S, Fujita H, et al. Prognostic implications of p21 (Waf1/Cip1) immunolocalization in multiple myeloma. Biomed Res 2005; 26: 91–8.
80. Filipits M, Pohl G, Stranzl T, et al. Low p27Kip1 expression is an independent adverse prognostic factor in patients with multiple myeloma. Clin Cancer Res 2003; 9:820–6.
81. Chen-Kiang S. Biology of plasma cells. Best Pract Res Clin Haematol 2005; 18:493–507.
82. Chauhan D, Auclair D, Robinson EK, et al. Identification of genes regulated by dexamethasone in multiple myeloma cells using oligonucleotide arrays. Oncogene 2002; 21:1346–58.
83. De Vos J, Couderc G, Tarte K, et al. Identifying intercellular signaling genes expressed in malignant plasma cells by using complementary DNA arrays. Blood 2001; 98:771–80.
84. Zhan F, Hardin J, Kordsmeier B, et al. Global gene expression profiling of multiple myeloma, monoclonal gammopathy of undetermined significance, and normal bone marrow plasma cells. Blood 2002; 99:1745–57.
85. Magrangeas F, Nasser V, Avet-Loiseau H, et al. Gene expression profiling of multiple myeloma reveals molecular portraits in relation to the pathogenesis of the disease. Blood 2003; 101:4998–5006.
86. Shaughnessy J, Jr, Zhan F, Barlogie B, et al. Gene expression profiling and multiple myeloma. Best Pract Res Clin Haematol 2005; 18:537–52.
87. Hideshima T, Bergsagel PL, Kuehl WM, et al. Advances in biology of multiple myeloma: clinical applications. Blood 2004; 104:607–18.
88. Bergsagel PL, Kuehl WM, Zhan F, et al. Cyclin D dysregulation: an early and unifying pathogenic event in multiple myeloma. Blood 2005; 106:296–303.
89. Bergsagel PL, Kuehl WM. Molecular Pathogenesis and a Consequent Classification of Multiple Myeloma. J Clin Oncol 2005; 23:6333–8.
90. Morgan RJ, Jr, Gonchoroff NJ, Katzmann JA, et al. Detection of hypodiploidy using multi-parameter flow cytometric analysis: a prognostic indicator in multiple myeloma. Am J Hematol 1989; 30:195–200.
91. Garcia-Sanz R, Orfao A, Gonzalez M, et al. Primary plasma cell leukemia: clinical, immunophenotypic, DNA ploidy, and cytogenetic characteristics. Blood 1999; 93:1032–7.

92. Shimazaki C, Gotoh H, Ashihara E, et al. Immunophenotype and DNA content of myeloma cells in primary plasma cell leukemia. Am J Hematol 1992; 39:159–62.

93. Tafuri A, Meyers J, Lee BJ, et al. DNA and RNA flow cytometric study in multiple myeloma. Clinical correlations. Cancer 1991; 67:449–54.

94. Garcia-Sanz R, Orfao A, Gonzalez M, et al. Prognostic implications of DNA aneuploidy in 156 untreated multiple myeloma patients. Castelano-Leones (Spain) Cooperative Group for the Study of Monoclonal Gammopathies. Br J Haematol 1995; 90:106–12.

95. San Miguel JF, Garcia-Sanz R, Gonzalez M, et al. DNA cell content studies in multiple myeloma. Leuk Lymphoma 1996; 23:33–41.

96. Chng WJ, Ketterling RP, Fonseca R. Analysis of genetic abnormalities provides insights into genetic evolution of hyperdiploid myeloma. Genes Chromosomes Cancer 2006.

97. Durie BG, Salmon SE, Moon TE. Pretreatment tumor mass, cell kinetics, and prognosis in multiple myeloma. Blood 1980; 55:364–72.

98. Joshua D, Petersen A, Brown R, et al. The labelling index of primitive plasma cells determines the clinical behaviour of patients with myelomatosis. Br J Haematol 1996; 94:76–81.

99. Greipp PR, Lust JA, O'Fallon WM, et al. Plasma cell labeling index and beta 2-microglobulin predict survival independent of thymidine kinase and C-reactive protein in multiple myeloma. Blood 1993; 81:3382–7.

100. Orfao A, Garcia-Sanz R, Lopez-Berges MC, et al. A new method for the analysis of plasma cell DNA content in multiple myeloma samples using a CD38/propidium iodide double staining technique. Cytometry 1994; 17: 332–9.

101. San Miguel JF, Garcia-Sanz R, Gonzalez M, et al. A new staging system for multiple myeloma based on the number of S-phase plasma cells. Blood 1995; 85:448–55.

102. Garcia-Sanz R, Gonzalez-Fraile MI, Mateo G, et al. Proliferative activity of plasma cells is the most relevant prognostic factor in elderly multiple myeloma patients. Int J Cancer 2004; 112:884–9.

103. Janssen-Heijnen ML, Houterman S, Lemmens VE, et al. Prognostic impact of increasing age and co-morbidity in cancer patients: a population-based approach. Crit Rev Oncol Hematol 2005; 55:231–40.

104. Lenhoff S, Hjorth M, Westin J, et al. Impact of age on survival after intensive therapy for multiple myeloma: a population-based study by the Nordic Myeloma Study Group. Br J Haematol 2006; 133:389–96.

105. Mileshkin L, Biagi JJ, Mitchell P, et al. Multicenter phase 2 trial of thalidomide in relapsed/refractory multiple myeloma: adverse prognostic impact of advanced age. Blood 2003; 102:69–77.

106. Mileshkin L, Prince HM. The adverse prognostic impact of advanced age in multiple myeloma. Leuk Lymphoma 2005; 46:951–66.

107. Ross FM, Ibrahim AH, Vilain-Holmes A, et al. Age has a profound effect on the incidence and significance of chromosome abnormalities in myeloma. Leukemia 2005; 19:1634–42.

108. San Miguel JF, Garcia-Sanz R. Prognostic features of multiple myeloma. Best Pract Res Clin Haematol 2005; 18:569–83.
109. Blade J, Kyle RA, Greipp PR. Presenting features and prognosis in 72 patients with multiple myeloma who were younger than 40 years. Br J Haematol 1996; 93:345–51.
110. Siegel DS, Desikan KR, Mehta J, et al. Age is not a prognostic variable with autotransplants for multiple myeloma. Blood 1999; 93:51–4.
111. Badros A, Barlogie B, Siegel E, et al. Autologous stem cell transplantation in elderly multiple myeloma patients over the age of 70 years. Br J Haematol 2001; 114:600–7.
112. Barlogie B, Jagannath S, Vesole D, et al. Autologous and allogeneic transplants for multiple myeloma. Semin Hematol 1995; 32:31–44.
113. Greipp PR, San Miguel JF, Durie BGM, et al. International staging system for multiple myeloma. J Clin Oncol 2005; 23:3412–20.
114. Modiano MR, Villar-Werstler P, Crowley J, et al. Evaluation of race as a prognostic factor in multiple myeloma. An ancillary of Southwest Oncology Group Study 8229. J Clin Oncol 1996; 14:974–7.
115. Saraf S, Chen YH, Dobogai LC, et al. Prolonged responses after autologous stem cell transplantation in African-American patients with multiple myeloma. Bone Marrow Transplant 2006; 37:1099–102.
116. Lincz LF, Scorgie FE, Robertson R, et al. Genetic variations in benzene metabolism and susceptibility to multiple myeloma. Leuk Res 2006.
117. Spink CF, Gray LC, Davies FE, et al. Haplotypic structure across the IkappaBalpha gene (NFKBIA) and association with multiple myeloma. Cancer Lett 2006;.
118. Morgan GJ, Adamson PJ, Mensah FK, et al. Haplotypes in the tumour necrosis factor region and myeloma. Br J Haematol 2005; 129:358–65.
119. Roddam PL, Rollinson S, O'Driscoll M, et al. Genetic variants of NHEJ DNA ligase IV can affect the risk of developing multiple myeloma, a tumour characterised by aberrant class switch recombination. J Med Genet 2002; 39: 900–5.
120. Parker KM, Ma MH, Manyak S, et al. Identification of polymorphisms of the IkappaBalpha gene associated with an increased risk of multiple myeloma. Cancer Genet Cytogenet 2002; 137:43–8.
121. Davies FE, Rollinson SJ, Rawstron AC, et al. High-producer haplotypes of tumor necrosis factor alpha and lymphotoxin alpha are associated with an increased risk of myeloma and have an improved progression-free survival after treatment. J Clin Oncol 2000; 18:2843–51.
122. Dasgupta RK, Adamson PJ, Davies FE, et al. Polymorphic variation in GSTP1 modulates outcome following therapy for multiple myeloma. Blood 2003; 102:2345–50.
123. Neben K, Mytilineos J, Moehler TM, et al. Polymorphisms of the tumor necrosis factor-alpha gene promoter predict for outcome after thalidomide therapy in relapsed and refractory multiple myeloma. Blood 2002; 100:2263–5.
124. Kay NE, Leong TL, Bone N, et al. Blood levels of immune cells predict survival in myeloma patients: results of an Eastern Cooperative Oncology

Group phase 3 trial for newly diagnosed multiple myeloma patients. Blood 2001; 98:23–8.

125. Kay NE, Leong T, Kyle RA, et al. Circulating blood B cells in multiple myeloma: analysis and relationship to circulating clonal cells and clinical parameters in a cohort of patients entered on the Eastern Cooperative Oncology Group phase III E9486 clinical trial. Blood 1997; 90:340–5.

126. Osterborg A, Nilsson B, Bjorkholm M, et al. Natural killer cell activity in monoclonal gammopathies: relation to disease activity. Eur J Haematol 1990; 45:153–7.

127. Garcia-Sanz R, Gonzalez M, Orfao A, et al. Analysis of natural killer-associated antigens in peripheral blood and bone marrow of multiple myeloma patients and prognostic implications. Br J Haematol 1996; 93:81–8.

128. Brown RD, Yuen E, Nelson M, et al. The prognostic significance of T cell receptor beta gene rearrangements and idiotype-reactive T cells in multiple myeloma. Leukemia 1997; 11:1312–17.

129. Sze DM, Giesajtis G, Brown RD, et al. Clonal cytotoxic T cells are expanded in myeloma and reside in the CD8(+)CD57(+)CD28(-) compartment. Blood 2001; 98:2817–27.

130. Drayson M, Begum G, Basu S, et al. Effects of paraprotein heavy and light chain types and free light chain load on survival in myeloma: an analysis of patients receiving conventional-dose chemotherapy in Medical Research Council UK multiple myeloma trials. Blood 2006; 108:2013–19.

131. Witzig TE, Gertz MA, Lust JA, et al. Peripheral blood monoclonal plasma cells as a predictor of survival in patients with multiple myeloma. Blood 1996; 88:1780–7.

132. Cuzick J, De Stavola BL, Cooper EH, et al. Long-term prognostic value of serum beta 2 microglobulin in myelomatosis. Br J Haematol 1990; 75:506–10.

133. Bataille R, Grenier J, Sany J. Unexpected normal serum beta-microglobulin (B2M) levels in multiple myeloma. Anticancer Res 1987; 7:513–15.

134. Garewal H, Durie BG, Kyle RA, et al. Serum beta 2-microglobulin in the initial staging and subsequent monitoring of monoclonal plasma cell disorders. J Clin Oncol 1984; 2:51–7.

135. Boccadoro M, Omede P, Frieri R, et al. Multiple myeloma: beta-2-microglobulin is not a useful follow-up parameter. Acta Haematol 1989; 82:122–5.

136. Greipp PR. Monoclonal gammopathies: new approaches to clinical problems in diagnosis and prognosis. Blood Rev 1989; 3:222–36.

137. San Miguel JF, Sanchez J, Gonzalez M. Prognostic factors and classification in multiple myeloma. Br J Cancer 1989; 59:113–18.

138. Klein B, Zhang XG, Jourdan M, et al. Paracrine rather than autocrine regulation of myeloma-cell growth and differentiation by interleukin-6. Blood 1989; 73:517–26.

139. Papadaki H, Kyriakou D, Foudoulakis A, et al. Serum levels of soluble IL-6 receptor in multiple myeloma as indicator of disease activity. Acta Haematol 1997; 97:191–5.

140. Pulkki K, Pelliniemi TT, Rajamaki A, et al. Soluble interleukin-6 receptor as a prognostic factor in multiple myeloma. Finnish Leukaemia Group. Br J Haematol 1996; 92:370–4.

141. Ohtani K, Ninomiya H, Hasegawa Y, et al. Clinical significance of elevated soluble interleukin-6 receptor levels in the sera of patients with plasma cell dyscrasias. Br J Haematol 1995; 91:116–20.

142. Bataille R, Boccadoro M, Klein B, et al. C-reactive protein and beta-2 microglobulin produce a simple and powerful myeloma staging system. Blood 1992; 80:733–7.

143. Merlini G, Perfetti V, Gobbi PG, et al. Acute phase proteins and prognosis in multiple myeloma. Br J Haematol 1993; 83:595–601.

144. Seidel C, Sundan A, Hjorth M, et al. Serum syndecan-1: a new independent prognostic marker in multiple myeloma. Blood 2000; 95:388–92.

145. Lovell R, Dunn JA, Begum G, et al. Soluble syndecan-1 level at diagnosis is an independent prognostic factor in multiple myeloma and the extent of fall from diagnosis to plateau predicts for overall survival. Br J Haematol 2005; 130: 542–8.

146. Moulopoulos LA, Gika D, Anagnostopoulos A, et al. Prognostic significance of magnetic resonance imaging of bone marrow in previously untreated patients with multiple myeloma. Ann Oncol 2005; 16:1824–8.

147. Baur-Melnyk A, Buhmann S, Durr HR, et al. Role of MRI for the diagnosis and prognosis of multiple myeloma. Eur J Radiol 2005; 55:56–63.

148. Orchard K, Barrington S, Buscombe J, et al. Fluoro-deoxyglucose positron emission tomography imaging for the detection of occult disease in multiple myeloma. Br J Haematol 2002; 117:133–5.

149. Durie BG, Waxman AD, D'Agnolo A, et al. Whole-body (18)F-FDG PET identifies high-risk myeloma. J Nucl Med 2002; 43:1457–63.

150. Pecherstorfer M, Seibel MJ, Woitge HW, et al. Bone resorption in multiple myeloma and in monoclonal gammopathy of undetermined significance: quantification by urinary pyridinium cross-links of collagen. Blood 1997; 90: 3743–50.

151. Hernandez JM, Suquia B, Queizan JA, et al. Bone remodelation markers are useful in the management of monoclonal gammopathies. Hematol J 2004; 5: 480–8.

152. Sfiridaki A, Miyakis S, Tsirakis G, et al. Systemic levels of interleukin-6 and matrix metalloproteinase-9 in patients with multiple myeloma may be useful as prognostic indexes of bone disease. Clin Chem Lab Med 2005; 43:934–8.

153. Demacq C, Montenegro MF. Systemic matrix metalloproteinase-9 (MMP-9) levels as prognostic indexes of bone disease in patients with multiple myeloma. Clin Chem Lab Med 2006; 44:232.

154. Zannettino AC, Farrugia AN, Kortesidis A, et al. Elevated serum levels of stromal-derived factor-1alpha are associated with increased osteoclast activity and osteolytic bone disease in multiple myeloma patients. Cancer Res 2005; 65:1700–9.

155. Terpos E, Szydlo R, Apperley JF, et al. Soluble receptor activator of nuclear factor kappaB ligand-osteoprotegerin ratio predicts survival in multiple myeloma: proposal for a novel prognostic index. Blood 2003; 102:1064–9.

156. Ladetto M, Vallet S, Trojan A, et al. Cyclooxygenase-2 (COX-2) is frequently expressed in multiple myeloma and is an independent predictor of poor outcome. Blood 2005; 105:4784–91.

157. Blade J, Lopez-Guillermo A, Bosch F, et al. Impact of response to treatment on survival in multiple myeloma: results in a series of 243 patients. Br J Haematol 1994; 88:117–21.

158. No authors listed. Combination chemotherapy versus melphalan plus prednisone as treatment for multiple myeloma: an overview of 6,633 patients from 27 randomized trials. Myeloma Trialists' Collaborative Group. J Clin Oncol 1998; 16:3832–42.

159. Attal M, Harousseau JL, Stoppa AM, et al. A prospective, randomized trial of autologous bone marrow transplantation and chemotherapy in multiple myeloma. Intergroupe Francais du Myelome. N Engl J Med 1996; 335:91–7.

160. Child JA, Morgan GJ, Davies FE, et al. High-dose chemotherapy with hematopoietic stem-cell rescue for multiple myeloma. N Engl J Med 2003; 348: 1875–83.

161. Palumbo A, Bringhen S, Caravita T, et al. Oral melphalan and prednisone chemotherapy plus thalidomide compared with melphalan and prednisone alone in elderly patients with multiple myeloma: randomised controlled trial. The Lancet 2006; 367:825–31.

162. Facon T, Mary JL, Hulin C, Benboubker L, Attal M, Renaud M, et al. Major Superiority of Melphalan – Prednisone (MP) + Thalidomide (THAL) over MP and autologous stem cell transplantation in the treatment of newly diagnosed elderly patients with multiple myeloma. Blood 2006; 106(11).

163. Kyle RA, Leong T, Li S, et al. Complete response in multiple myeloma: clinical trial E9486, an Eastern Cooperative Oncology Group Study not involving stem cell transplantation. Cancer 2006; 106:1958–66.

164. Lahuerta JJ, Martinez-Lopez J, Serna JD, et al. Remission status defined by immunofixation vs. electrophoresis after autologous transplantation has a major impact on the outcome of multiple myeloma patients. Br J Haematol 2000; 109:438–46.

165. Barlogie B, Jagannath S, Desikan KR, et al. total therapy with tandem transplants for newly diagnosed multiple myeloma. Blood 1999; 93:55–65.

166. Alexanian R, Weber D, Giralt S, et al. Impact of complete remission with intensive therapy in patients with responsive multiple myeloma. Bone Marrow Transplant 2001; 27:1037–43.

167. Durie BG, Jacobson J, Barlogie B, et al. Magnitude of response with myeloma frontline therapy does not predict outcome: importance of time to progression in southwest oncology group chemotherapy trials. J Clin Oncol 2004; 22: 1857–63.

168. Barlogie B, Tricot G, Anaissie E, et al. Thalidomide and hematopoietic-cell transplantation for multiple myeloma. N Engl J Med 2006; 354:1021–30.

169. Facon T, Menard JF, Michaux JL, et al. Prognostic factors in low tumour mass asymptomatic multiple myeloma: a report on 91 patients. The Groupe d'Etudes et de Recherche sur le Myelome (GERM). Am J Hematol 1995; 48: 71–5.

170. Weber DM, Dimopoulos MA, Moulopoulos LA, et al. Prognostic features of asymptomatic multiple myeloma. Br J Haematol 1997; 97:810–14.

171. Perez-Persona E, Vidriales MB, Mateo G, et al. New criteria to identify risk of progression in monoclonal gammopathy of uncertain significance and

smoldering multiple myeloma based on multiparameter flow cytometry analysis of bone marrow plasma cells. Blood 2006; Jun 18 [Epub ahead of print].

172. Kyle RA, Therneau TM, Rajkumar SV, et al. A long-term study of prognosis in monoclonal gammopathy of undetermined significance. N Engl J Med 2002; 346:564–9.

173. Knobel D, Zouhair A, Tsang RW, et al. Prognostic factors in solitary plasmacytoma of the bone: a multicenter rare cancer network study. BMC Cancer 2006; 6:118.

8

Novel Agents for Previously Untreated Multiple Myeloma

Sheeba Thomas, Tiffany Richards, and Donna M. Weber

Department of Lymphoma and Myeloma, The University of Texas M.D. Anderson Cancer Center, Houston, Texas, U.S.A

For decades, chemotherapy for multiple myeloma has consisted of standard combinations of alkylating agents, anthracyclines, and steroids with or without hematopoietic stem cell rescue. While these therapies can provide rapid responses and result in modest gains for patients, the disease eventually relapses in all patients and becomes resistant to treatment. More recently, agents with novel mechanisms of action, such as the proteasome inhibitor, bortezomib and immunomodulatory drugs like thalidomide and its derivative lenalidomide, have shown promise for treatment of patients with not only refractory and relapsed disease, but also for those with previously untreated multiple myeloma. Recent combinations of these agents (thalidomide, bortezomib, lenalidomide) with or without alkylating agents, anthracyclines, and steroids have produced rapid remissions (within 1–3 cycles) resulting in improved overall response rates of 75–95% and complete response rates of 5–25% in patients receiving induction therapy (1–11). Initial data with the combination of melphalan-prednisone-thalidomide demonstrates improved overall survival in elderly patients compared with melphalan-prednisone and reduced intensity myeloablative therapy with autologous stem cell support, and provides the first suggestion that the improvement in overall response rates with novel agent combinations for induction therapy is likely to translate into an overall survival benefit for many patients with multiple myeloma (12). Thus, these regimens may provide a useful alternative or adjunct to myeloablative therapy with stem cell transplant in the future. This chapter will focus on the role of bortezomib, thalidomide and lenalidomide in induction therapy of multiple myeloma.

THALIDOMIDE

Initially developed as a sedative, thalidomide was found to be an effective antiemetic for women with morning sickness in the 1950s. It was removed from the market in the early 1960s, when its teratogenic effects (phocomelia) became known, but re-emerged in the 1980s, when early investigation in erythema nodosum leprosy, Behçet's syndrome, and graft versus host disease led to subsequent approval of the drug by the U.S. Food and Drug Administration (1998) for the treatment of erythema nodosum leprosy (13–18).

The in vitro antiangiogenic properties of thalidomide led researchers at the University of Arkansas to evaluate thalidomide's clinical efficacy in patients with multiple myeloma (MM). A pilot study was initiated, and one of five patients treated, achieved near complete remission (19). The subsequent phase II clinical trial, in patients with relapsing or refractory disease confirmed a partial response rate of 25% (20). Multiple studies have since confirmed single agent response rates between 24% and 36% in relapsing/refractory patients and 34–36% in previously untreated patients with MM (21,22).

MECHANISM OF ACTION

The mechanism of action of thalidomide is not clearly understood; however, it is thought to act both directly on myeloma cells and indirectly on the bone marrow microenvironment (23). In preclinical models, granulation tissue from animals treated with thalidomide has demonstrated decreased microvascular density suggesting that the drug has potent antiangiogenic properties, perhaps related to inhibition of bFGF and VEGF (24,25).

In vitro, thalidomide also enhances degradation of TNF-α mRNA, and may bind to and potentiate the effect of α1-acid glycoproteins, which have intrinsic anti-TNF activity (26). Inhibition of TNF-α decreases secretion of IL-6, a potent promoter of myeloma cell proliferation, and also decreases expression of IL-8 in endothelial cells, an important regulator of angiogenesis (27–29). Thalidomide may further act by decreasing NF-κB DNA binding activity through suppression of IκB activity and inhibition of cyclooxygenase 1 and 2 (28,30).

Other potential mechanisms of antitumor activity include, induction of G1 growth arrest and activation of caspase 8, stimulation of cytotoxic T cells, thereby inducing IL-2 and IFN-γ, and modulation of cell adhesion molecules (31–34). The degree to which thalidomide's antiangiogenic properties contribute to its anti-myeloma effects is unclear and it is likely that these and many other mechanisms of action play a substantial role in the drug's activity.

TOXICITY

Thalidomide is teratogenic and, therefore, contraindicated in pregnant women (35). All patients treated in the United States must be registered on the System for Thalidomide Education and Prescribing Safety (STEPS) program before thalidomide can be prescribed and dispensed (36). Women of childbearing potential (premenopausal and <2 years postmenopausal) must take a pregnancy test, use two effective forms of birth control, and have repeated pregnancy tests every four weeks for the duration of treatment with thalidomide (36). Men receiving thalidomide must either abstain from sex or use a latex condom (36). Since sedation is a frequent side effect, thalidomide is taken at bedtime (20,37–39). Constipation, can often be avoided with hydration, stool softeners, and laxatives, and dry skin and pruritus can be managed with the use of nonalcohol based lubricants. However, the development of an erythematous macular skin rash requires cessation of thalidomide until resolution (20,37–39). Rarely, cases of Stevens-Johnson syndrome have been reported in patients treated with thalidomide and concurrent dexamethasone, and are a contraindication to further therapy with thalidomide (38). While thromboembolic events are uncommon with single agent thalidomide, the incidence is 17–25% in patients treated with the combination of thalidomide and dexamethasone (TD), or with steroid-anthracycline combinations (39–41). Although most investigators agree that some form of therapeutic anticoagulation is appropriate for all patients receiving thalidomide in high-risk combinations, controversy still exists regarding the ideal agent for prevention of thrombosis. Aspirin has lowered the incidence of thrombotic events in some studies (usually with lower dose or less frequent dexamethasone), while others have advocated use of warfarin or low molecular weight heparin (39,41,42). Sensorimotor peripheral neuropathy, most commonly of the hands and feet, is seen in up to 75% of patients, particularly after prolonged exposure to thalidomide (43). Less commonly, peripheral edema, tremors, bradycardia, hypothyroidism, and rarely neutropenia and hepatic enzyme elevation have been observed (20,37–39,42).

CLINICAL TRIALS

Single Agent Thalidomide

The University of Arkansas first reported thalidomide's activity in MM in 1998 (19). Since then, numerous studies have confirmed its activity in both the relapsed and previously untreated setting (20,22,37–39). In asymptomatic patients at risk for early disease progression, clinical trials have demonstrated overall response rates of 34–36% in patients treated with daily doses of 200–800 mg (22,38,39). While thalidomide monotherapy may produce responses in asymptomatic patients, its impact on prolonging time to disease progression (TTP) and later drug resistance when thalidomide-based combination therapy is indicated for control of symptomatic disease, remains unknown. In addition, the development of neuropathy in asymptomatic patients treated with thalidomide may limit its use, as well as that of other potentially neuropathic drugs, when symptomatic disease develops. Thus, until benefits for patients with asymptomatic disease are clearly demonstrated, the use of thalidomide in these patients is considered investigational and should be performed only in conjunction with a clinical trial.

Thalidomide Combinations

In previously untreated patients with symptomatic myeloma, combination therapy with thalidomide–dexamethasone (TD) was initially evaluated in two phase II single institution clinical trials conducted at the Mayo Clinic and the University of Texas M.D. Anderson Cancer Center (39,44). Partial response rates of 64% and 72% were observed, with a complete response rate of 16% noted in one of the trials (39,44). These results were confirmed in a phase III trial of 207 patients, comparing TD with dexamethasone (D) alone (RR 63% vs. 41%, $p=0.0017$), suggesting superiority for TD (42). The ability to harvest stem cells was excellent in both arms of the study (>90% of patients in either arm). Data regarding survival in patients either proceeding to, or not receiving consolidative myeloablative therapy with stem cell support has not been reported (42). Similar results were seen in a placebo-controlled, double-blind trial of 470 patients randomized to receive either TD or placebo-D (overall response TD 59% vs. D 42%, $p < 0.01$) (45). An improvement in progression-free survival (PFS) was seen with TD (not reached) compared with dexamethasone-placebo (8.1 months, $p < 0.01$) and the trial was stopped early and unblinded. Subsequently, TD was approved in the United States for first line therapy in patients with myeloma (45).

Although the benefit of TD in terms of response and progression-free survival appears clear compared with D, until recently TD had not been compared with vincristine-doxorubicin-dexamethasone (VAD). A recent randomized trial compared induction TD with VAD and subsequent myeloablative therapy with autologous stem cell transplant (AuSCT), in previously untreated patients with myeloma (46). Prior to AuSCT, 34.7% of patients treated with TD achieved a very good partial response (VGPR) compared with 12.6% of patients treated with VAD. However, by 6 months post-AuSCT this difference in VGPR was no longer evident (44.4% of TD patients vs. 41.7% of VAD patients, p. 87). Peripheral neuropathy developed in 17.4% of patients treated with TD and 12.9% of patients treated with VAD ($p=0.42$). The incidence of thromboembolic events was higher in patients treated with TD (22.8%) than in patients treated with VAD (7.5%) ($p=0.004$); however, it is unclear if prophylactic anticoagulation was used (46).

Thalidomide (50 mg daily increasing as tolerated to a maximum of 400 mg × 1 dose) has also been combined with pegylated liposomal doxorubicin (40 mg × 1 dose) (47), vincristine (2 mg IV × 1 dose), and dexamethasone (40 mg daily × 4 days) resulting in overall response rates of 87%

for 53 previously untreated patients, 36% of whom achieved complete response (47). At 50 months of follow-up, the median overall survival had not been reached. The most common grade 3–4 adverse events seen were thromboembolic events (25%), peripheral neuropathy (22%), and neutropenia (14%) (47).

A similar study of 39 previously untreated patients who received vincristine 2 mg, pegylated liposomal doxorubicin 40 mg/m^2 on day 1, dexamethasone on days 1–4 and 15–18, and concurrent thalidomide (200 mg continuously once daily for 28 days) confirmed high response rates with this combination (48). Seventy-four percent of patients responded and 10% achieved CR; response was rapid with 80% of patients responding by 2 months. In patients for whom stem cell transplant was planned, there was no difficulty collecting an adequate number of stem cells. Grade 3–4 toxicities included neutropenic infection, constipation, deep venous thrombosis, neutropenia, and thrombocytopenia. Peripheral neuropathy developed in 46% of patients and 10% developed palmar-plantar erythrodysesthesia (48).

Preliminary results of an ongoing phase II trial combining standard VAD plus thalidomide (200 mg) for 4 cycles every 28 days in treatment-naïve MM patients has shown similarly promising results, with 3 complete remissions and 7 partial remissions in the initial 11 patients (49). Fatigue was the most common side effect, and thrombosis was noted in 12% of patients. Adequate stem cells were harvested in all patients eligible for transplant (49).

In an effort to develop effective therapies for patients not eligible for autologous stem cell transplant, investigators have looked at combining thalidomide (100 mg daily) with melphalan-prednisone (MPT) (11,50). In a study of 49 previously untreated patients with symptomatic myeloma who received 6 courses of MPT, 55% of patients achieved a partial response (PR) and 18% achieved a complete response (CR) resulting in a median event-free survival (EFS) of 30 months (50). Major toxicities included peripheral neuropathy (39%), constipation (33%), infections (29%), and deep venous thrombosis (20%). When compared with melphalan-prednisone (MP) given to patients between the age of 65 and 85, MPT showed an improved response (76% vs. 47%) and 2-year, event-free survival (54% vs. 27%, $p = <0.001$) (11). Longer follow-up is necessary to assess the impact of adding thalidomide to MP on overall survival (OS).

Based on the promising results of the MPT regimen reported by Palumbo et al., Facon reported results of a subsequent study (IFM 99-06) that compared MP (12 courses at 6 weeks intervals), MPT (maximum tolerated dose up to 400 mg/day) and melphalan 100 mg/m^2 (MEL 100), with autologous stem cell support (AuSCT) in patients aged 65–75 years (11,12,50). In those receiving MEL 100, patients received induction therapy with VAD $\times$ 2 followed by cyclophosphamide 3 g/m^2 for stem cell mobilization, then proceeded to intensive therapy with MEL 100 and AuSCT $\times$ 2.

Progression free survival and OS were significantly prolonged in patients treated with MPT (29.5 mos, and not reached at 56 mos, respectively) compared with MP (17.2 mos, and 30.3 mos, respectively) and MEL 100 (19.0 mos, and 38.6 mos, respectively) (PFS, HR=2.4, $p<0.0001$; OS, HR= 1.9, $p = 0.0008$) (12). No significant difference in PFS or OS was noted between the MP and MEL 100 arms. Although this trial demonstrated superiority of MPT compared with either MP or MEL 100 in patients >65 years, the question of equivalence of the less intense MEL 100 tandem AuSCT compared with the standard melphalan 200 mg/m^2 tandem AuSCT (MEL 200) is of some concern. Although there has been no prospective randomized trial comparing MPT with MEL 200, preliminary results of a trial comparing MEL 100 versus MEL 200 demonstrated no difference in PFS (51%, 33%, respectively, $p=0.31$) or OS (86%, 71%, respectively, $p=0.51$) at 3 years (51). These early results suggest that MEL 100 may be equivalent to MEL 200 and may infer superiority of MPT in patients >65 years; however, with a median follow-up of only 26.5 months, it may be too premature to detect significant differences in the tandem regimens. Nevertheless, the results of these trials are promising and suggest that further well-designed direct comparisons of novel agent combinations and myelo-intense regimens are warranted to determine the role of both approaches, in not only elderly nontransplant candidates, but younger patients as well.

Other studies have attempted to improve on these response rates by combining thalidomide with various chemotherapeutic drugs including cyclophosphamide and bortezomib. In untreated patients, response rates for these varying combination therapies range from 50% to 90% with complete response rates remaining low in the range from 10% to 26% (Table 1) (11,12,39,42,44,45–50,52–55).

LENALIDOMIDE

Mechanism of Action

Lenalidomide is a structural analogue of thalidomide created by adding an amino group to the fourth carbon of the phthaloyl ring of thalidomide (54). Although the mechanism of action of lenalidomide is not fully understood, in vitro it is up to 50,000 times more potent in inhibiting tumor necrosis factor alpha than its parent molecule. Like thalidomide, it down regulates interleukin-6 and NFκB, activates caspase 8, may promote natural killer cell-mediated myeloma cell death and directly induces apoptosis of myeloma cells (33,55–59). Such in vitro activity was confirmed clinically by the 20–25% PR rate seen in 2 phase I trials among patients with relapsing or refractory myeloma and a follow-up phase II trial which identified that a daily dose of 30 mg was well tolerated (58,60,61). An additional 29% of

(Text continues on page 150)

Table 1 Selected Thalidomide-Based Combination Therapy for Previously Untreated MM

Study (Study acronym)	Regimen	No. of pts.	PR (%)	CR (%)	EFS/PFS/TTP (med. mos)	OS (med. mos)
Weber (39) (Thal-dex)	T: 100–600 mg daily po D: 20 mg/m²/day × 4 day po (days 1–4, 9–12, 17–20)	40	56	16	NA	NA
Rajkumar (44) (Thal-dex)	T: 200 mg daily po D: 40 mg/day × 4d po (days 1–4, 9–12, 17–20, odd cycles, days 1–4, even cycles)	50	64		NA	NA
Rajkumar (45) (Thal-dex vs. Dex)	T: 200 mg daily po D: 40 mg/day × 4 days po (days 1–4, 9–12, 17–20, odd cycles, days 1–4, even cycles)	235	59	0	NR	NA
	D: 40 mg/day × 4d po (days 1–4, 9–12, 17–20, odd cycles, d1–4, even cycles)	235	42	0	TTP 8.1	NA
Rajkumar (42) (Thal-dex vs. Dex)	T: 200 mg daily po D: 40 mg/day × 4days po (days 1–4, 9–12, 17–20, odd cycles, days 1–4, even cycles)	99	68	4	NA	NA
	D: 40 mg/day × 4days po (days 1–4, 9–12, 17–20, odd cycles, days 1–4, even cycles)	100	50	0	NA	NA
Macro (46) (TD vs. VAD)	T: 200 mg daily po D: 40 mg/day × 4days po q 2 wks 2 mos then q mo	100	35	0	NA	NA
	V: 0.4 mg/day × 4 days by CI (max 2 mg) A: 9 mg/m²/day × 4days by CI D: 40 mg/day × 4 days po q2 wk for 2 mos then q mo	104	13	0	NA	NA

(Continued)

Table 1 Selected Thalidomide-Based Combination Therapy for Previously Untreated MM (*Continued*)

Study (Study acronym)	Regimen	No. of pts.	PR (%)	CR (%)	EFS/PFS/TTP (med. mos)	OS (med. mos)
Palumbo (50) (MPT)	M: 4 mg/m² /day po × 7d/mo P: 40 mg/m² /day po × 7d/mo T: 100 mg /day daily po	41	55	18	EFS 30	NR
Facon (12) (MP-THAL vs. MP vs. MEL 100)	M: 4 mg/m² /day po × 7 days/mo P: 40 mg/m² /day po × 7 days/mo M: 4 mg/m² /day po × 7 days/mo P: 40 mg/m² /day po × 7 days/mo T: 100–400 mg daily po M: 100 (VAD × 2, Cy 3g/m² iv) M: 100 mg/m² iv × 2 courses				PFS 17.2 PFS 29.5 PFS 19	30.3 NR 38.6
Chanan-Khan (49) (VAD-T)	V: doses not specified A: D: T:	11	63	27	NA	NA
Hussein (47) (DVd-T)	T: 50–400 mg /day po Do: 40 mg/m² IV, day 1 V: 2 mg IV, day 1 D: 40 mg /day po × 4 day	53	47	36	PFS 28.2	NR
Zervas (48) (T-VAD doxil)	T: 200 mg /day po V: 2 mg IV, day 1 Do: 40 mg/m² IV, day 1 D: 40 mg /day po × days 1–4 (and days 15–18 on cycle 1)	39	64	10	PFS 55% at 22 m	74% at 22 mos

					Projected PFS at 3 yrs, 57%	Projected at 3 yrs, 74%
Offidani (52) (ThaDD)	T: 100 mg daily po Do: 40 mg/m² IV, day 1 D: 40 mg/day, days 1–4, 9–12	50	54	34	NA	NA
Hassoun (53) (AD-TD)	A: 9 mg/m²/day × 4 days IV bolus D: 40 mg/day × 4 day po days 1–4, 9–12, 17–20 pts with ≥ SD received 3 cycles then received 2 cycles TD as below T: 100 increased to 200 mg daily po D: 40 mg/day × 4 day po days 1–4, 9–12, 17–20	42	69	16		

Abbreviations: Drugs: A, doxorubicin; D, dexamethasone; Do, pegylated liposomal doxorubicin; M, melphalan; P, prednisone; T, thalidomide; V, vincristine. Route of administration: CI, continuous infusion; IV, intravenous; po, oral.

patients in the phase II trial that had not responded to lenalidomide as a single agent, achieved partial remission with the addition of intermittent pulses of dexamethasone (61). These observations provided the rationale for the use of lenalidomide-dexamethasone and other combinations in previously untreated patients with multiple myeloma.

TOXICITY

The side effect profile of lenalidomide appears to differ somewhat from thalidomide; however, since the teratogenic effects in humans are unknown, precautions must be taken to avoid pregnancy in patients and their sexual partners. Neuropathy appears to be much less frequent than with thalidomide (grade 3–4, <10% of patients), and although grade 3–4 myelosuppression is seen more frequently in 38–69% (61–63) of patients with refractory or relapsing myeloma, the incidence in previously untreated patients appears to be less frequent 12–21% (2,64). An Eastern Cooperative Oncology Group (ECOG) trial of lenalidomide-dexamethasone in previously untreated patients revealed an 18% frequency of thrombotic events (66,67). A subsequent phase II trial demonstrated the somewhat surprising efficacy of aspirin prophylaxis for prevention of thrombotic events, despite their venous origin (2). Others, however, have reported less successful results with aspirin (3,4,66). Additionally in two phase III trials for refractory or relapsing myeloma, a higher incidence of thromboembolic events occurred in patients taking concomitant erythropoietin or darbepoietin (63,68). If this association is confirmed in future trials, additional studies seem warranted to determine whether concomitant erythropoietic agents should be avoided, or a hemoglobin threshold should be determined for their use. Studies are also needed to determine which and which antithrombotic/ anticoagulant and dose should be recommended for patients receiving the combination of lenalidomide and dexamethasone. Other side effects of lenolidomide include fatigue, constipation, and less frequently, anxiety, pneumonitis, muscle weakness, rash, diarrhea, occasional elevation of liver enzymes, and infections (2,56,60–62).

Lenolidomide Combinations

In a phase 2 trial, 34 patients received lenalidomide 25 mg/day × 21 days with dexamethasone 40 mg/day on days 1–4, 9–12, and 17–20 of each 28 day cycle for 4 cycles. All patients received low-dose aspirin once daily for thromboembolic prophylaxis (2). In a recent update of this data (64), the overall response rate was 91% and complete remission was documented in 18% of patients. Among those patients who did not receive stem cell transplant, the CR/VGPR rate was 67%. The median TTP, PFS, and OS had not been reached at the time of publication, but adequate stem cells were harvested from all 13 patients proceeding to high dose chemotherapy supported by autologous stem cell infusion (64). Most hematologic toxicities were grade 1–2 and only 3% of patients who received aspirin prophylaxis developed deep venous thrombosis (2,64).

The ECOG has initiated a randomized phase III trial of lenalidomide with either concomitant "high-dose" dexamethasone (40 mg on days 1–4, 9–12, 17–20) or "low-dose" dexamethasone (40 mg on days 1, 8, 15, 20) (67). Available results indicate a higher rate of grade 3–4 toxicities in the "high-dose" dexamethasone arm compared with the "low-dose" dexamethasone arm, including infections/pneumonitis (15.7% vs. 7.5%, respectively), thromboembolism (22.1% vs. 6.1%, respectively), and hyperglycemia (9.7% vs. 6.6%, respectively), but the incidence of ≥ grade 3 neuropathy was similar with both regimens (< 1%). While data regarding response and PFS of this trial have not yet been reported, survival at one year was significantly higher for the "low-dose" dexamethasone group (96.5%) than the "high-dose" dexamethasone group (86%) (p < 0.001). This prolongation of survival in the face of decreased toxicity, if confirmed, represents a major improvement in induction therapy for myeloma (67).

Based on the success of MPT, recent studies have explored the combination of lenalidomide with MP (R-MP). Palumbo et al. (4) evaluated the efficacy of MPR in a dose escalation study of 54 patients. The maximum tolerated dose (MTD) was reached with melphalan 0.18 mg/kg/day × 4 days, lenalidomide 10 mg/day × 21 days, and prednisone 2 mg/kg/day × 4 days. Cycles were repeated every 4–6 weeks and all patients received ciprofloxacin and aspirin prophylaxis. After treatment with a median of seven cycles at the MTD, 85.6% of patients achieved at least PR, 52.3% achieved at least VGPR, and 23% achieved CR. With a median 9.6 months of follow-up, the 16-month PFS was 87%. No difference in response rate or PFS was noted in 42 patients with deletion of chromosome 13q by FISH; however karyotypic analysis, which generally has more prognostic significance, was not available (4). Major grade 3–4 toxicities observed in this study, included neutropenia (66%), thrombocytopenia (34%), anemia (17%), and skin eruption (10%). Three patients had thromboembolic events, however, two of these occurred after discontinuation of aspirin (4). Roy et al. (5) conducted a similar study of MPR in patients ineligible for stem cell transplant. At the MTD (melphalan at 5 mg/ m^2/day × 4 days, prednisone 60 mg/m^2/day × 4 days, lenalidomide 10 mg/ day × 21 days), 82% patients achieved at least PR. Major toxicities observed were similar to those previously described by Palumbo et al. (4,5).

In an attempt to decrease the frequency of dexamethasone dosing, while increasing its bioavailability, the use of concurrent clarithromycin has been investigated. Niesvizky et al. (3) recently reported results of the BiRD regimen (clarithromycin 500 mg b.i.d., lenalidomide 25 mg/day × 21 days, dexamethasone 40 mg weekly) in previously untreated patients. Within 3–4 months, 95% of 40 evaluable patients achieved at least a PR, 43% achieved a VGPR, 5% a near CR, and 25% a CR. Thromboembolism was noted in 15% (7 patients) of these patients who received aspirin prophylaxis (81 mg/day), although 4 events occurred while patients were off aspirin, illustrating, once again, the need for further study of the best prophylactic management of thromboembolism for patients receiving combination therapy with lenalidomide and steroids (3).

Based on these results, the role of lenalidomide for treatment of previously untreated patients with myeloma is promising, particularly when the potential for minimizing or delaying neuropathy is considered. Thus many studies of lenalidomide in combination with the aforementioned drugs, and other agents, such as melphalan, liposomal doxorubicin and bortezomib are currently underway (Table 2).

BORTEZOMIB

Bortezomib is a dipeptide boronic acid analog that inhibits the function of the 26S proteasome complex (69,70). Each human cell contains approximately 30,000 proteasome complexes which are responsible for protein degradation, and subsequent regulation of cellular functions such as transcription, cell cycle progression, DNA repair, growth arrest, and apoptosis (69,70).

MECHANISM OF ACTION

Bortezomib, a proteasome inhibitor, is part of a class of drugs that block protein degradation, leading to accumulation of misfolded/damaged proteins which, in turn, may trigger a heat shock response within the cell resulting in apoptosis (69–72). In vitro, malignant cells are more sensitive to proteasome inhibition than normal cells, perhaps because of an increased number of altered or defective cell cycle proteins and subsequent dependence on the proteasome for elimination of these accumulated products (69,70,72–74).

Bortezomib is thought to produce many of its effects by inhibiting NFκB signaling. In multiple myeloma cells, NFκB is thought to mediate many functions, such as immune response, growth, and survival (60,75), and inhibition of NF-κB by bortezomib results in subsequent apoptosis (76,77). Preclinical studies of bortezomib demonstrate decreases in cytokines (IL-6), angiogenesis factors (VEGF), and growth factors (IGF-1) which also inhibit adhesion of myeloma cells to bone marrow stromal cells (70,77–80). These in vitro effects were successfully translated clinically when a phase I and subsequent phase II (SUMMIT) and III (APEX) trials in patients with refractory or relapsing myeloma revealed an overall single agent response rate of 25–30% (81–83). Furthermore, additive, and possibly synergistic, effects with dexamethasone had been noted in preclinical investigations, and in patients not responsive to bortezomib alone, providing the framework for investigation of this combination for induction therapy of myeloma (78,84).

Table 2 Lenalidomide-Based Combination Therapy for Previously Untreated MM

Study (Study acronym)	Regimen	No. of pts.	PR (%)	CR (%)	EFS/PFS/TTP (med. mos)	OS (med. mos)
Palumbo (4) (RMP)	L: 5–10 mg/day × 21 day po M: 0.18–0.25 mg/kg/day po × 4day P: 2 mg/kg/day po × 4days Cycles repeated q 4–6 wks	54	52	23	87% at 16 mos	NA
Rajkumar (2) Lacy (64) (Len-dex)	L: 25 mg/day × 21 day po D: 40 mg/day × 4 day po days1–4, 9–12, 17–20	34	79 73	6 18	Projected 2 yr 74%	Projected 2 yr 91%
Roy (5) (MPR)	L: 10 mg/day × 21 day po M: 5–8 mg/m²/day × 4day po P: 60 mg/m²/day × 4day po	7	57	14	NA	NA
Niesvizky (3) (BiRD)	Bi: 500 mg/day b.i.d. po L: 25 mg/day × 21 day po D: 40 mg × 1 day q wk po	40	70	25	NA	NA

Abbreviations: Drugs: Bi, clarithromycin; D, dexamethasone; L, lenalidomide; M, melphalan; P, prednisone. Route of dmin;stration: po, oral.

TOXICITY

Approximately one-third of patients treated with bortezomib will develop constipation, diarrhea, nausea, vomiting, and/or transient cytopenias (1,85). Thrombocytopenia secondary to bortezomib is somewhat unique among chemotherapeutic agents since it does not appear to result from decreased megakaryocytes or from peripheral destruction, but instead appears to be secondary to a transient, reversible impairment of megakaryocyte function and subsequent decrease in platelet budding, making reductions in platelets self-limited and short-lived (86). Other side effects may include fatigue, myalgias and transient hypotension, usually seen shortly after infusion of bortezomib (81–83). An increased incidence of varicella zoster has also been noted, thus antiviral prophylaxis may be warranted, although its efficacy in this regard with bortezomib remains unproven (6,87).

Perhaps the most troublesome side effect of bortezomib is peripheral neuropathy which affects up to 30–50% of patients receiving the drug (7,81,82,88). Improvement in neuropathic symptoms is often seen with prompt dose reduction or temporary cessation of bortezomib followed by dose reduction (82,89). The mechanism of neuropathy remains unclear. However, correlative studies conducted in conjunction with a trial of bortezomib in previously untreated patients with myeloma demonstrated that 52% of patients had subclinical small fiber neuropathy and 9% had large fiber neuropathy prior to the initiation of any chemotherapy (85). This may explain why myeloma patients are particularly susceptible to neurotoxicity, not only with bortezomib, but with other agents as well.

CLINICAL TRIALS

Single Agent Bortezomib +/– Dexamethasone

The use of single agent bortezomib ($1.3\,mg/m^2$ on days 1, 4, 8, 11 repeated on day 21 for a maximum of 6 cycles) for induction therapy of myeloma was originally reported by Jagannath et al. (1). In this phase II study, oral dexamethasone 40 mg (days 1, 2, 4, 5, 8, 9, 11, 12) was added if patients had not achieved at least a PR after two cycles or CR after four cycles of therapy. The long-term follow-up data of 48 evaluable patients was recently updated and demonstrated an overall response rate ($\geq$ PR) of 90%, CR/nCR of 19%, with an additional 8% of patients achieving a minor response (MR) (88). After cycle 2 (bortezomib alone), ORR was 50% and CR was 10%. Dexamethasone was added in 75% of patients and improved the best response in 64% of those treated with the bortezomib-dexamethasone combination. With a median follow-up of 24 months, the 1-year survival (1 year OS) for all patients was 90%, median overall survival had not been reached, and the median time to an alternate treatment was seven months. In patients who did not proceed onto stem cell transplant, the 1-year survival rate was 80%, median overall survival had not been reached, and the median time to alternate therapy was 22 months. In contrast, patients who received myeloablative therapy with stem cell support had 1-yr OS of 90% and median time to alternative therapy and overall survival had not been reached. Although this trial was not designed with the power to detect differences in patients treated with novel agents without AuSCT compared with those who received autologous transplant, with time, if large differences in PFS and OS become apparent, a randomized trial seems justified. The most common > grade 2 toxicities were, as expected, neuropathic pain (37%), fatigue (20%), constipation (16%), nausea (12%), and neutropenia (12%) (88) (Table 3).

Anderson et al. (85) have also reported results of a phase II trial of single agent standard dose bortezomib given for eight cycles as induction therapy for previously untreated myeloma. Among 60 evaluable patients the overall response was 38% and CR was 10% (85); these results appear consistent with those of Jagannath et al. where the addition of dexamethasone in 64% of patients increased the best response resulting in an overall response rate of 90% (Table 3) (88).

Combination Therapy Including Steroids

Preclinical studies of bortezomib not only indicated additive or synergistic activity with dexamethasone, but also suggested potential for numerous agents including doxorubicin, melphalan, thalidomide, and lenalidomide (78,90). Subsequent clinical trials of bortezomib in combination with other novel drugs and/or conventional chemotherapeutic agents have confirmed excellent activity, producing response rates of 55–95% in refractory/relapsing patients with myeloma, giving promise for these same regimens in previously untreated patients (1,6–10,91–99).

Considering the success of thalidomide-dexamethasone for front-line therapy of myeloma, and in vitro data suggesting synergy of this combination with bortezomib, it is not surprising that the combination of bortezomib-thalidomide-dexamethasone produced responses in over 50% of patients with resistant myeloma (96). On the basis of these results, investigators at the M.D. Anderson Cancer Center reported a retrospective review of this regimen which induced an ORR of 92% (CR 19%) in previously untreated, symptomatic patients with myeloma (100,101). The median time to remission was rapid (0.6 months) and in 21 patients who underwent AuSCT, adequate collection proceeded without difficulty. Grade 3–4 nonhematologic toxicities of neuropathy, infections, and venous thromboembolism all occurred in < 10% of patients (100,101).

The combination of bortezomib and doxorubicin was also ideal for clinical investigation based not only on preclinical synergy, but also on the in vitro restoration of doxorubicin sensitivity in previously doxorubicin

Table 3 Bortezomib-Based Combination Therapy for Previously Untreated MM

Study (Study acronym)	Regimen	No. of pts.	PR (%)	CR (%)	EFS/PFS/TTP (med. mos)	OS (med. mos)
Jagannath (1,88)	B: 1.3 mg/m²/day IV, days 1, 4, 8, 11 D: 40 mg/day po days 1, 2, 4, 5, 8, 9, 11, 12	48	71	19 CR/nCR	NR	NR
Anderson (85)	B: 1.3 mg/m²/day IV, days 1, 4, 8, 11	60	28	10	NA	NA
Wang (100,101) (VTD)	B: 1.3 mg/m²/day IV, days 1, 4, 8, 11 T: 100–200 mg/day po D: 40 mg/day × 4day po, days 1–4, 9–12, 17–20 × 2 then days 1–4 only	38	73	18	NA	NA
Oakervee (7) (PAD)	B: 1.3 mg/m²/day IV, days 1, 4, 8, 11 A: 4.5–9 mg/m²/day × 4day CI D: 40 mg/day × 4day po, days 1–4, 8–11, 15–18 × 1 then days 1–4 only	21	71	24	NA	NA
Popat (8) (reduced-dose PAD)	B: 1.0 mg/m²/day IV, days 1, 4, 8, 11 A: 9 mg/m²/day × 4day CI D: 40 mg/day × 4day po, days 1–4, 8–11, 15–18 × 1 then days 1–4 only	18	78	11	NA	NA

Study	Regimen				EFS	Projected 2 yr
Mateos (6) (VMP)	B: 1.0–1.3 mg/m²/day IV, days 1, 4, 8, 11, 22, 25, 29, 32 M: 9 mg/m²/day × 4 day po P: 60 mg/m²/day × 4 day po	60	56	32	EFS 83% 16 mo PFS 91%	86%
Jakubowiak (102) (VDD)	B: 1.3 mg/m²/day IV, days 1, 4, 8, 11 Do: 30 mg/m² IV, day 4 D: 40 mg/day × 4 day po, days 1–4 20 mg/day po, days 1, 2, 4, 5, 8, 9, 11, 12	10 18	57	32 CR/nCR	NA	NA
Borrello (9) (VT)	B: 1.3 mg/m²/day IV, days 1, 4, 8, 11 T: 50 mg increased to 150 mg/day po	27	51	31	NA	NA
Orlowski (10)	B: 1.3 mg/m²/day IV, days 1, 4, 8, 11 Do: 30 mg/m² IV, day 4	57	58	16 CR/nCR	NA	NA

Abbreviations: Drugs: A, doxorubicin; D, dexamethasone; Do, pegylated liposomal doxorubicin; P, prednisone; T, thalidomide; V, vincristine. Route of administration: CI, continuous infusion; IV, intravenous; po, oral.

resistant cell lines (78,84). Oakervee et al. (7) subsequently reported results of a phase I/II study of bortezomib-doxorubicin-dexamethasone (PAD) (Bortezomib 1.3 mg/m^2 day 1, 4, 8, 11, doxorubicin as continuous infusion for 4 days at 4.5 or 9 mg/m^2/day, dexamethasone days 1–4, 8–11, 15–18 on cycle 1 and days 1–4 on cycles 2–4 repeated every 21 days) for induction therapy of myeloma. Time to remission was rapid, and after 1 cycle 71% of patients achieved at least PR. After 2 cycles nearly all patients were in remission (ORR, 95%, 71% PR, 24% CR) (7). Stem cells were successfully collected in all but one patient, who had previously received radiation therapy to the spine. Toxicities were, as expected, similar to those previously reported for these agents with mild neuropathy, usually grade I, noted in 48% (Gr 3, 1 pt) of patients; only 1 cardiac was event reported (atrial fibrillation) (7). A subsequent trial of reduced intensity PAD (bortezomib 1 mg/m^2/day) decreased the incidence of peripheral neuropathy to 16%; however, response was also mildly diminished at 89% (8).

Given the previous success of novel agents combined with melphalan-prednisone, and preclinical data to support the combination of bortezomib and MP (BMP), clinical evaluation of this combination was certainly worthy of study in symptomatic, newly diagnosed elderly patients who were not considered candidates for stem cell supported therapy. In a Phase I-II study, patients received 1 or 1.3 mg/m^2 of bortezomib on days 1, 4, 8, 11, 22, 25, 29, 32 and melphalan 9 mg/m^2/day with prednisone 60 mg/m^2/day, both on days 1–4 (cycles repeated q6 weeks × 4) (6). Patients then received less intense maintenance with BMP. Eighty-nine percent of patients responded (>PR), and 32% achieved CR, but the median time to response of 2.7 months was somewhat slower than noted previously with more intensive dexamethasone-based regimens (6,100,101). Event-free survival was 83% and 16 month PFS was 91%. Grade 3 and 4 toxicities included thrombocytopenia (51%), neutropenia (43%), peripheral neuropathy (17%), and diarrhea (16%). Herpes zoster was observed in 13% of the first 38 patients, prompting subsequent patients to be placed on prophylactic antiviral therapy with acyclovir (Table 3) (6).

Combination Therapy Without Steroids

Among the most exciting new combinations for induction therapy are recent combinations that produce response in more than 75% of patients in the absence of steroids and myeloablative doses of therapy. The combination of thalidomide and bortezomib reported by Borrello et al. (9) produced a response in 82% of patients and CR in 31% of previously untreated patients. The median time to response was slower than usually noted with steroid based combinations and occurred at 5 cycles (100,101). Peripheral neuropathy was observed in all patients by the fifth cycle of therapy; however, only 19% developed grade 3 or higher neuropathy. Additional toxicities included fatigue (57%), constipation (52%), generalized pain (44%), and leg cramps (23%) (9).

The preliminary results of a CALGB study of bortezomib and pegylated liposomal doxorubicin (PLD) were also recently reported and appear promising (10). Patients received standard 21 day cycles of bortezomib with PLD 30 mg/m^2 on day 4, for a maximum of 8 cycles. Preliminary response data was available for 57 patients, 58% of whom achieved at least PR (CR/ nCR, 16%) and final response data was available for 29 patients, 79% of whom achieved ≥ PR (CR/nCR, 28%). The most frequent grade 3–4 hematologic toxicities included neutropenia (18%), thrombocytopenia (14%), and lymphopenia (13%) and the most common grade 3–4 non-hematologic toxicities included fatigue (16%), sensory neuropathy (13%), hand-foot syndrome (9%), syncope (9%), motor neuropathy (7%), and dehydration (7%). Stem cell collection was possible for 6 patients in which it was attempted (10).

Based on a striking response rate of 59% in a phase I trial of borte-zomib-lenalidomide in patients with refractory/relapsing myeloma, trials of this promising combination are currently underway in patients with previously untreated myeloma (103).

If response rates are consistent, and benefits in PFS and overall survival demonstrated, these novel, steroid-free regimens hold much promise for improved quality of life for patients with the potential for minimizing or eliminating complications of steroids such as weight gain, hypertension, ulcer disease and diabetes (Table 3).

SUMMARY

Although myeloma remains an incurable disease, the discovery of new agents with novel mechanisms of action, has provided many new options for treatment, not only for patients with resistant disease, but also for those with newly diagnosed symptomatic disease. Additionally, in vitro studies with thalidomide, lenalidomide, and bortezomib have led to a better understanding of the molecular biology of malignant plasma cells, unmasked potential targets for rational combinations of conventional and novel agents, and fostered discovery of both second generation drugs and new potential targets for thoughtful drug development.

Until the late 1990s, standard induction therapy for myeloma consisted of various combinations of steroids, alkylating agents, and anthra-cyclines. Although these regimens induced response in 45–65% of patients, complete remissions usually occurred in less than 15% of patients and the disease eventually relapsed in all patients. Despite many investigations of new combinations and/or schedules of these agents, none proved superior to melphalan and prednisone and the median survival of patients with myeloma remained unchanged. Subsequently, data from the IFM-90 trial of myeloablative therapy with autologous stem cell support, and the IFM-94 trial demonstrating superiority of tandem transplant compared with single autologous transplant provided the only consistent survival benefits compared with conventional chemotherapy for myeloma patients in recent years (104,105). Not all patients, however, qualify for, or benefit from, these intensive therapies and improvements in survival have remained modest.

Since the introduction of thalidomide for treatment of myeloma in the late 90's, lenalidomide, thalidomide and bortezomib have been approved by the FDA for treatment of patients with multiple myeloma in the United States. Since employing these agents with novel mechanisms of action for treatment of previously untreated patients, partial remission has become a reality for more than 90% of newly diagnosed patients with symptomatic myeloma, CR rates due to induction therapy have nearly doubled, high response rates without steroids are now achievable, and for the first time, without myeloablative therapy, a hint of an improved future has been realized with a demonstrated survival benefit in elderly patients treated with MPT compared with, not only MP, but reduced intensity AuSCT as well.

There is still much to be discovered regarding the use of this new generation of drugs in myeloma. Well designed studies to determine which combinations of novel and/or conventional agents provide the greatest gains in response, PFS, and ultimately, overall survival for all previously untreated patients are necessary. Additionally, randomized trials comparing the best combinations with, and without, myeloablative therapy followed by AuSCT are essential to clarify the best treatments, not only for elderly patients, but for all patients with multiple myeloma. With these, and appropriately designed quality of life studies, further refinements of novel induction therapy to minimize or delay side effects like neuropathy and diabetes, and maximize benefits are likely to translate into improved survival for all patients with myeloma.

REFERENCES

1. Jagannath S, Durie BG, Wolf J, et al. Bortezomib therapy alone and in combination with dexamethasone for previously untreated symptomatic multiple myeloma. Br J Haematology 2005; 129(6):776–83.
2. Rajkumar SV, Hayman SR, Lacy MQ, et al. Combination therapy with lenalidomide plus dexamethasone (Rev/Dex) for newly diagnosed myeloma. Blood 2005; 106(13):4050–3.
3. Niesvizky R, Jayabalan D, Jr,. Furst R, et al. Clarithromycin, lenalidomide and dexamethasone combination therapy as primary treatment of multiple myeloma. J Clin Oncol 2006; 24(18S).
4. Palumbo A, Falco P, Falcone A, et al. Oral Revlimid(R) Plus Melphalan and Prednisone (R-MP) for Newly Diagnosed Multiple Myeloma: Results of a Multicenter Phase I/II Study. ASH Annual Meeting Abstracts 2006; 10811:800.

5. Roy V, Leif BP, Jacob A, Philip GR. Melphalan (M), Prednisone (P) and Lenalidomide (R) Combination (MPR) for Newly Diagnosed Multiple Myeloma Patients Who Are Not Candidates for Stem Cell Transplantation. ASH Annual Meeting Abstracts 2006; 108(11):3558.

6. Mateos M-V, Hernandez J-M, Hernandez M-T, et al. Bortezomib plus melphalan and prednisone in elderly untreated patients with multiple myeloma: results of a multicenter phase 1/2 study. Blood 2006; 108(7):2165–72.

7. Oakervee HE, Popat R, Curry N, et al. PAD combination therapy (PS-341/ bortezomib, doxorubicin and dexamethasone) for previously untreated patients with multiple myeloma. Br J Haematol 2005; 129(6):755–62.

8. Popat R, Oakervee HE, Curry N, et al. Reduced Dose PAD Combination Therapy (PS-341/Bortezomib, Adriamycin and Dexamethasone) for Previously Untreated Patients with Multiple Myeloma. ASH Annual Meeting Abstracts 2005; 106(11):2554.

9. Borrello I, Ferguson A, Huff CA, et al. Bortezomib and Thalidomide Treatment of Newly Diagnosed Patients with Multiple Myeloma—Efficacy and Neurotoxicity. ASH Annual Meeting Abstracts 2006; 108(11):3528.

10. Orlowski RZ, Peterson BL, Sanford B, et al. Bortezomib and Pegylated Liposomal Doxorubicin as Induction Therapy for Adult Patients with Symptomatic Multiple Myeloma: Cancer and Leukemia Group B Study 10301. ASH Annual Meeting Abstracts 2006; 108(11):797.

11. Palumbo A, Bringhen S, Caravita T, et al. Oral melphalan and prednisone chemotherapy plus thalidomide compared with melphalan and prednisone alone in elderly patients with multiple myeloma: randomised controlled trial. Lancet 2006; 367(9513):825–31.

12. Facon T, Mary J, Harousseau J, et al. Superiority of melphalan-prednisone (MP) + thalidomide (THAL) over MP and autologous stem cell transplantation in the treatment of newly diagnosed elderly patients with multiple myeloma. J Clin Oncol 2006; 24(18S).

13. FDA. Thalidomide approved for erythema nodosum leprosum. J Am Med Assoc 1998; 280:872.

14. Hamza MH. Treatment of Behcet's disease with thalidomide. Clin Rheumatol 1986; 5:365–71.

15. Lenz W. Thalidomide and congenital abnormalities. Lancet 1962; 729(7219 (6)):45–6.

16. Pearson JM, Vedagiri M. Treatment of moderately severe erythema nodosum leprosum with thalidomide—a double-blind controlled trial. Lepr Rev 1969; 40(2):111–6.

17. Saylan T, Saltik I. Thalidomide in the treatment of Behçet's syndrome. Arch Dermatol 1982; 118:536.

18. Vogelsang GB, Farmer ER, Hess AD, et al. Thalidomide for the treatment of chronic graft-versus-host disease. N Engl J Med 1992; 326(16):1055–8.

19. Singhal S, Mehta J, Eddlemon P, et al. Marked anti-tumor effect from anti-angiogenesis therapy with thalidomide in high risk refractory multiple myeloma. Blood 1998; 92(318a).

20. Singhal S, Mehta J, Desikan R, et al. Antitumor activity of thalidomide in refractory multiple myeloma. N Engl J Med 1999; 341(21):1565–71.

21. Dimopoulos MA, Anagnostopoulos A, Weber D. Treatment of plasma cell dyscrasias with thalidomide and its derivatives. J Clin Oncol 2003; 21(23): 4444–54.

22. Glasmacher A, Hahn C, Hoffmann F, et al. A systematic review of phase-II trials of thalidomide monotherapy in patients with relapsed or refractory multiple myeloma. Br J Haematol 2006; 132(5):584–93.

23. Gupta D, Treon SP, Shima Y, et al. Adherence of multiple myeloma cells to bone marrow stromal cells upregulates vascular endothelial growth factor secretion: therapeutic applications. Leukemia 2001; 15(12):1950–61.

24. D'Amato RJ, Loughnan MS, Flynn E, Folkman J. Thalidomide is an inhibitor of angiogenesis. Proc Nat Acad Sci USA 1994; 91(9):4082–5.

25. Kenyon BM, Browne F, D'Amato RJ. Effects of thalidomide and related metabolites in a mouse corneal model of neovascularization. Exp Eye Res 1997; 64(6):971–8.

26. Moreira AL, Sampaio EP, Zmuidzinas A, Frindt P, Smith KA, Kaplan G. Thalidomide exerts its inhibitory action on tumor necrosis factor alpha by enhancing mRNA degradation. J Exp Med 1993; 177(6): 1675–80.

27. Hideshima T, Chauhan D, Podar K, Schlossman RL, Richardson P, Anderson KC. Novel therapies targeting the myeloma cell and its bone marrow microenvironment. Seminars Oncol 2001; 28(6):607–12.

28. Keifer JA, Guttridge DC, Ashburner BP, Baldwin AS, Jr. Inhibition of NF-kappa B activity by thalidomide through suppression of IkappaB kinase activity. Journal of Biol Chem 2001; 276(25):22382–7.

29. Marriott JB, Clarke IA, Dredge K, Muller G, Stirling D, Dalgleish AG. Thalidomide and its analogues have distinct and opposing effects on TNF-alpha and TNFR2 during co-stimulation of both CD4(+) and CD8(+) T cells. Clin Exp Immunol 2002; 130(1):75–84.

30. Noguchi T, Shimazawa R, Nagasawa K, Hashimoto Y. Thalidomide and its analogues as cyclooxygenase inhibitors. Bioorganic Med Chem Lett 2002; 12(7):1043–6.

31. Kumar S, Rajkumar SV. Thalidomide and lenalidomide in the treatment of multiple myeloma. Eur J Cancer 2006; 42(11):1612–22.

32. Mitsiades N, Mitsiades CS, Poulaki V, et al. Apoptotic signaling induced by immunomodulatory thalidomide analogs in human multiple myeloma cells: therapeutic implications. Blood 2002; 99(12):4525–30.

33. Davies FE, Raje N, Hideshima T, et al. Thalidomide and immunomodulatory derivatives augment natural killer cell cytotoxicity in multiple myeloma. Blood 2001; 98(1):210–6.

34. Geitz H, Handt S, Zwingenberger K. Thalidomide selectively modulates the density of cell surface molecules involved in the adhesion cascade. Immunopharmacology 1996; 31(2–3):213–21.

35. Fabro S, Smith RL, Williams RT. Toxicity and teratogenicity of optical isomers of thalidomide. Nature 1967; 215(5098):296.

36. Zeldis JB, Williams BA, Thomas SD, Elsayed ME. S.T.E.P.S.: a comprehensive program for controlling and monitoring access to thalidomide. Clin Therap 1999; 21(2):319–30.

37. Alexanian R, Weber D, Anagnostopoulos A, et al. Thalidomide with or without dexamethasone for refractory or relapsing multiple myeloma. Semin Hematol 2003; 40(4):3–7.

38. Rajkumar SV, Dispenzieri A, Fonseca, R, et al. Thalidomide for previously untreated indolent or smoldering multiple myeloma. Leukemia 2001; 15(8):1274–6.

39. Weber D, Rankin K, Gavino M, et al. Thalidomide alone or with dexamethasone for previously untreated multiple myeloma. J Clin Oncol 2003; 21:16–19.

40. Osman K, Comenzo R, Rajkumar SV. Deep venous thrombosis and thalidomide therapy for multiple myeloma. N Engl J Med 2001; 344(25):1951–2.

41. Baz R, Li L, Kottke-Marchant K, et al. The role of aspirin in the prevention of thrombotic complications of thalidomide and anthracycline-based chemotherapy for multiple myeloma. Mayo Clinic Proc 2005; 80(12):1568–74.

42. Rajkumar SV, Blood E, Vesole D, Fonseca R, Greipp PR, Eastern Cooperative Oncology G. Phase III clinical trial of thalidomide plus dexamethasone compared with dexamethasone alone in newly diagnosed multiple myeloma: a clinical trial coordinated by the Eastern Cooperative Oncology Group. J Clin Oncol 2006; 24(3):431–6.

43. Tosi P, Zamagni E, Cellini C, et al. Neurological toxicity of long-term (>1 yr) thalidomide therapy in patients with multiple myeloma. Eur J Haematol 2005; 74(3):212–6.

44. Rajkumar SV, Hayman S, Gertz MA, et al. Combination therapy with thalidomide plus dexamethasone for newly diagnosed myeloma. J Clin Oncol 2002; 20(21):4319–23.

45. Rajkumar SV, Hussein M, Catalano J, et al. A randomized, double-blind, placebo-controlled trial of thalidomide plus dexamethasone versus dexamethasone alone as primary therapy for newly diagnosed multiple myeloma. Blood 2006; 108:795.

46. Macro M, Divine M, Uzunhan Y, et al. Dexamethasone + thalidomide (dex/thal) compared to vad as a pre-transplant treatment in newly diagnosed multiple myeloma (MM): a randomized trial. Blood 2006; 108(57).

47. Hussein MA, Baz R, Srkalovic G, et al. Phase 2 study of pegylated liposomal doxorubicin, vincristine, decreased-frequency dexamethasone, and thalidomide in newly diagnosed and relapsed-refractory multiple myeloma. Mayo Clinic Proc 2006; 81(7):889–95.

48. Zervas K, Dimopoulos MA, Hatzicharissi E, et al. Primary treatment of multiple myeloma with thalidomide, vincristine, liposomal doxorubicin and dexamethasone (T-VAD doxil): a phase II multicenter study. Ann Oncol 2004; 15(1):134–8.

49. Chanan-Khan AA, Miller KC, McCarthy P, et al. VAD-t (vincristine, adriamycin, dexamethasone and low-dose thalidomide) is an effective initial therapy with high response rates for patients with treatment naïve multiple myeloma (MM). Blood 2004; 104.

50. Palumbo A, Bertola A, Musto P, et al. Oral melphalan, prednisone, and thalidomide for newly diagnosed patients with myeloma. Cancer 2005; 104: 1428–33.

51. Palumbo A, Bringhen S, Petrucci MT, et al. A Prospective, Randomized, Phase III Study of Melphalan 200 mg/m2 (MEL200) Versus Melphalan

100 mg/m2 (MEL100) in Newly Diagnosed Myeloma Patients. ASH Annual Meeting Abstracts 2006; 108(11):55.

52. Offidani M, Corvatta L, Piersantelli, M-N, et al. Thalidomide, dexamethasone, and pegylated liposomal doxorubicin (ThaDD) for patients older than 65 years with newly diagnosed multiple myeloma. Blood 2006; 108:2159–64.

53. Hassoun H, Reich L, Klimek VM, et al. Doxorubicin and dexamethasone followed by thalidomide and dexamethasone is an effective well tolerated initial therapy for multiple myeloma. Br J Haematol 2006; 132(2):155–61.

54. Muller GW, Chen R, Huang SY, et al. Amino-substituted thalidomide analogs: potent inhibitors of TNF-alpha production. Bioorganic Med Chem Lett 1999; 9(11):1625–30.

55. Knight R. IMiDs: a novel class of immunomodulators. Semin Oncol 2005; 32(4 Suppl 5):S24–30.

56. Richardson P, Schlossman R, Edie Weller E, et al. Immunomodulatory drug cc-5013 overcomes drug resistance and is well tolerated in patients with relapsed multiple myeloma. Blood 2002; 100:3063–7.

57. Hideshima T, Chauhan D, Shima Y, et al. Thalidomide and its analogs overcome drug resistance of human multiple myeloma cells to conventional therapy. Blood 2000; 96(9):2943–50.

58. Chauhan D, Uchiyama H, Akbarali Y, et al. Multiple myeloma cell adhesion-induced interleukin-6 expression in bone marrow stromal cells involves activation of NF-kappa B. Blood 1996; 87(3):1104–12.

59. Hayashi T, Hideshima T, Akiyama M, et al. Molecular mechanisms whereby immunomodulatory drugs activate natural killer cells: clinical application. Br J Haematol 2005; 128(2):192–203.

60. Zangari M Tricot G, Zeldis J, et al. Results of phase I study of CC-5013 for the treatment of multiple myeloma (MM) patients who relapse after high dose chemotherapy (HDCT). Blood 2001; 775a.

61. Richardson PG, Blood E, Mitsiades CS, et al. A randomized phase 2 study of lenalidomide therapy for patients with relapsed or relapsed and refractory multiple myeloma. Blood 2006; 108(10):3458–64.

62. Dimopoulos MA, Spencer A, Attal M, et al. Study of lenalidomide plus dexamethasone versus dexamethasone alone in relapsed or refractory multiple myloma (MM): Results of a Phases study (MM010). ASH Annual Meeting Abstracts 2005 November 16, 2005; 106(11):6.

63. Weber DM, Chen C, Niesvizky R, et al. Lenalidomide plus high-dose dexamethasone provides improved overall survival compared to high-dose dexamethasone alone for relapsed or refractory multiple myeloma (MM): results of a North American phase III study (MM-009. J Clin Oncol 2006; 24(18S).

64. Lacy M, Gertz M, Dispenzieri A, et al. Lenalidomide plus dexamethasone (Rev/Dex) in newly diagnosed myeloma: response to therapy, time to progression, and survival. Blood 2006; 108.

65. Rajkumar SV. Lenalidomide and venous thrombosis in multiple myeloma. N Engl J Med 2006; 354(19):2079.

66. Zonder JA, Barlogie B, Durie BGM, et al. Thrombotic complications in patients with newly diagnosed multiple myeloma treated with lenalidomide and dexamethasome: benefit of aspirin prophylaxis. Blood 2006; 108:403–4.

67. Rajkumar SV, Jacobus S, Callander N, et al. Phase III trial of lenalidomide plus high-dose dexamethasone versus lenalidomide plus low-dose dexamethasone in newly diagnosed multiple myeloma (E4A03): a trial coordinated by the eastern cooperative oncology group. J Clin Oncol, 2007 ASCO Annual meeting proceedings, Part I. Vol 25, No 185 (June 20 Supplement) 2007; LBA8025.

68. Knight R. Lenalidomide and venous thrombosis in multiple myeloma. N Engl J Med 2006; 354(19):2079.

69. Chauhan D, Hideshima T, Anderson KC. Proteasome inhibition in multiple myeloma: therapeutic implication. Annu Rev Pharmacol Toxicol 2005; 45: 465–76.

70. Adams J. Development of the proteasome inhibitor PS-341. Oncologist 2002; 7(1):9–16.

71. Adams J. The development of proteasome inhibitors as anticancer drugs. Cancer Cell 2004; 5(5):417–21.

72. Goldberg AL. Protein degradation and protection against misfolded or damaged proteins. Nature 2003; 426(6968):895–9.

73. Drexler HC. Activation of the cell death program by inhibition of proteasome function. Proc Nat Acad Sci USA 1997; 94(3):855–60.

74. Delic J, Masdehors P, Omura S, et al. The proteasome inhibitor lactacystin induces apoptosis and sensitizes chemo- and radioresistant human chronic lymphocytic leukaemia lymphocytes to TNF-alpha-initiated apoptosis [see comment]. Br J Cancer 1998; 77(7):1103–7.

75. Feinman R, Koury J, Thames M, Barlogie B, Epstein J, Siegel DS. Role of NF-kappaB in the rescue of multiple myeloma cells from glucocorticoid-induced apoptosis by bcl-2. Blood 1999; 93(9):3044–52.

76. Mitsiades N, Mitsiades CS, Poulaki V, et al. Biologic sequelae of nuclear factor-kappaB blockade in multiple myeloma: therapeutic applications. Blood 2002; 99(11):4079–86.

77. Hideshima T, Chauhan D, Richardson P, et al. NF-kappa B as a therapeutic target in multiple myeloma. J Biol Chem 2002; 277(19):16639–47.

78. Hideshima T, Richardson P, Chauhan D, et al. The proteasome inhibitor PS-341 inhibits growth, induces apoptosis, and overcomes drug resistance in human multiple myeloma cells. Cancer Res 2001; 61(7):3071–6.

79. Mitsiades N, Mitsiades CS, Poulaki V, et al. Molecular sequelae of proteasome inhibition in human multiple myeloma cells. Proc Nat Acad Sci USA 2002; 99(22):14374–9.

80. Rajkumar SV, Richardson PG, Hideshima T, Anderson KC. Proteasome inhibition as a novel therapeutic target in human cancer. J Clin Oncol 2005; 23(3):630–9.

81. Richardson PG, Sonneveld P, Schuster MW, et al. Bortezomib or high-dose dexamethasone for relapsed multiple myeloma. N Engl J Med 2005; 352(24): 2487–98.

82. Richardson PG, Barlogie B, Berenson J, et al. A phase 2 study of bortezomib in relapsed, refractory myeloma. N Engl J Med 2003; 348(26):2609–17.

83. Richardson PG, Barlogie B, Berenson J, et al. Extended follow-up of a phase II trial in relapsed, refractory multiple myeloma: final time-to-event results from the SUMMIT trial. Cancer 2006; 106(6):1316–19.

84. Mitsiades N, Mitsiades CS, Richardson PG, et al. The proteasome inhibitor PS-341 potentiates sensitivity of multiple myeloma cells to conventional chemotherapeutic agents: therapeutic applications. Blood 2003; 101(6):2377–80.

85. Anderson K, Richardson P, Chanan-Khan A, et al. Single-agent bortezomib in previously untreated multiple myeloma (MM): results of a phase II multicenter study. J Clin Oncol 2006; 24(18S).

86. Lonial S, Waller EK, Richardson PG, et al. Risk factors and kinetics of thrombocytopenia associated with bortezomib for relapsed, refractory multiple myeloma. Blood 2005; 106(12):3777–84.

87. Chanan-Khan AA, Sonneveld P, Schuster MW, et al. Analysis of Varicella Zoster Virus Reactivation among Bortezomib-Treated Patients in the APEX Study. ASH Annual Meeting Abstracts 2006; 108(11):3535.

88. Jagannath S, Durie BGM, Wolf JL, et al. Long-Term Follow-Up of Patients Treated with Bortezomib Alone and in Combination with Dexamethasone as Frontline Therapy for Multiple Myeloma. ASH Annual Meeting Abstracts 2006; 108(11):796.

89. Miguel JFS, Richardson P, Sonneveld P, et al. Frequency, Characteristics, and Reversibility of Peripheral Neuropathy (PN) in the APEX Trial. ASH Annual Meeting Abstracts 2005; 106(11):366.

90. Lenz HJ. Clinical update: proteasome inhibitors in solid tumors. Cancer Treatment Reviews 2003; 29 Suppl 1:41–8.

91. Terpos E, Anagnostopoulos A, Heath D, et al. The Combination of Bortezomib, Melphalan, Dexamethasone and Intermittent Thalidomide (VMDT) is an Effective Regimen for Relapsed/Refractory Myeloma and Reduces Serum Levels of Dickkopf-1, RANKL, MIP-1α and Angiogenic Cytokines. ASH Annual Meeting Abstracts 2006; 108(11):3541.

92. Reece DE, Piza G, Trudel S, et al. A Phase I-II Trial of Bortezomib Plus Oral Cyclophosphamide and Prednisone for Relapsed/Refractory Multiple Myeloma. ASH Annual Meeting Abstracts 2006; 108(11):3536.

93. Popat R, Williams C, Cook M, et al. A Phase I/II Trial of Bortezomib, Low Dose Intravenous Melphalan and Dexamethasone for Patients with Relapsed Multiple Myeloma. ASH Annual Meeting Abstracts 2006; 108(11):3542.

94. Palumbo A, Ambrosini MT, Benevolo G, et al. Combination of Bortezomib, Melphalan, Prednisone and Thalidomide (VMPT) for Relapsed Multiple Myeloma: Results of a Phase I/II Clinical Trial. ASH Annual Meeting Abstracts 2006; 108(11):407.

95. Orlowski RZ, Zhuang SH, Parekh T, et al. The Combination of Pegylated Liposomal Doxorubicin and Bortezomib Significantly Improves Time to Progression of Patients with Relapsed/Refractory Multiple Myeloma Compared with Bortezomib Alone: Results from a Planned Interim Analysis of a Randomized Phase III Study. ASH Annual Meeting Abstracts 2006; 108(11):404.

96. Zangari M, Barlogie B, Jacobson J, et al. VTD Regimen Comprising Velcade (V) + Thalidomide (T) and Added DEX (D) for Non-Responders to V + T Effects a 57% PR Rate among 56 Patients with Myeloma (M) Relapsing after Autologous Transplant. Blood 2003; 102(11).

97. Ciolli S, Leoni F, Gigli F, Rigacci L, Bosi A. Low dose Velcade, thalidomide and dexamethasone (LD-VTD): an effective regimen for relapsed and refractory multiple myeloma patients. Leukemia & Lymphoma 2006; 47(1):171–3.

98. Chanan-khan AA, Padmanabhan S, Miller KC, et al. Final Results of a Phase II Study of Bortezomib (Velcade) in Combination with Liposomal Doxorubicin (Doxil) and Thalidomide (VDT) Demonstrate a Sustained High Response Rates in Patients (pts) with Relapsed (rel) or Refactory (ref) Multiple Myeloma. ASH Annual Meeting Abstracts 2006; 108(11):3539.

99. Chanan-Khan A, Miller KC. Velcade, Doxil and Thalidomide (VDT) is an effective salvage regimen for patients with relapsed and refractory multiple myeloma. Leukemia & Lymphoma 2005; 46(7):1103–4.

100. Wang LM, Weber DM, Delasalle KB, Alexanian R. VTD (Velcade, Thalidomide, Dexamethasone) as Primary Therapy for Newly-Diagnosed Multiple Myeloma. ASH Annual Meeting Abstracts 2004; 104(11):210.

101. Wang M, Delasalle K, Giralt S, Alexanian R. Rapid Control of Previously Untreated Multiple Myeloma with Bortezomib-Thalidomide-Dexamethasone Followed by Early Intensive Therapy. ASH Annual Meeting Abstracts 2005; 106(11):784.

102. Jakubowiak A, Kendall T, Al-Zoubi A, et al. High Rate of Complete and near Complete Responses (CR/nCR) after Initial Therapy with Bortezomib (Velcade(R)), Doxil(R), and Dexamethasone (VDD) Is Further Increased after Autologous Stem Cell Transplantation (ASCT). *ASH Annual Meeting Abstracts* 108(11):3093.

103. Richardson PG, Jagannath S, Avigan DE, et al. Lenalidomide Plus Bortezomib (Rev-Vel) in Relapsed and/or Refractory Multiple Myeloma (MM): Final Results of a Multicenter Phase 1 Trial. ASH Annual Meeting Abstracts 2006; 108(11):405.

104. Attal M, Harousseau JL. Standard therapy versus autologous transplantation in multiple myeloma. Hematology—Oncology Clinics of North America 1997; 11(1):133–46.

105. Attal M, Harousseau J-L, Facon T, et al. Single versus double autologous stem-cell transplantation for multiple myeloma. N Engl J Med 2003; 349(26): 2495–502.

9

Novel Therapeutic Options for the Treatment of Relapsed and Relapsed, Refractory Myeloma

Melissa Alsina
H. Lee Moffitt Cancer Center & Research Institute, Tampa, Florida, U.S.A.

Paul Richardson
Dana-Farber Cancer Institute, Harvard Medical School, Boston, Massachusetts, U.S.A.

INTRODUCTION

Despite major advances in the treatment of newly diagnosed multiple myeloma (MM), the vast majority of patients relapse after induction therapy and therefore require further treatment. Historically, the mainstay of therapy for patients with relapsed MM has been high dose dexamethasone or dexamethasone-based regimens, but these have failed to impact survival. Fortunately, in the past eight years there have been significant advances in the treatment of relapsed and relapsed, refractory MM through the development, and U.S. Food and Drug Administration (FDA) approval, of two major new classes of therapeutic agents; lenalidomide and thalidomide as immunomodulatory drugs, and bortezomib as a first-in-class proteasome inhibitor (1,2). These drugs represent a new paradigm of antitumor agent which not only target the MM cell directly, but also have significant activity against key tumor cell interactions with the bone marrow microenvironment (3). Both lenalidomide and bortezomib have been shown to be superior to high dexamethasone in the relapsed setting and confer significant survival advantage to patients with relapsed MM (4,5). Preclinical and clinical studies to date have also shown that the combination of these agents, in particular bortezomib, with targeted therapy and conventional chemotherapy enhances their anti-MM activity (6). Furthermore, there continues to be progress in the development of additional novel immunomodulatory drugs and second generation proteasome inhibitors, with potentially enhanced activity. In this chapter, we will review the role of these agents, both as monotherapy and as combinations in the treatment of relapsed MM, as well as other emerging novel agents that are currently in development.

DEFINITIONS OF RELAPSED AND RELAPSED, REFRACTORY MYELOMA

Relapsed or progressive myeloma has been defined by the European bone marrow tansplant (EBMT) response criteria and more recently in the International uniform response criteria (7,8). In the former, the term progression is used to describe an increase in disease activity in patients in partial remission or with stable disease (CR), whereas the term relapse refers to recurrent disease after complete remission. More specifically, progression is defined as and increased of 25% in serum or urinary paraprotein, or on the basis of increasing marrow infiltration, skeletal disease, and/or hypercalcemia. Relapse is defined as the reappearance of detectable paraprotein or other manifestation of disease in patients previously in CR. This definition includes the appearance of immunofixation positivity even in the absence of measurable levels of paraprotein with the caveat that relapse does not necessarily become an indication to institute therapy as recurrence of IF positivity is not always followed by an immediate increase in paraprotein levels and/or symptoms. The international uniform response criteria defines progressive disease and relapse in the same way as the EBMT criteria but introduces a new category of clinical relapse defined as the presence of one or more indicators of increasing disease activity and/or end organ dysfunction, sometimes referred to as "CRAB" features (namely hypercalcemia, renal dysfunction, anemia, and bone disease).

Relapsed and refractory disease describes patients who must achieve minor response (MR) or better followed by relapse and then become nonresponsive to salvage therapy, or experience progression within 60 days of their last therapy. Characteristically, they have poor prognosis (i.e., median overall survival of 6–9 months, especially in the face of ineffective therapy).

A Mayo Clinic study showed that in a cohort of patients from 1985 to 1998, the median survival was 29 months from diagnosis, and from first relapse to death median survival was just 17 months (9). The analysis of data showed that a decrease in response duration with increasing lines of treatment was an important feature.

IMMUNOMODULATORY DRUGS

Thalidomide and the analogues lenalidomide (CC-5013, Revlimid) and pomalidomide (CC-4047, Actimid), belong to the family of immunomodulatory drugs (known as IMiDs). These agents have a broad spectrum of activity which include antiangiogenic properties, cytokine secretion modulation, stimulation of T cells and NK cell toxicity as well as direct anti-MM effects (10,11). These characteristics have made them promising drugs for the treatment of relapsed and relapsed, refractory MM. These agents have shown high responses in all phases of MM therapy and these responses are enhanced when used in combination with dexamethasone, conventional chemotherapy and other novel agents. The data that has led to the widespread use of these drugs in the setting of relapsed or refractory MM is discussed below.

THALIDOMIDE AND THALIDOMIDE-BASED COMBINATIONS

Single Agent Thalidomide

Thalidomide is effective as a single agent in approximately 30% of patients with refractory MM. Singhal et al conducted the first trial that showed activity in patients with relapsed or relapsed and refractory MM (12). In this phase II study, 84 patients (76 progressing after high dose chemotherapy), received oral thalidomide 200–800 mg/day as monotherapy. Responses ($\geq 50\%$ reduction in paraprotein levels) were seen in 25% of patients. Median time to response was 29 days. Longer follow-up in twice as many patients studied by the same group confirmed the activity of thalidomide in relapsed MM, with 2-year event free survival and overall survival of 26% and 54%, respectively (13). We evaluated the effects of thalidomide in patients with relapsed MM after high-dose chemotherapy (HDC) and stem cell transplantation (SCT) (14). In this phase II study 31 patients were treated with single agent thalidomide at doses from 200 to 600 mg/day over 12 weeks and a subsequent maintenance phase of 200 mg/day for up to one year. The response rate [partial response (PR) plus minor response (MR)] was 43% with a median duration of six months. Dose escalation to 600 mg/day was achieved in only 50% of patients and toxicities included constipation, fatigue, rash, and neuropathy, which were dose limiting in 27% of patients and cumulative, with 200 mg/day being tolerated best. Several other phase II studies have shown similar results but to date there is no randomized studies of single agent thalidomide in relapsed MM (15,16). Glasmacher et al. conducted a systematic review of phase II trials of thalidomide monotherapy in relapsed myeloma. They reviewed published data from 42 trials involving 1674 patients. Thalidomide doses varied from 50 to 800 mg/day (17). The intention to treat population for efficacy was 1629 patients and the response rate (PR + CR) reported was 29%, with an additional 25% of patients achieving MR or stable disease. The median overall survival from all trials was 14 months and grade III–IV toxicities included somnolence (11%), constipation (16%), neuropathy (6%), rash (3%), thromboembolism (3%), and cardiac events (2%). While toxicity was

Table 1 Pharmacologic Treatment of Patients with Relapsed Multiple Myeloma in Phase II and III Clinical Trials: Activity/Efficacy

Study	Phase	No. of pts.	Regimen	Outcome								
				CR+PR (%)	CR (%)	TTR[a] (mos)	DOR[a] (mos)	TTP[a] (mos)	Follow-up[a] (mos)	ORR (%)	OS[a] (mos)	1-year survival (%)
Jagannath et al. (32) (CREST)	II	54	Bortezomib 1.0 mg/m^2[b]	30[c]		1.3	9.5	7	26.2			
Richardson et al. (33,36)	II	202	Bortezomib 1.3 mg/m^2[b] (SUMMIT)	38[d]		1.5	13.7	11	26.1			
Bortezomib 1.3 mg/m^2[b]		27	1.3	12.7	7		35	17				
Richardson et al. (35) (APEX)	III	669	Bortezomib 1.3 mg/m^2 twice wk × 2 wks day 1, 4, 8, and 11 (eight 21-day cycles) followed by bortezomib 1.3 mg/m^2 days 1, 18, 15, and 22 (three 35-day cycles)	38	6	43[d](CR + PR)		6.2				80
			Dexamethasone 40 mg day 1–4, 9–12, 17–20, every 5 wks × four cycles + five cycles d 1–4 every 28 days	18	1	43[d](CR + PR)		3.5				66

[a] Median values.

[b] Days 1, 4, 8, and 11 plus dexamethasone 20 mg days 1, 2, 4, 5, 8, and 12 if PD after two cycles or SD after four cycles. Maximum of eight 21-day cycles.

[c] Thirty-seven percent when administered with dexamethasone.

[d] Fifty percent when administered with dexamethasone.

Abbreviations: APEX, assessment of proteasome inhibition for extending remissions; CR, complete response; CREST, clinical response and efficacy study of bortezomib in the treatment of relapsing multiple myeloma; DOR, duration of response; ORR, overall response rate; OS, overall survival; PD, progressive disease; PR, partial response; SD, stable disease; SUMMIT, study of uncontrolled multiple myeloma managed with proteasome inhibition therapy; TTP, time-to-progression; TTR, time-to-response.

Source: Ref. 57.

Table 2 Pharmacologic Treatment with Bortezomib (± Dexamethasone) in Relapsed Multiple Myeloma in Phase II Clinical Trials: Safety

Study (Study acronym)	Reported adverse events	
	Grade 3	Grade 4
Jagannath et al. (32) (CREST)	Peripheral neuropathy (4%, $1.0 \, mg/m^2$; 15%, $1.3 \, mg/m^2$); pain in limb (11%, 8%); thrombocytopenia (29%, 19%); weakness (4%, 12%); neutropenia (11%, 23%); lymphopenia (11%, 12%); pneumonia (15%, $1.3 \, mg/m^2$); hyponatremia (11%, $1.0 \, mg/m^2$; 8%, $1.3 \, mg/m^2$)	Peripheral neuropathy (4%, $1.0 \, mg/m^2$); thrombocytopenia (4%, $1.3 \, mg/m^2$)
Richardson et al. (33) (SUMMIT)	Thrombocytopenia (28%); fatigue (12%); neuropathy (12%); neutropenia (11%); vomiting (8%); diarrhea (7%); dehydration (7%); pain in limb (7%); nausea (6%); weakness (5%); headache (3%); anorexia (2%); constipation (2%); dizziness (1%); rash (<1%)	Thrombocytopenia (3%); neutropenia (3%); diarrhea (1%); vomiting (<1%); weakness (<1%)

Abbreviations: CREST, clinical response and efficacy study of bortezomib in the treatment of relapsing multiple myeloma; SUMMIT, study of uncontrolled multiple myeloma managed with proteasome inhibition therapy.
Source: Ref. 57.

dose related and cumulative, the authors were not able to show conclusively a dose-response effect. This data shows that thalidomide monotherapy is active and relatively well tolerated in relapsed MM, with the caveat of some of its non-hematologic adverse effects. It suggests a role for single agent thalidomide in the treatment of selected patients with relapsed disease and supports combination approaches being pursued.

Thalidomide-Based Combinations

The clinical benefit of thalidomide increases when it is combined with other agents. For example, thalidomide in combination with dexamethasone has become one of the most commonly used front-line regimens in the US for patients with MM and also shows significant activity in relapsed disease (18). A recent retrospective analysis of patients with relapsed or refractory MM indicates that the combination is superior to thalidomide alone.

(Text continues on page 182)

Table 3 Activity of Emerging Therapies for Patients with Relapsed Multiple Myeloma: Preliminary Results in Phase I, Phase I/II, and Phase II Trials

Study	Phase	No. of pts.	Regimen	Outcome
Reece et al. (43)	I/II	16	Bortezomib 0.7–1.5 mg/m², days 1, 8, and 15; cyclophosphamide 150–300 mg, days 1, 8, 15, and 22; prednisone 50–100 mg	CR = 6%; PR = 25%; MR = 25%; SD = 31%
Kropff et al. (44)	II	50	Bortezomib 1.3 mg/m², days 1, 4, 8, and 11; cyclophosphamide 50 mg/day; dexamethasone 20 mg	CR = 5 pts (10%); PR = 33 pts (66%); MR = 6 pts (12%); ORRR = 44 pts (88%) median EFS = 10 mos
Berenson et al. (45)	I/II	34 evaluable	Bortezomib 0.7 mg/m², days 1, 4, 8, and 11 (dosage increased to 1.0 mg/m²if no DLT); melphalan 0.025, 0.05, 0.10, 0.15, or 0.25 mg/kg, days 1–4 (eight 28-day cycles)	RR = 68%; CR = 6%; PR = 32%; PFS = 8 mos
Popat et al. (46)	I/II	16 evaluable	Bortezomib 1.3 mg/m², days 1, 4, 8, and 11 and melphalan 2.5–10 mg/m², days 2 for up to eight 4-wk cycles; dexamethasone added after two or four cycles for PD or SD, respectively	CR + PR + MR = 50%
Hollmig et al. (47)	I/II	37 (27 evaluable for response)	Bortezomib 1.0 or 1.3 mg/m² given 4 and 1 days before SCT, prior to melphalan; melphalan 100–250 mg/m² in fractionated doses or as a single dose prior to SCT	CR + PR >35%

Palumbo et al. (48)	II	20	Bortezomib $1.0–1.6\,\mathrm{mg/m^2}$, days 1, 4, 15, and 22; melphalan $6\,\mathrm{mg/m^2}$, days 1–5; predisone $60\,\mathrm{mg/m^2}$, days 1–5; thalidomide $100\,\mathrm{mg/day}$	RR $\geq 50\% = 67\%$
Terpos et al. (49)	II	25 evaluable	Bortezomib $1.0\,\mathrm{mg/m^2}$, days 1, 4, 8, and 11; melphalan $0.15\,\mathrm{mg/kg}$; thalidomide $100\,\mathrm{mg/day}$; dexamethasone $12\,\mathrm{mg/m^2}$, days 1–4 and 17–20	RR (CR + PR) $= 56\%$; MR $= 8\%$; SD $= 20\%$
Zangari et al. (50)	I/II	85	Bortezomib $1.0/1.3\,\mathrm{mg/m^2}$, days 1, 4, 8, and 11 of a 3-wk cycle; thalidomide (incremental dosages of 50, 100, 150 or $200\,\mathrm{mg/day}$) starting on day 1 of cycle 2; dexamethasone $20\,\mathrm{mg}$, days 1, 2, 4, 5, 8, 9, 11, and 12 from cycle 4 in pts not achieving PR or better	CR + PR $= 55\%$; median EFS $= 9\,\mathrm{mo}$; median OS $= 22\,\mathrm{mo}$
Hollmig et al. (51)	I/II	20 (14 evaluable)	Bortezomib 1.0 or $1.3\,\mathrm{mg/m^2}$, days 1, 4, 9, and 11; doxorubicin $2.5–10\,\mathrm{mg/m^2}$, days 1–4 and 9–12; thalidomide 50 or $100\,\mathrm{mg}$, days 1–12; dexamethasone 20 or $40\,\mathrm{mg}$, days 1–4 and 9–12	PR $= 50\%$
Jakubowiak et al. (52)	II	20	Bortezomib $1.3\,\mathrm{mg/m^2}$, days 1, 4, 8, and 11; PLD $30\,\mathrm{mg/m^2}$, day 4; dexamethasone $40\,\mathrm{mg}$, days 1–4	RR $= 83\%$; CR + nCR $= 33\%$

(Continued)

Table 3 Activity of Emerging Therapies for Patients with Relapsed Multiple Myeloma: Preliminary Results in Phase I, Phase I/II, and Phase II Trials (*Continued*)

Study	Phase	No. of pts.	Regimen	Outcome
Orlowski et al. (53)	I	24 with multiple myeloma (22 evaluable); total population = 42 with hematologic malignancies	Bortezomib 0.90–1.50 mg/m², days 1, 4, 8, and 11; PLD 30 mg/m², day 4 (21-day cycles)	ORR = 73%; CR = five pts.; nCR = three pts.; PR = eight pts.
Chanan-Khan et al. (54)	II	16 evaluable	Bortezomib 1.3 mg/m², days 1, 4, 15, and 18; PLD 20 mg/m², days 1 and 15; thalidomide 200 mg/day (four to six 4-wk cycles)	CR + PR >57%
Singhal et al. (15)	II	84	Thalidomide 200–800 mg/day, escalated over 12 wks	CR + PR = 25%
Richardson et al. (16)	II	30 (26 evaluable) pts. who had relapsed after HDT/SCT	Thalidomide 200–600 mg/day, escalated over 12 wks; thalidomide maintenance 200 mg/day up to 1 yr	12-week PFS = 67%; ORR (PR + MR) = 43%; PR = 33%; MR = 10%; SD = 17%; PD = 27%
Almhanna et al. (21)	II	105	Vincristine 2 mg; PLD 40 mg/m²; dexamethasone 40 mg; thalidomide 50–400 mg	ORR = 89%; CR/nCR = 49%; median PFS = 28 mos
Lee et al. (23)	II	236	Dexamethasone 40 mg × 4 day; thalidomide 400 mg/day; 4-day continuous infusion: cisplatin 10 mg/m²/day, doxorubicin 10 mg/m²/day, cyclophosphamide 400 mg/m²/day, and etoposide 40 mg/m²/day	After two cycles: CR = 7%; nCR = 9%; PR = 16%; improvement = 54%

Study	Phase	Treatment	N	Results
Hovenga et al. (24)	II	Thalidomide 100–400 mg/day (median dose 100 mg/day); cyclophosphamide 100–150 mg/day (median dose 95 mg/day)	38	ORR (CR + PR + MR = 84%; PR = 64%; median PFS = 30 mos; median OS = 20 mos; median time to maximum response = 3 mos; median DOR = 9 mos; median TTP = 4.5 mos
Richardson et al. (55)	I	Lenalidomide 5, 10, 25, and 50 mg/day (dose-finding study)	27 (24 evaluable)	≥PR = 29%; median time to best response = 2 mos; median DOR = 6 mos
Richardson et al. (56)	II	Lenalidomide 30 mg/day	222	TTP = 22.4 wk; ≥PR = 25%
Richardson et al. (57)	I	Bortezomib 1.0–1.3 mg/m^2, days 1, 4, 8, and 11; lenalidomide 5–20 mg/day, days 1–14	19	CR + PR = 59%
Baz et al. (58)	II	Lenalidomide 10 mg/day; vincristine 2 mg; PLD 40 mg/m^2; dexamethasone 40 mg	45 evaluable	CR = 13%; PR = 35%; SD = 24%; PD = 15%
Schey et al. (59)	I	CC-4047 1, 2, 5, and 10 mg/day (dose-finding study)	24	CR = 17%; VGPR = 13%; PR = 25%; MR = 17%; SD = 25%; PD = 4%; median time to best response = 21 wks; median EFS = 28 wks; median PFS = 39 wks; median OS = 90 wks

(Continued)

Table 3 Activity of Emerging Therapies for Patients with Relapsed Multiple Myeloma: Preliminary Results in Phase I, Phase I/II, and Phase II Trials (*Continued*)

Study	Phase	No. of pts.	Regimen	Outcome
Borad et al. (60)	Pilot	10	Melphalan 0.1 mg/kg; arsenic trioxide 0.25 mg/kg twice wk; ascorbic acid 1 g twice wk after arsenic trioxide (4 pts. received arsenic trioxide and ascorbic acid on the same 4 days as melphalan during the first wk, instead of twice wk) (6-wk cycles)	Reduction in serum M-protein levels = 29–90%; reduction in urine M-protein levels = 34–71%; sustained response = 60%

Abbreviations: CR, complete response; DLT, dose-limiting toxicity; DOR, duration of response; EFS, event-free survival; HDT, high-dose chemotherapy; MR, minimal response; nCR, near complete response; NS, not stated; ORR, overall response rate; OS, overall survival; pts., patients; PD, progressive disease; PEG, polyethylene glycol; PFS, progression-free survival; PLD, PEGylated liposomal doxorubicin; PR, partial response; RR, response rate; SCT, stem cell transplantation; SD, stable disease; TTP, time-to-progression; VGPR, very good partial remission.
Source: Ref. 57.

Table 4 Safety of Emerging Therapies for Relapsed Multiple Myeloma: Preliminary Results in Phase I, I/II, and II Trials

Study	Regimen	Reported adverse events (%)
Kropff et al. (44)	Bortezomib + cyclophosphamide + dexamethasone	Grade 4: thrombocytopenia (17); neutropenia (2). Grade 3/4: infections (26); peripheral neuropathy (25); fatigue (15); cardiac events (11)
Berenson et al. (45)	Bortezomib + melphalan	Peripheral neuropathy (new or worsening of existing) Grade 3/4: anemia; neutropenia; thrombocytopenia
Popat et al. (46)	Bortezomib + low-dose melphalan	Grade 3/4: thrombocytopenia (63); neutropenia (38)
Hollmig et al. (47)	Bortezomib + high-dose melphalan	Mucositis (14); diarrhea (30); febrile neutropenia (14); pneumonia/sepsis (38); fatigue (59)
Palumbo et al. (48)	Bortezomib + melphalan + prednisone + thalidomide	Grade 1 and 2: constipation; infection; fatigue; rash
Terpos et al. (49)	Bortezomib + doxorubicin + thalidomide + dexamethasone	Grade 3/4: thrombocytopenia (12); neutropenia (8%) anemia (grade 3 = 8)
Jakubowiak et al. (52)	Bortezomib + PEGylated liposomal doxorubicin + dexamethasone	Grade 3 or 4: thrombocytopenia (35); neutropenia (35); pneumonia (25)
Chanan-Khan et al. (54)	Bortezomib + PEGylated liposomal doxorubicin + thalidomide	Grade 2: plantar-palmar erythrodysthesia (14) Grade 3: cellulitis (6)
Orlowski et al. (53)	Bortezomib + PEGylated liposomal doxorubicin[a]	Grade 3 or 4: thrombocytopenia (43); lymphopenia (40); neutropenia (17); fatigue (14); pneumonia (14); peripheral neuropathy (12); febrile neutropenia (10); diarrhea (10)

(Continued)

Table 4 Safety of Emerging Therapies for Relapsed Multiple Myeloma: Preliminary Results in Phase I, I/II, and II Trials (*Continued*)

Study	Regimen	Reported adverse events (%)
Richardson et al. (16)	Thalidomide	Grade 1 and 2: constipation (43); fatigue (37); rash (33); neuropathy (30). Grade 3: neuropathy (7); rash (3); somnolence (3); constipation (3); muscle cramps (3); impotence (3)
Lee et al. (23)	DTPACE	Grade ≥2: neutropenia (65% of cycles); thrombocytopenia (11% of cycles) Nonhematologic toxicities: nausea and vomiting (21); mucositis (19); hypophosphatemia (17)
Hovenga et al. (24)	Thalidomide + cyclophosphamide	Grade 1–2: neurotoxicity (51). Grade 3: neurotoxicity (16); constipation (13). Grade 3–4: drowsiness and dizziness (20); deep venous thrombosis (3)
Richardson et al. (55)	Lenalidomide (CC-5013)	Grade 3: neutropenia (60); thrombocytopenia (20). Grade 4: neutropenia (16)
Richardson et al. (56)	Lenalidomide	≥10%: upper respiratory tract infection; neutropenia; thrombocytopenia
Baz et al. (58)	Lenalidomide + vincristine + PEGylated liposomal doxorubicin + dexamethasone	Grade 3: leukopenia (24); infection (26); thrombocytopenia (20). Grade 4: leukopenia (15); infection (3)

Schey et al. (59)	CC-4047	Grade 1: skin toxicity (21); gastrointestinal toxicity (17); neuropathy (13); orthostatic hypotension (8). Grade 1 and 2: edema (8) Grade 2: gastrointestinal toxicity (17). Grade 3: neutropenia (33); thrombocytopenia (13). Grade 4: neutropenia (25); deep venous thrombosis (17)
Borad et al. (60)	Melphalan + arsenic trioxide + ascorbic acid	Grade 1–2: sensory neuropathy (40); gastrointestinal symptoms (40). Grade 1–3: anemia (70); leukopenia (70); thrombocytopenia (40). Grade 1: fatigue (70); headache (20); QTc interval prolongation (50). Grade 2: reactivation of herpes zoster (20); skin rash (30). Grade 3: pulmonary peripheral edema (20)

[a] Results for 42 patients with hematological malignancies, 24 of whom had multiple myeloma.
Abbreviations: DTPACE, dexamethasone, thalidomide, cisplatin, doxorubicin, cyclophosphamide, and etoposide; PEG, polyethylene glycol; QTc, corrected QT.
Source: Ref. 57.

Thalidomide monotherapy resulted in a response rate of 29%, and this increased to 51% with the addition of dexamethasone (19).

The addition of dexamethasone to thalidomide also has activity in patients who are resistant to dexamethasone, thalidomide monotherapy or standard chemotherapy. In heavily pretreated patients, thalidomide and dexamethasone were combined as salvage therapy in a study by Dimopoulous et al. (20). Fifty-five percent of patients achieved PR, with a median time to response of 1.3 months. Median survival for all patients was 12.6 months. The combination was equally effective regardless of previous resistance to dexamethasone, or prior HDC/SCT. Mild to moderate toxicity was observed, consisting primarily of constipation, morning somnolence, tremor, xerostomia, and peripheral neuropathy. In another study by Terpos et al. (21) intermediate dose thalidomide (thal) plus dexamethasone (dex) and zoledronic acid was also shown to be effective in 35 patients with refractory/relapsed MM, with a response rate of 66% and a median survival of 20 months.

In order to examine and compare several treatment options for patients with MM relapsing after HDC/SCT, Palumbo et al., compared the outcome of 90 MM patients treated at diagnosis with induction therapy followed by HDC/SCT and then salvaged with thal/dex (43 patients), a second autologous transplant (28 patients) or conventional chemotherapy (19 patients) (22). The major prognostic factors, the median times between diagnosis and start of salvage treatment and the progression-free survival (PFS) from diagnosis were similar among the three groups. The response rate was higher after salvage autologous transplant and after thal/dex, and lower after conventional chemotherapy ($p < 0.001$). Thal/dex significantly prolonged PFS from first relapse ($p < 0.0001$). Median PFS was 20.3 months after thal/dex, nine months after autologous transplant, and 4.5 months after chemotherapy. Overall survival (OS) from first relapse was significantly improved by thal/dex (median 55.5 months) but not by autologous transplant (15 months) or chemotherapy (27.5 months) ($p = 0.008$). Multivariate analysis indicated that thal/dex and age were the only independent risk factors associated with improved outcome.

Thalidomide has also been evaluated in combination with chemotherapy in the relapsed setting, and these combinations have achieved significant rates of CR. For example, the efficacy and safety of thalidomide in combination with the DVd regimen (DVd-T) was evaluated in 49 patients with relapsed myeloma (23). Thalidomide was given at 50 mg/day orally and the dose increased to a maximum of 400 mg/day. At the time of best response, patients received maintenance prednisone, 50 mg orally every other day, and daily thalidomide at the maximum tolerated dose for each patient. The primary end point was the rate of CR plus very good partial response (VGPR). The CR plus VGPR rate was 45%, with an overall response rate (ORR) of 90%. Furthermore, better responses were associated with improved PFS and OS. The most common grade 3 and 4 adverse events were thromboembolic events, peripheral neuropathy and neutropenia. The authors concluded that the addition of thalidomide to the DVd regimen significantly improved the response rate and quality of responses compared with the DVd regimen alone.

A regimen of thal, dex plus pulsed cyclophosphamide has been shown to have significant activity in patients with relapsed MM: 60% of patients achieved a partial response with median time-to-progression for responding patients of 12 months, and a median overall survival for all patients of 17.5 months (24). Toxicities were mild or moderate and the cumulative incidence of deep vein thrombosis and peripheral neuropathy was 4% and 2% respectively. Two other studies have evaluated the efficacy of cyclophosphamide in combination with thalidomide in patients with relapsed MM. Garcia-Sanz et al. combined escalating doses of thal (up to 800 mg/day), oral cyclophosphamide 50 mg/day and dex 40 mg/day for 4 days every 3 weeks. Partial responses were observed in 53% of patients and the 2-year PFS and OS were 57 and 62% respectively (25). Similarly, Kyriakou et al. evaluated the efficacy and tolerability of low dose thal up to 300 mg/day in combination with dex 40 mg for four days per month and cyclophosphamide at 300 mg/m^2 weekly: ORR was 79% with a CR rate of 17%. The most common nonhematologic toxicities were constipation and neuropathy, and 25% of patients developed grade 3 or lower neutropenia (26).

Clearly thalidomide in combination with other chemotherapeutic agents is active in patients with relapsed MM. Special attention should be given to side effects, including neuropathy, and in particular deep vein thrombosis, especially when given in combination with chemotherapy and dexamethasone.

Lenalidomide

Lenalidomide is an immunomodulatory derivative of thalidomide with higher in vitro potency and greater activity than thalidomide in myeloma cell lines (27,28).

A phase I dose-finding trial of lenalidomide 5, 10, 25, and 50 mg/day determined that MTD was 25 mg/day. Dose limiting toxicity was defined as grade >2 cardiac arrhythmia, grade 3 nonhematologic toxicity or grade 4 hematologic toxicity during the first 4 weeks. Patients ($n = 27$) had relapsed or refractory disease with median of three prior therapies, including 16 patients who had received prior thalidomide. Partial responses were seen in 29% of patients. The DLT was myelosuppresion with grade 3/4 myelosuppresion seen in 12/13 patients treated at the 50 mg/day dosage levels beyond 28 days, resulting in dosage reduction to 25 mg/day and growth factor support in all 12 patients. However, in contrast with thalidomide, no significant somnolence, constipation, or neuropathy was observed at any dose level (29).

In another Phase I/II study by Zangari et al., lenalidomide was evaluated at doses of 5, 10, 25 and 50 mg/day in 15 patients with relapsed myeloma. Eight of the patients had a reduction of 25% or more in the paraprotein and, all at dose levels of 25 mg or higher. No responses were observed at the 5 or 10 mg dose (30).

We conducted a multicenter, open-label, randomized phase 2 study to evaluate two dose regimens of lenalidomide for relapsed, refractory myeloma (31). Seventy patients were randomized to receive either 30 mg once daily or 15 mg twice a day versus daily oral lenalidomide for 21 days of every 28-day cycle. Patients with progressive or stable disease after two cycles received dexamethasone at low dose. Analysis of the first 70 patients showed increased grade 3/4 myelosuppresion in patients receiving 15 mg twice daily (41% vs. 13%, $p = 0.03$). An additional 32 patients received 30 mg once daily. Responses were evaluated according to the modified European Group for Blood and Marrow Transplantation (EBMT) criteria. Overall response rate (complete, partial, or minor) to lenalidomide alone was 25% (24% for once-daily and 29% for twice-daily lenalidomide). Median overall survival in 30 mg once-daily and twice-daily groups was 28 and 27 months, respectively. Median progression-free survival was 7.7 months on once daily versus 3.9 months on twice-daily lenalidomide ($p = 0.2$). Dexamethasone was added in 68 patients and 29% responded. Time to first occurrence of clinically significant grade 3/4 myelosuppresion was shorter in the twice-daily group (1.8 vs. 5.5 months, $p = 0.05$). Significant peripheral neuropathy and deep vein thrombosis each occurred in only 3%, and venous thromboembolism only occurred when dexamethasone was added.

These findings confirm the activity of single agent lenalidomide in relapsed myeloma and support the evaluation of lenalidomide in combination therapy.

Lenalidomide-Based Combinations

Weber et al. and Dimopoulous et al. conducted two multicenter double-blind randomized trials concomitantly in North America and Europe, respectively (32). Over 300 patients with relapsed or relapsed refractory myeloma were randomized to lenalidomide in combination with dexamethasone or dexamethasone alone. Patients were treated with dex 40 mg/day on days 1–4, 9–12, and 17–20 every 28 days with or without lenalidomide 25 mg daily on days 1–21 every 28 days or placebo. Dexamethasone was reduced to only days 1–4 on cycle 5. Overall response rate was greater in patients that received the combination than in patients that received dex alone in both trials (58% vs. 22%, European trial, 59.1% vs. 21.1%, North American trial). The median time-to-progression for patients treated with the combination was 13.3 months compared with 5.1 months in the European trial and 11.1 months compared with 4.7 months in the North American trial? The striking difference in TTP between the two arms surpassed the prespecified boundary for stopping the trial and the Independent data monitoring committee recommended the data to be released to all study participants and lenalidomide was offered to the patients randomized to dexamethasone and placebo. Both grade 3–4 neutropenia and thromboembolic events were more commonly seen with the combination; however, the rate of infection was similar between both regimens. Niesvizky et al. (33) further explored the increased incidence of thrombosis observed with the combination. The investigators performed sub group analysis of both randomized studies and reported thrombotic events in 11.3% of patients treated with lenalidomide and dexamethasone compared to 3.8% of patients treated with dexamethasone alone. A multivariate analysis showed this combination and the use of erythropoietin to be independent factors for thrombosis. Interestingly, none of the 23 patients using aspirin during initiation of therapy developed thrombosis. The authors concluded that Epo administration must be minimized when using lenalidomide and dexamethasone, and that antithrombotic prophylaxis therapy should be considered with aspirin, coumadin, or low molecular weight heparin.

Lenalidomide has also been tested in combination with conventional chemotherapy in patients with relapsed myeloma. In combination with doxyl and dexamethasone, responses were observed in 59% of patients including 24% rate of CR and nCR (34). Knop et al conducted a trial of lenalidomide, adriamycin and dexamethasone in patients with relapsed myeloma. The study established doses of 25 mg lenalidomide daily, 9 mg/m^2 Adriamycin days 1–4 and 40 mg of dexamethasone on days 1–4 and 17–20 of a 21-day cycle. The overall response rate was 84% in 37 valuable patients (35).

We conducted a phase I trial to evaluate the tolerability and efficacy of lenalidomide in combination with the proteasome inhibitor bortezomib in 38 patients with relapsed myeloma (36). The combination was well tolerated and resulted in a 58% response rate in 36 valuable patients, with treatment ongoing in responding patients for up to three years. The maximum tolerated dose was defined at 15-mg/day lenalidomide plus 1.0 mg/m^2 bortezomib in the standard 21-day cycles. Although 15 patients also received low dose dexamethasone when they progressed on the doublet with response seen in most and no unexpected added toxicity to date, the lenalidomide plus bortezomib combination offers a "steroid sparing" approach. Interestingly, overall, there were few thromboembolic events reported in this study, and no grade 3 or worse peripheral neuropathy has been seen, despite the prolonged courses of treatment given. Currently, phase II trials are ongoing in the relapsed and refractory setting, as well as in newly diagnosed patients.

Pomalidomide

Pomalidomide is another immunomodulatory thalidomide analog. In vitro studies suggest markedly increased stimulation of T-cell proliferation, IL-2 secretion, and IFN-g production (37). Schey et al. (38) conducted a Phase I study to evaluate the safety, efficacy, and immunomodulatory effects of pomalidomide in relapsed or refractory myeloma. Twenty-four patients were treated with a dose-escalating regimen. Pomalidomide was tolerated with no serious nonhematologic adverse events. The treatment-related incidence of thrombosis was high at 12.5%. Dose-limiting hematologic neutropenia was observed in six patients, but it resolved in all patients except one with progressive disease. All the patients were able to restart treatment at lower dose. There was no grade 4 limiting thrombocytopenia observed. The oral maximum tolerated dose of pomalidomide was 2 mg/day. Treatment resulted in greater that 25% reduction in paraprotein in 67% of patients, with 17% of patients achieving a complete remission. This study demonstrated the activity and tolerability of this novel agent in relapsed MM and phase II studies are now starting in this population.

Proteasome Inhibitors

Through their unique mechanism of action, proteasome inhibitors have markedly extended the treatment armamentarium for MM (39). Bortezomib [(PS-341) Velcade®], a boronic acid dipeptide, is a first-in-class, selective, and reversible proteasome inhibitor and was the lead compound to undergo clinical testing. It was approved by the FDA for the treatment of relapsed and refractory MM, with accelerated approval given in 2003 and full approval in 2005.

Carfilzomib (PR-171), a selective, irreversible proteasome inhibitor, is now under-going evaluation in early phase clinical trials, as is another potent agent, a marine-derived small molecule, NPI-0052.

Specifically, proteasome inhibitors exert their effects through the inhibition of the nuclear factor (NF)-κB pathway. These compounds inhibit the chymotrypsin-like protease activity of the 20S proteasome (40).

Bortezomib reversibly inhibits the active-site N-terminal threonine residue located within the multi-unit 26S proteasome (41,42). Carfilzomib is a tetrapeptide ketoepoxide-based irreversible inhibitor of the chymotrypsin-like protease activity of the 20S proteasome (43). NPI-0052 is a small molecule derived from the fermentation of Salinospora, an acinomycete found in the Pacific Ocean, which is orally bioactive and is also selective but irreversible in its effects on the proteasome (44).

The NF-κB pathway has been shown to be an important target in MM. NF-κB is a transcription factor located within the cytoplasm of eukaryotic cells. I-κB is a family of cytoplasmic inhibitory proteins that contain multiple ankyrin repeats. I-κB binds to NF-κB in the cell cytoplasm, and thereby inhibits the ability of NF-κB to induce nuclear transcription (45). Particular cell signals that are released due to inflammation, stress, and radiation regulate I-κB serine phosphorylation, ubiquitination, and ultimate degradation by the proteasome (46).

Importantly, bortezomib has additional activity in refractory MM through its ability to resensitize malignant plasma cells to the effects of cytotoxic chemotherapy (4).

Bortezomib

Bortezomib gained accelerated approval in May 2003 for the treatment of patients with relapsed and refractory MM who had received at least two prior regimens. The FDA then approved its use for the treatment of relapsed disease following treatment with one prior regimen in 2005.

In a non-randomized, multicenter, Phase II trial evaluating the efficacy of bortezomib in patients with relapsed, refractory MM, 193 patients were evaluated after having received bortezomib $1.3 \, mg/m^2$ on days 1, 4, 8, and 11 every 21 days for a median duration of treatment of 3.8 months (47). Ninety-two percent of these patients had received three or more prior therapies, and almost all were refractory to their most recent therapy. Follow-up after 24 weeks of treatment revealed an OR which included MRs of 35%. Moreover, 27% of patients who received bortezomib achieved either a CR or PR. Of these responses, 4% developed CR and 6% achieved a near-CR (nCR) (myeloma protein only demonstrable by immunofixation) (47). The median overall survival and duration of response were 16 months and 12 months, respectively. Grade 4 toxicities included thrombocytopenia (3%), diarrhea, and neutropenia (3%), while grade 3 toxicities included but were not limited to: thrombocytopenia (28%), neutropenia (11%), and peripheral neuropathy (12%).

In a second Phase II study, 54 MM patients who progressed or relapsed after first-line therapy were evaluated (48). Two doses of bortezomib (1.0 and $1.3 \, mg/m^2$) were given twice weekly, of a 3-week cycle, for eight cycles. The CR and PR rates among those who received bortezomib $1.3 \, mg/m^2$ were 38%, while the CR and PR rate among those who received bortezomib $1.0 \, mg/m^2$ was 30%.

In the largest Phase III trial performed in patients with relapsed MM to date, bortezomib was compared with high dose dexamethasone in relapsed patients that had received up to three prior therapies (49). A total of 669 patients were enrolled and treated with ether bortezomib monotherapy ($n = 333$), at the usual dose and schedule for eight months or high dose dexamethasone ($n = 336$) at 40 mg orally on days 1–4, 9–12, and 17–20 for four cycles followed by treatment on days 1–4 for five cycles. Patients progressing on high-dose dexamethasone (dex) were allowed to crossover to the bortezomib on a companion study. The ORR at initial analysis was 38%

in the bortezomib arm versus 18% in the high-dose dex group, with a median TTP of 6.22 and 3.49 months for the bortezomib and high-dose dex arms, respectively. At 1-year follow up, the patients who received bortezomib had a statistically significant higher rate of overall survival than those who received high dose dex (80% vs. 66%). In terms of toxicity, grade 3 or 4 adverse events were higher in the bortezomib arm (primarily thrombocytopenia) but serious adverse events (including grade 3 or above infections and bleeding) were similar in both arms (49). This data confirmed the activity of bortezomib in this patient population and set the basis for its evaluation both in newly diagnosed disease and in combination with other novel agents, as well as conventional chemotherapeutic agents.

Bortezomib-Based Combinations

Given the improved response obtained when bortezomib is combined with dexamethasone and the results in vitro showing the bortezomib sensitize resistant MM cells to chemotherapy, bortezomib has been studied in combination with chemotherapy in multiple phase I and II studies.

The combination of oral cyclophosphamide, prednisone and bortezomib has been used to treat patients with relapsed/refractory MM (50). Response rates in 16 evaluable patients were around 50% including one complete remission. In another Phase II trial bortezomib was combined with cyclophosphamide and high dose dexamethasone. Fifty patients with relapsed MM were treated with this combination and ORR was 88% with a median event-free survival of 10 months (4).

Berenson et al. (51) reported results of a Phase I-II clinical trial evaluating the combination of bortezomib and melphalan in patients with relapsed myeloma. Bortezomib at doses of $1.0 \, mg/m^2$ given on days 1, 4, 8, and 11 every 28 days were combined with oral melphalan in escalating doses from 0.025 to 0.25 mg/kg on days 1–4 for a total of 8 cycles. The maximum tolerated dose was defined at $1.0 \, mg/m^2$ of bortezomib and 0.10 mg/kg of melphalan. Overall response was 68% in 34 evaluable patients with a progression free survival of 8 months. Adverse events included myelosuppresion and grade 1–2 neuropathy. The investigators concluded that bortezomib plus melphalan is an active combination with acceptable toxicity. This has led to the evaluation of this combination both in the newly diagnosed as well as in the peritransplant setting as conditioning regimen (4).

In another phase I/II trial, bortezomib was given at doses of 1.0 or $1.3 \, mg/m^2$ on the regular schedule, in combination with thalidomide in escalating doses from 50 to 200 mg daily (52). Patients who did not achieve at least a PR after 4 cycles were treated with dexamethasone 20 mg the day of and the day after the bortezomib. This regimen resulted in response rates of 55% in patients with relapsed myeloma. The combination was well tolerated and there was no significant development or worsening of neuropathy reported.

In another study doxorubicin was added to this combination and resulted in similar response rates (53). A randomized trial to compare these two combinations is ongoing.

Bortezomib-based treatment is also safe in high risk populations such as patients with renal failure, as well as in elderly patients and those with negative prognostic factors such as B2 microglobulin >2.5 mg/L and refractoriness to prior treatment (54).

The promising results obtained using bortezomib and combinations in this patient population have led to multiple studies evaluating these regimens in the upfront setting.

PR-171 (CARFILZOMIB)

There has been much research effort to develop more potent and selective proteasome inhibitors. This research has led to the development of carfilzomib (PR-171) (Proteolix, Inc.). carfilzomib is a potent and selective irreversible inhibitor of the chymotrypsin-like protease activity of the 20S proteasome that results in rapid proteasome inhibition, accumulation of ubiquinated proteins, and apoptosis of tumor cells. Carfilzomib inhibits the chymotrypsin-like activity of the proteasome with comparable potency of bortezomib. However, carfilzomib exhibits greater selectivity for the chymotrypsin-like activity and little activity against the trypsin-like or post-glutamyl peptide hydrolase (PGPH) activities of the proteasome, whereas bortezomib shows significant inhibition of the PGPH activity (55).

We evaluated the effects of carfilzomib on human MM cell survival, proteasome activity, and drug resistance (56). We found that carfilzomib directly inhibits proteasome activity, proliferation, and induces apoptosis in human MM sensitive and resistant cell lines, induces apoptosis in isolated MM cells from newly diagnosed and relapsed refractory patients, and overcomes de novo drug resistance. These studies provided the foundation for clinical investigations of carfilzomib to improve the outcome of patients with MM and other hematologic malignancies.

Two phase I dose-escalation studies have been initiated, aimed at determining the safety, tolerability, and clinical response to PR-171 in hematologic malignancies. Two different dose-intensive schedules are being used in these phase I studies. In PX-171-001, PR-171 is administered on a two-week cycle, QDx5 with nine days rest, while in PX-171-002; PR-171 is administered on a four-week cycle, QDx2 weekly for three weeks with 12 days rest. Both studies were initiated with a dose of 1.2 mg/m^2. On an update presented at ASH 2006, a total of 15 and 23 subjects have been enrolled in PX-171-001 and -002, respectively (57). PR-171 has been well tolerated at the highest doses thus far, 8.4 and 15 mg/m^2, respectively. Proteasome inhibition in whole blood at the highest dose levels exceeded 75%, and in peripheral blood mononuclear cells inhibition exceeded 65%, one hour after the first dose. There were no dose-limiting toxicities reported and no incidence of painful peripheral neuropathy on either study. Although transient renal dysfunction has been seen. The minium forward dose has not yet been identified on either study, but preliminary evidence of activity has been observed with reduction in myeloma paraprotein levels and symptomatic improvement in some patients on both protocols. These studies are ongoing and remain preliminary, but PR-171 data looks promising in terms of anti-MM activity and the tolerability in particular of the drug is encouraging. Phase II trials are being developed.

NPI-0052

NPI-0052 is a novel proteasome inhibitor shown to inhibit proteasome activity both in vitro and in vivo in clinically achievable doses. It has been shown to be a more potent inhibitor of NF-κB and related cytokine secretion than bortezomib, and it induces apoptosis in MM cell lines resistant to conventional chemotherapy and bortezomib (44). Importantly, it has been shown to overcome drug resistance conferred by the microenvironment. In vivo studies using human MM xenogratfs shows that NPI-0052 is well tolerated, prolongs survival, and reduces tumor recurrences. These studies provided the basis for the clinical evalution of this agent in MM. A Phase I study evaluating the safety and tolerability of NPI-0052 in relapsed, refractory MM is currently ongoing.

OTHER NOVEL THERAPIES

The pathophysiology of myeloma is now understood in significant detail at the molecular level. This knowledge has led to the development and testing of agents that target specific signaling pathways shown to be important for myeloma cell survival. Several examples of these agents and their target are included in Figure 1. Given the complexity of MM pathogenesis, it is unlikely that any of these agents alone will induce significant response, but it is very likely that they will have a significant impact when combined with backbone agents such as bortezomib, lenalidomide, or thalidomide. Currently there are multiple studies ongoing evaluating these combinations.

CONCLUSION

The better understanding of MM pathogenesis has undoubtedly led to major advances in treatment for these patients that have impacted survival and quality of life positively. While significant progress has been made, MM remains incurable and ongoing studies are trying to combine chemotherapy agents with novel therapies. Further understanding of the mechanism of drug resistance and the contribution of the microenvironment to MM

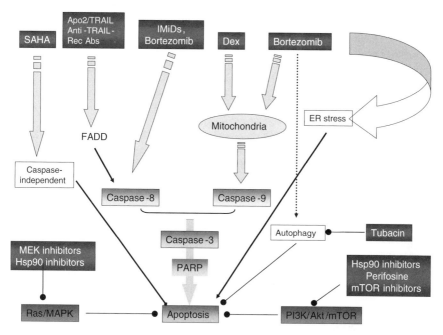

Figure 1 Agents that target specific signaling pathways that are important for myeloma cell survival. Current studies evaluating these agents in combination with bortezomib, lanalidomide, and thalidomide may yield significant results in the future. *Source*: Ref. 58.

pathogenesis is likely to result in the development of novel therapies or combinations that would ultimately lead to the cure of this disease.

REFERENCES

1. Anderson KC. Lenalidomide and thalidomide: mechanisms of action–similarities and differences. Semin Hematol 2005; 42(4 Suppl 4):S3–8.
2. Kalmadi S, Baz R, Mahindra A. Lenalidomide: the emerging role of a novel targeted agent in malignancies. Drugs Today (Barc) 2007; 43(2):85–95.
3. Anderson KC. Targeted therapy of multiple myeloma based upon tumor-microenvironmental interactions. Exp Hematol 2007; 35(4 Suppl 1):155–62.
4. Richardson PG, Mitsiades C, Ghobrial I, et al. Beyond single-agent bortezomib: combination regimens in relapsed multiple myeloma. Curr Opin Oncol 2006; 18(6):598–608.
5. Voorhes PM, Orlowski RZ. Emerging role of novel combinations for induction therapy in multiple myeloma. Clin Lymphoma Myeloma 2006; 7(1):33–41.
6. Ghobrial IM, Leleu X, Hatjijarissi E, et al. Emerging Drugs in Multiple Myeloma. Expert Opin Emerg Drugs 2007; 12(1):155–63.
7. Blade J, Samson D, Reece D, et al. Br J Haematol 1998 Sep; 102(5):1115–23.

8. Durie BG, Harrousseau JL, Miguel JS, et al. International uniform response criteria for multiple myeloma. Leukemia 2006; 20(9):1467–73. Epub 2006 July 20.

9. Kumar SK, Thernau TM, Gertz MA, et al. Clinical Course of patients with relapsed MM. Mayo Clin Proc 2004; 79:867–874.

10. Crane E. List A Immunomodulatory drugs. Cancer Invest 2005; 23(7):625–34.

11. Haslett PAJ, Corral LG, Albert M, et al. Thalidomide costimulates primary T lymphocytes, preferentially inducing proliferation, cytokine production, and cytotoxic responses in the CD 8+ subset. J Exp Med 1998; 187:1855–1892.

12. Singhal S, Mehta J, Desikan R, et al. Antitumor activity of thalidomide in refractory multiple myeloma. N Engl J Med 1999; 41:1565–1571.

13. Barlogie B, Desikan R, Eddlemon P, et al. Extended survival in advanced and refractory multiple myeloma after single agent thalidomide: identification of prognostic factors in a Phase 2 study of 169 patients. Blood 2001; 98(2):492–494.

14. Richardson P, Schlossman R, Jagannath S, Alsina M, et al. Thalidomide for patients with relapsed multiple myeloma after high-dose chemotherapy and stem cell transplantation: results of an open-label multicenter phase 2 study of efficacy, toxicity, and biological activity. Mayo Clin Proc 2004 Jul; 79(7):875–82.

15. Alexanian R, weber D, Anagnostopoulos A, et al. Thalidomide with or without dexamethasone for refractory or relapsing multiplemyeloma. Semin Hematol 2003; 40(4 suppl 4):3–7.

16. Palumbo A. Giaccone L, bertola A, et al. Low-dose thalidomide plus dexamethasone is an effective salvage regimen for advance dyeloma. Haematologica 2001; 86:399–403.

17. Glasmacher A, Hahn C, Hoffmann F et al. A systematic review of Phase II trials of thalidomide monotherapy in patients with relapsed or refractory multiple myeloma. Br J Haematol 2006; 132(5):584–593.

18. Rajkumar SV, Hayman S, Gertz MA, et al. Combination therapy with thalidomide plus Dexamethasone for newly diagnosed myeloma. J Clin Oncol 2006; 20(21):4319–4323.

19. Glasmacher A, Hahn C, Hoffmann F, et al. Thalidomide in relapsed or refractory patients with multiple myeloma:monotherapy or combination therapy? A report from systematic review. Blood 2005; 106:364b.

20. Dimopoulos MA, Zervas K, Kouvatseas G, et al. Thalidomide and dexamethasone combination for refractory multiple myeloma Ann Oncol 2001; 12:991–995.

21. Terpos E, Mihou D, Szydlo R, et al. The combination of intermediate doses of thalidomide with dexamethasone is an effective treatment for patients with relapsed/refractory multiple myeloma and normalizes abnormal bone remodeling through the reduction of s RANKL/osteoprotegerin ratio. Leukemia 2005; 19:1969–76.

22. Palumbo A, Falco P, Ambrosini MT, et al. Thalidomide plus dexamethasone is an effective salvage regimen for myeloma patients relapsing alter autologous transplant. Eur J Haematol 2005; 75(5):391–395.

23. Almhanna K, Suppiah R, Baz R, et al. Doxil, vincristine, rediced frequesncy Dexamethasone in combination with thalidomide(DVd-T), is associated with higher overall survival and progression free survival as compared to DVd in patients with multiple myeloma. Blood 2005; 106:718a.

24. Kropff MH, Lang N, Bisping G, et al. Hyperfractionated cyclophosphamide in combination with pulsed Dexamethasone and thalidomide in primary refractory or relapsed multiplemyeloma. Br J Haematol 122, 607–616.

25. Garcia-Sanz R, Gonzalez-Porras JR, Hernandez JM, et al. The oral combination of thalidomide, cyclophosphamide and dexamethasone (Thal CyDex) is effective in relapsed/refractory multiplemyeloma. Leukemia 2004; 18:856–863.

26. Kyriakou C. Thompson K, D'Sa S, et al. Low dose Thalidomide in combination with oral weekly cyclophosphamide and pulsed dexamethasone is a well tolerated and effective regimen in patients with relapsed and refractory multiple myeloma Br J Haematol 2005; 129:763–770.

27. Davies FE, Raje N, Hideshima T, et al. Thalidomide and immunomudalotory derivatives augment natural killer cell cytotoxicity in multiple myeloma. Blood 2001; 98(1):210–216.

28. Kumar S, Rajkumar SV. Thalidomide and lenalidomide in the treatment of multiple myeloma. Eur J Cancer 2006; 42(11):1612–22.

29. Richardson PG, Schlossman RL, Weller E, et al. Immunomodulatory drug CC-5013 overcomes durg resistance and is well tolerated in patients with relapsed multiple myeloma. Blood 2002; 100(9):3063–3067.

30. Zangari M, Tricot G, Zeldis J et al. Results of Phase I study of CC-5013 for the treatment of multiplemyeloma patienst who relapse after high dose chemotherapy (HDCT). Blood 2001; 98(11):775A (abstract 3226).

31. Richardson PG, Blood E, Mitisiades CS, et al. A randomized phase 2 study of lenalidomide therapy for patients with relapsed or relapsed and refractory multiple myeloma. Blood 2006; 108(10):3458–64.

32. Dimopoulos MA, Spencer A, Attal M, et al. Study of lenalidomide plus dexamethasone versus Dexamethasone alone in relapsed or refractory multiple myeloma: results of a Phase III study. Blood 2005; 106(11):6A.

33. Niesvizky R, Spencer A, Wang M, et al. Increased risk of thrombosis with lenalidomide in combination with Dexamethasone and erythropoietin. J Clin Oncol 2006; 24(18S):423 S (abstract 7506).

34. Baz R, Walker E, Karam MA, et al. Lenalidomide and pegylated liposomal doxorubicin-based chemotherapy for relapsed or refractory multiple myeloma: safety and efficacy. Ann Oncol 2006; 17(12):1766–71.

35. Knop S, Gerecke C, Topp MLenalidomide (Revlimid), Adriamycin and Dexamethasone Chemotherapy (RAD) is Safe and Effective in Treatment of Relapsed Multiple Myeloma—First Results of a German Multicenter Phase I/II Trial. Blood 108(11):Aabstract 408.

36. Richardson PG, Jagannath S, Avigan DE, Alsina M. Lenalidomide plus bortezomib (rev-vel) in relapsed and/or refractory multiple myeloma (MM): Final results of a multicenter phase 1 Trial. Blood 2006; 108(11):abstract 405.

37. Payvandi F, Wu L, Haley M, et al. Immunomodulatory drugs inhibit expression of cyclooxygenase-2 from TNF-alpha, IL-1beta, and LPS-

stimulated human PBMC in a partially IL-10-dependent manner. Cell Immunol 2004; 230(2):81–8.

38. Schey SA, Fields P, Barlett JB, et al. Phase I study of an immunomodulatory thalidomide analog, CC-4047, in relapsed or refractory multiple myeloma. J Clin Oncol 2004; 22(16):3269–76.

39. Adams J, Palombella VJ, Sausville EA, et al. A novel class fopotent adn effective antitumor agents. Cancer Res 1999; 59:2615–2622.

40. Goldberg AL, Stein R, Admas J. New insights into proteasome function: from Archaebacteria to drug development. Chem Biol 1995; 2(8):503–8.

41. Roccaro AM, Hideshima T, Richardson PG, et al. Bortezomib as an antitumor agent. Curr Pharm Biotechnol 2006; 7(6):441–8.

42. Teicher BA, Ara G, Herbst R, et al. The proteasome inhibitor PS-341 in cancer therapy. Clin Cancer Res 1999; 5(9):2638–45.

43. Ivancsits D, Nimmanapali R, Sun M, et al. The proteasome inhibitor PR-171 inhibits cell growth, induces apoptosis, and overcomes de novo and acquired drug resistance in human multiple myeloma cells. Blood 2005; 106(11):Abstract 1575.

44. Chauhan D, Hideshima T, Anderson KC. A novel proteasome inhibitor NPI-0052 as an anticancer therapy. Br J Cancer 2006; 95:961–965.

45. Hideshima T, Mitisiades C, Akiyama M, et al. Molecular mechanisms mediating antimyeloma activity of proteasome inhibitor PS-341. Blood 2003 Feb 15; 101(4):1530–4.

46. Adams J. The proteasome: structure, function, and role in the cell. Cancer Treat Rev 2003 May; 29(Suppl 1):3–9.

47. Richardson PG, Barlogie B, Berenson J, et al. A phase 2 study of bortezomib in relapsed, refractory myeloma. N Engl J Med 2003 Jun 26; 348(26):2609–17.

48. Jagannath S. Barlogie B, Berenson J, et al. A phase 2 study of two doses of bortezomib in relapsed or refractory myeloma. Br J Haematol 2004; 127(2): 165–172.

49. Richardson PG, Sonneveld P, Schister MW, et al. Bortezomib or high-dose Dexamethasone for relapsed multiple myeloma. N Eng J Med 2005; 352: 2487–2498.

50. Reece DE, Piza G, Trudel S, et al. A phase I-II trial of bortezomib and oral cyclophosphamide plus prednisone fro relapsed/refractory multiplemyeloma. Blood 2005; 106:718a.

51. Berenson J, Yang HH, Sadler K, et al. Phase I/II trial assessing bortezomib and melphalan combination therapy for the treatment of patients with relapsed or refractory multiple myeloma. J Clin Oncol 2006; 24(6):937–944.

52. Zangari M, Barlogie B, Burns MJ, et al. velcade-(V), Thalidomide(T), Dexamethasone(D) for advanced and refractory multiple myeloma(MM): long term follow up of phase I-II trial UARK 2001-37: superior outcome in patients with normal cytogenetic and no prior T. Blood 2005; 106:717a.

53. Holming K, Stover J, Talamo G, et al. Bortezomib (Velcade), + Adriamycin + Thalidomide + Dexamethasone, (VATD), as an effective regimen in patients with refractory or relapsed multiple myeloma (MM). Blood 2004; 104:659a.

54. Chanan-Khan A, Richardson P, Lonial S, et al. Safety and efficacy of bortezomib in multiple myeloma patients with renal failure requiring dialysis. Blood 2005; 106:716a.

55. Stapnes C, Doskelan AP, Hatfield K, et al. The proteasome inhibitors bortezomib and PR-171 have antiproliferative and proapoptotic effects on primary human acute myeloid leukaemia cells. Br J Haematol 2007; 136(6): 814–28.
56. Owen A. O'Connor, Robert Z. Orlowski. Melissa Alsina multicenter phase I studies to evaluate the safety, tolerability, and clinical response to intensive dosing with the proteasome inhibitor PR-171 in patients with relapsed or refractory hematological malignancies. Blood 2006; 108(11):Abstract 2430.
57. Richardson PG. Schlossman R, Munshi N, Anderson KC. Management Strategies for Relapsed Multiple Myeloma. Amer J Canc 2006; 5(6): 393–406.
58. Ghobrial IM. Ghobrial J, Mitsiades C, Leleu X, Hatjiharissi E, Moreau A, Roccaro A, Schlossman R, Hideshima T, Anderson KC, Richardson PG. Novel therapeutic avenues in myeloma: changing the treatment paradigm. Oncology June 2007; in press.

10

High-Dose Therapy in Multiple Myeloma

Jean-Luc Harousseau

Hospitalier Universitaire de Nantes, Nantes, France

INTRODUCTION

Bone marrow transplantation (BMT) was introduced in the treatment of multiple myeloma (MM) in the eighties. Twenty five years later, the role of BMT remains a matter of controversy.

In the autologous setting, the use of peripheral blood stem cells instead of bone marrow has markedly improved feasibility. Since randomized studies have shown the superiority of autologous stem cell transplantation (ASCT) compared to conventional chemotherapy (CC), ASCT has become the standard of care, at least for younger patients (up to the age of 65) without renal failure. However, ASCT is currently challenged again by the introduction of novel agents such as thalidomide, bortezomib or, lenalidomide.

In the allogeneic setting, the immunological effect of donor's lymphoid cells, the so-called graft versus myeloma effect explains some long remissions and possible cures. However, the major issue is transplant-related mortality related to graft versus host disease (GVHD) and infection. Reduced intensity conditioning (RIC) allogeneic SCT has been developed with the objective of reducing transplant-related mortality while harnessing the graft versus myeloma effect.

Autologous Stem Cell Transplantation

Autologous Stem Cell Transplantation Versus Conventional Chemotherapy

Two randomized studies from France and UK showed that ASCT is superior to CC in terms of response rate, event-free survival (EFS) and overall survival

(OS) (1,2). As a consequence, until now, ASCT has been considered the standard of care and is usually proposed initially to younger patients (less than 65 years of age) or even to older fit patients. Another important finding from these studies was that OS is strongly dependent on the achievement of complete remission (CR) or at least very good partial remission (VGPR) (1). This led to two changes in the management of patients with MM.

1. CR achievement is now considered one of the objectives of any treatment, specially for newly diagnosed patients.
2. It appeared necessary to redefine response criteria in order to introduce these types of response which were rarely obtained previously with CC (3,4).

However, ASCT cannot be proposed to all patients with MM. Usually it is limited to patients up to 65 years of age, with a performance status 0–2 and a normal renal function (5). The issue of age limits is important since the median age of MM at diagnosis is currently over 65 years. ASCT is feasible in selected older patients (6) but the usual dose of melphalan (200 mg/m^2) is probably too toxic for patients over the age of 70 (7). The Turin group has evaluated two to three courses of intermediate doses of Melphalan (100 mg/m^2) supported by ASCT. They first showed that this approach was feasible even on an outpatient basis in patients up to 75 years of age and that the outcome was apparently superior to the historical results achieved with CC (8). They then performed a randomized study comparing this approach to the classical melphalan-prednisone (MP) oral regimen in patients aged 50–70 years (9) and showed that intermediate dose melphalan was superior to MP in terms of CR progression-free survival (PFS) and OS, even in the subgroup of patients aged 65–70.

The IFM recently completed a three-arm randomized study comparing this regimen with MP and with MP plus thalidomide (MPT) in patients aged 65–75 (10). Although the CR-VGPR rate achieved with 2 courses of melphalan 100 mg/m^2 was comparable to that achieved with MPT (43% vs. 50%) and dramatically superior to MP (8%), relapses were rapid. Median PFS and OS were not significantly different between MP and melphalan 100 mg/m^2 (17.2 vs. 19 months and 30.3 vs. 38.6 months, respectively). One possible explanation for this discrepancy between the Italian and the French study is that, in the Italian study, maintenance therapy with interferon plus dexamethasone was administered. Another difference is the upper age limit since in the Italian study patients over 70 years of age were not eligible. However, results of the IFM study do not support the use of ASCT in older patients out of a clinical trial.

Recent Concerns Regarding the Role of ASCT

Two recently published randomized studies raised concerns due to the lack of significant benefit from ASCT as compared to CC (11,12). In the first one from Spain, only patients responding to their initial chemotherapy were randomized between ASCT and further CC (11). Although the CR rate was significantly higher in the ASCT arm (30% vs. 11%) there was no difference as regards EFS and OS. Compared to other randomized studies where randomization was performed at diagnosis, the design of this trial introduced a selection bias, and, indeed, only 75% of the patients entering the study were randomized. This could be of importance since ASCT is a useful salvage treatment for patients with primary refractory MM. Moreover, although there was no significant difference in PFS between ASCT and CC, the median PFS was better in the ASCT arm (42 vs. 33 months). With more patients, this difference might have become significant.

In the large US Intergroup trial, 516 patients up to the age of 70 were randomized after induction therapy with VAD between CC and ASCT (12).

There was no difference between the two groups in terms of response rate, PFS, and OS.

How can we explain these discrepancies between this trial and the French and British trials? First, as in the Spanish study, patients were randomized only after the induction CC, and only 63% of patients who entered the study were actually randomized, which may again represent a selection bias. Second, a significant number of patients allocated to the CC arm did actually receive ASCT at the time of progression. Fermand et al. (13) have published a randomized trial showing no difference in OS between early (upfront) and late (at the time of progression) ASCT. But the most probable explanation is that, while results achieved with ASCT in this trial are quite comparable to those achieved in the other ones, results achieved with CC are much better, as shown in Table 1. Interestingly, the CR rates achieved with CC and ASCT were almost identical.

Table 1   Comparison of U.S. Intergroup Trial with the IFM 90 and MRC 7 Trials

	No. of Patients	CR rate		EFS		OS	
		CC (%)	ASCT (%)	CC	ASCT	CC	ASCT
IFM 90 (updated results in 5)	200	5	22	Median: 18 mos 7-year: 8%	28 mos 16%	44 mos 27%	57 mos 43%
MRC 7 (2)	401	8	44	Median: 19 mos	31 mos	42 mos	54 mos
U.S. Intergroup S 9321 (12)	516	17	17	7-year: 16%	17%	42%	37%

Abbreviations: ASCT, autologous stem cell transplantation; CC, conventional chemotherapy; CR, complete remission; EFS, event-free survival; OS, overall survival.

The lessons from these randomized studies are the following:

- ASCT should not be restricted to patients responding to their initial chemotherapy but should also be offered to patients with primary refractory MM.
- ASCT improves the outcome mostly by increasing the CR+VGPR rate.
- ASCT is superior to standard CC. But when results of CC are improved (specially with CR rates comparable to those achieved with high-dose therapy), the benefit of ASCT is no more significant.

However, comparison of CC and ASCT is no longer a relevant question since results of ASCT have already been improved compared to those achieved in the nineties. Two different approaches have contributed to this improvement in the past few years: further dose intensification and introduction of novel agents.

Further Dose-Intensification

Double ASCT

The first step in this context was the introduction of double intensive therapy (14), with the objective of increasing the CR rate. The Arkansas group developed a double ASCT program both in newly diagnosed patients and in relapsed patients (15). In newly diagnosed patients, the CR rate increased at each step of the procedure. This better tumor cell reduction was translated into encouraging median EFS and OS of 43 and 68 months, respectively (16).

The IFM was the first to conduct a randomized trial comparing simple and double ASCT in 399 patients up to 60 years of age (17). The 7-year EFS and OS were significantly improved in the double ASCT arm (respectively 20% vs. 10% and 42% vs. 21%). Two other recently published, randomized studies show a longer EFS (18,19) and the preliminary results of two other randomized studies are also in favor of double ASCT (20–21).

The feasibility of double ASCT was confirmed by the IFM 94 trial since 75% of patients did receive the second ASCT, and the toxic death rate was <5% (17). However, many investigators considered the benefit of this approach as marginal and were concerned by the issues of cost and morbidity. Therefore, it appeared important to define the population of patients who benefit more from this aggressive management. In the IFM 94 trial, the only parameter that could define a group of patients who did not benefit for double ASCT was the response to the first ASCT (17). Patients with less than 90% reduction of their M-component after one ASCT had a longer OS in the double ASCT arm, while patients in CR or VGPR after the first had the same OS with or without the second.

In the Arkansas and the IFM experience, patients with favorable prognostic factors (low β2 microglobulin or high albumin levels, no cytogenetics abnormalities) could enjoy very long remissions while patients with high β2 microglobulin level and/or cytogenetic abnormalities have a poor prognosis even with double ASCT (22–24).

In an attempt to further improve results of double ASCT, Barlogie and colleagues have evaluated a more intensive regimen termed "Total Therapy 2" with 4 consecutive phases: increased intensity induction treatment (including combination chemotherapy with dexamethasone, cyclophosphamide, etoposide, and platinum), tandem ASCT, consolidation chemotherapy, and maintenance with interferon and dexamethasone (25). In this trial, patients were randomized to receive or not thalidomide from initiation of the treatment. Comparison of 345 patients treated with the Total Therapy 2 arm without thalidomide and 231 patients previously treated with the Total Therapy 1 program showed that although the CR rates were identical (43% vs. 41%), the 5-year probability of continuous CR (45% vs. 32%, $p < 0.001$) and the 5-year EFS (43% vs. 28%, $p < 0.001$) were superior in the Total Therapy 2 program. This was translated into a trend for improved OS (62% vs. 57%, $p = 0.11$). Although not randomized, this comparison is in favor of the more intensive regimen and specially of post-ASCT consolidation.

The IFM also proposed a more intensive regimen in the IFM 99 trial but only to patients with poor-risk factors (high β2 microglobulin level + del 13 by FISH analysis) (26). This subgroup of 219 patients received double ASCT with an increased dose of melphalan (220 mg/m^2) prior to the second. The CR + VGPR rate increased from 34% after one ASCT to 51% after 2 ASCT, which translated into encouraging median EFS and OS (30 and 41 months), respectively. These results appeared to be superior to those previously achieved in poor-risk patients.

In conclusion, dose-intensification including double ASCT is a relatively safe procedure and apparently improves the outcome as compared to single ASCT. However, it is considered a cumbersome strategy by many patients and physicians and induces significant morbidity. Moreover, results in patients with poor-risk MM remain unsatisfactory, which explains the recent interest in the evaluation of novel agents in combination with ASCT.

Novel Agents in Combination with ASCT

The second way to improve results of ASCT is to use novel agents which do not have the same mode of action as cytotoxic chemotherapy agents. In the past few years three agents (thalidomide, bortezomib, and lenalidomide) have been introduced in the therapy of MM. Although their mechanism of action is not currently fully understood, they are not only active on the myeloma cells but also on the microenvironment and on the interactions between the myeloma clone and the bone marrow stromal cells. Immediately after the stimulating results obtained in relapsed/refractory patients with thalidomide (27), bortezomib (28,29), and lenalidomide (30,31), these agents have been tested in newly diagnosed patients both in older patients and in the context of ASCT. Currently, the most mature data have been obtained with thalidomide.

The impact of adding thalidomide to a double ASCT program was evaluated in the randomized Total Therapy 2 program (32). In this study, 323 patients were randomly assigned to receive thalidomide from the onset until disease progression or adverse effects while 345 patients did not receive thalidomide. The thalidomide arm was significantly superior in terms of CR rate (62% vs. 43%, $p < 0.001$) and of five-year EFS (56% vs. 41%, $p = 0.01$). However there was no difference in the 5-year OS (65% in both groups) due to a shorter survival after relapse (median 1.1 vs. 2.7 years $p = 0.001$). Relapses in the thalidomide arm appeared to be more resistant than in the control arm. Patients in the no-thalidomide arm had an obvious benefit from thalidomide salvage treatment at relapse. Since in this arm, 85% of patients received thalidomide after relapse, this study was actually a comparison between thalidomide upfront and thalidomide as rescue treatment in the context of a double ASCT program. Moreover, the combination of chemotherapy and thalidomide during induction treatment, induced a high incidence of deep-vein thrombosis (30%) and peripheral neuropathy grade >2 was observed in 27% of patients.

This study shows the potential interest of adding thalidomide but also raises the issue of the optimal timing, dose, and duration of treatment.

In the IFM 99-02 trial, thalidomide was evaluated as maintenance therapy after double ASCT in patients under the age of 65 and with standard prognosis (0 or 1 adverse prognostic factors defined as was β2 microglobulin >3mg/L or del 13 by FISH analysis) (33). In this 3-arm study, 597 patients responding to double ASCT were randomly allocated to receive no further treatment, pamidronate or pamidronate plus thalidomide (up to 400 mg/day).

The 3-year EFS was 52% in the thalidomide arm versus 36% in the control arm and 37% in the pamidronate arm. This was converted into a longer 4-year OS (87% in the thalidomide arm versus 77% and 74% in the other 2 arms). However, the benefit was significant only in patients who had not achieved CR or VGPR after the second ASCT and was therefore mostly due to an increase of the CR + VGPR rate (from 50% after two ASCT to 68%). Although deep vein thrombosis was rare (2%) due to the use of thalidomide alone, peripheral neuropathy was noted in 68% of patients and was the main reason for drug discontinuation. In this study, the median dose of thalidomide was 200 mg/day, and the median duration of treatment was 15 months.

The difference in OS benefit between the two studies raises the issue of the value of prolonged maintenance therapy. Since in the IFM study, patients in CR or VGPR after double ASCT did not benefit from thalidomide maintenance, the interest of post-ASCT thalidomide could be mostly to increase the CR rate. If this hypothesis is true, thalidomide could be used only as a consolidation treatment and could be prescribed for a limited period since responses with thalidomide usually occur rapidly. This strategy could also reduce the risk of side effects specially of peripheral neuropathy.

The impact of bortezomib or lenalidomide as post-ASCT maintenance is currently evaluated in randomized trials that are ongoing in the US and in Europe.

Novel agents could also be used as part of the induction treatment prior to ASCT. In the US, the combination of thalidomide plus dexamethasone has already replaced dexamethasone alone or combined to chemotherapy like in the VAD regimen and has recently been approved by the FDA. This is partly based on the results of a randomized study showing that thalidomide + dexamethasone yielded more responses than thalidomide alone but at the expense of a greater toxicity (34).

In a retrospective analysis, the remission rate achieved with thalidomide plus dexamethasone was also superior to that achieved with VAD (35). However in both studies, the CR rate was not superior in the thalidomide/dexamethasone group. Whether the higher remission rate will be translated into a higher post-ASCT CR rate and into a longer remission duration is still unknown. Preliminary results of two multicenter randomized trials suggest that, despite a higher response rate after induction treatment with thalidomide plus dexamethasone, the post-ASCT CR rates are not superior to those achieved with VAD (36,37). Moreover, in all these studies the increased incidence of deep-vein thrombosis in the groups of patients receiving thalidomide was a concern (34–37).

Several Phase II trials have also evaluated the impact of Bortezomib given prior to ASCT in combination with dexamethasone (38,39) or chemotherapy (40,41). Preliminary results are encouraging in terms of efficacy and safety. High CR rates are achieved and since stem cell collection is feasible, these combinations are currently tested prior to ASCT in randomized trials. The combination of lenalidomide with dexamethasone is also an attractive induction regimen (42). Combinations of thalidomide plus bortezomib with dexamethasone (43) or with multiagent chemotherapy (44) have also been evaluated. The CR rates are impressive but, in the absence of randomized trials, the impact of these combinations compared to simpler regimens like thalidomide or bortezomib plus dexamethasone is still unknown.

Are Novel Agents Going to Replace ASCT?

In the IFM study for patients aged 65–75 years, the MPT arm was superior to the other 2 arms (MP, and intermediate dose melphalan + ASCT) (10). The high CR + VGPR achieved with MPT was translated into PFS and OS significantly longer than in the intensive arm (median PFS 29.5 vs. 19 months; median OS not reached at 56 vs. 38.6 months).

Palumbo et al. (45) have also compared MP and MPT in a recently published randomized trial. Their results are quite comparable to those achieved in the IFM 9906 trial with a significant superiority of MPT in terms of CR rate and EFS. The absence of significant OS benefit is possibly due to the short follow-up time.

Although there are still some concerns regarding the toxicity of this regimen, MPT represents the first improvement over MP in this age group and should currently be considered the standard of care for elderly patients. Moreover MPT yields CR+ VGPR and survival rates that are comparable to those achieved with single ASCT (Table 2).

Impressive preliminary results have also been obtained with bortezomib or lenalidomide combined with MP (46,47). In a phase I/II study of bortezomib plus MP in 60 untreated MM patients aged at least 65 years, Mateos et al. (46) have obtained 89% response rate including 32% immunofixation-negative CR and a very encouraging 83% EFS at 16 months. A high response rate has also been observed with Lenalidomide + MP in 54 patients older than 55 years at the expense of frequent grade 3–4 hematologic toxicity (47).

These combinations have been evaluated in older patients but would probably have obtained at least similar response rates in younger patients. Therefore, some investigators already consider that ASCT could be replaced by one of these combinations, or at least that new randomized studies should compare again ASCT and CC including novel agents. However, while in the past the arguments against ASCT have been cost and morbidity, it should be noted that these new combinations will be expensive and carry the risk of acute complications like thromboembolism or chronic sequelae like peripheral neuropathy. Moreover, as already stated, results of ASCT

Table 2 Comparison of Conventional Chemotherapy + Thalidomide with Single and Double ASCT Programs

	MPT		ASCT		Double ASCT	
	Palumbo (45)	Facon (10)	Attal (1)	Child (2)	IFM 99	TT2 Thal (32)
CR (%)	16	15	22	44	54.5[a]	62
Median EFS	29	29.5 mos	27 mos	31 mos	36 mos	5-year, 56%
Median OS		NR at 56 mos	57 mos	54 mos	NR at 66 mos	5-year, 65%

[a] Iincluding VGPR.

Abbreviations: ASCT, autologous stem cell transplantation; CR, complete remission; EFS, event-free survival; MPT, melphalan=prednisome+thalidomide; NR, not reached; OS, overall survival; VGPR, very good partial remission.

have recently improved and appear to be superior to those achieved with MP + novel agents (Table 2). Rather that opposing ASCT and novel agents, it should be more useful to combine them with the objective of increasing the CR rate, prolonging the remission duration, and decreasing the need for a second ASCT.

ALLOGENEIC STEM CELL TRANSPLANTATION

Standard Allogeneic Stem Cell Transplantation

Allogeneic SCT with a conventional myeloablative preparative regimen has a limited role in MM. Although it is probably the only curative treatment, its use is limited by toxicity. It can be proposed only to patients aged less than 55 years with an Hla identical donor which represents a small minority of patients. Even in younger patients, transplant-related mortality remains high as a consequence of GVHD and infections.

A retrospective analysis of the European experience had suggested that results could be improved by earlier transplants (48). However two multicenter trials with upfront allogeneic ASCT yielded poor results (12,49).

Therefore the great majority of investigators have stopped standard allogeneic SCT in MM.

Reduced Intensity Conditioning Allogeneic Stem Cell Transplantation

The so-called graft versus myeloma effect of the allogeneic graft has been demonstrated by donor lymphocytes injections in patients relapsing after allogeneic SCT. Non-myeloablative or RIC regimens prior to allogeneic SCT represent a new hope.

The objective is to reduce transplant-related toxicity while harnessing graft versus myeloma effect related to the donor immune system.

Non-myeloablative RIC are associated with a much lower transplant-related mortality and can be proposed to older patients (up to 65 years of age) even with unrelated donors (50).

However, relapses are frequent when tumor burden at transplantation is high (51,52).

Therefore, a strategy combining tumor burden reduction with high-dose therapy plus ASCT and RIC allogeneic transplantation has been developed in the past few years.

Several groups have published their experience with this approach (53–55). The short-term results shown are encouraging, but these studies raise several concerns:

1. Although this strategy is considerably less toxic than myeloablative allogeneic SCT, 1-year transplant-related mortality remains at 10–15%.
2. Chronic GVHD remains a frequent complication, which causes added morbidity and mortality and can seriously impair quality of life.

3. In the majority of studies follow-up time is still short. With more follow-up the relapse rate increases. It appears that relapse rate is decreased in patients with chronic GVHD. Therefore, attempts to reduce GVHD incidence and severity could increase post transplantation relapse.

With these results and knowing the results of less dangerous approaches like ASCT or even CC combined with novel agents it appears difficult to propose this tandem approach ASCT/RIC allogeneic SCT to all patients. The IFM group has compared tandem ASCT/RIC also SCT and double ASCT in patients with high-risk MM (b2 microglobulin level >3 mg/L and del 13 by FISH analysis). There was no significant difference between the two treatments. However, while in the RIC allo group, transplant-related mortality was acceptable, the major cause of failure was relapse (56). Relapse rate might be decreased by the use of different preparative regimens and graft versus host prophylaxis or by introducing novel agents after RIC allo SCT (57,58). Although recently published results from Italy look very encouraging, clinical trials evaluating the impact of tandem auto-RIC allo in selected patients with MM are still necessary.

REFERENCES

1. Attal M, Harousseau JL, Stoppa AM, et al. A randomized prospective trial of autologous bone marrow transplantation and chemotherapy in multiple myeloma. N Engl J Med 1996; 335:91–7.
2. Child JA, Morgan GJ, Davies FE, et al. High-dose chemotherapy with Hematopoietic stem-cell rescue for multiple myeloma. N Engl J Med 2003; 348: 1875–83.
3. Blade J, Samson D, Reece D, et al. Criteria for evaluating disease response and progression in patients with multiple myeloma treated with high-dose therapy and haematopoietic stem cell transplantation. Br J Haematol 1998; 102:1115–23.
4. Durie BGM, Harousseau JL, San Miguel J, et al. International uniform response criteria for multiple myeloma. Leukemia 2006; 20:1467–73.
5. Harousseau JL. Role of Transplantation in Myeloma. Hematology 2002. ASH Educational Program Book 221–7.
6. Siegel DS, Desikan KR, Nehta J, et al. Age is not a prognostic variable with autotransplants for multiple myeloma. Blood 1999; 93:51–4.
7. Badros A, Barlogie B, Siegel E, et al. Autologous stem cell transplantation in elderly multiple myeloma patients over the age of 70 years. Br J Haematol 2001; 114:600–7.
8. Palumbo A, Triolo S, Argentin C. Dose intensive melphalan with stem-cell support is superior to standard treatment in elderly myeloma patients. Blood 1999; 94:1248–53.
9. Palumbo A, Bringhen S, Petrucci MT, et al. Intermediate-dose Melphalan improves survival of myeloma patients aged 50–70: results of a randomized controlled trial. Blood 2004; 3052–57.
10. Facon T, Mary JY, Harousseau JL. Superiority of melphalan and prednisone plus thalidomide over melphalan and prednisone alone or autologous stem cell

transplantation in the treatment of newly diagnosed elderly patients with multiple myeloma. J Clin Oncol 2006; 24:1s (abstract).

11. Blade J, Rosinol L, Sureda A, et al. High-dose therapy intensification compared with continued standard chemotherapy in multiple myeloma patients responding to the initial chemotherapy; long-term results from a prospective randomized trial from the Spanish cooperative group PETHEMA. Blood 2005; 106:3755–9.

12. Barlogie B, Kyle RA, Anderson KC, et al. Standard chemotherapy compared with high-dose chemoradiotherapy for multiple myeloma: final results of Phase III US Intergroup trial S9321. J Clin Oncol 2006; 24:929–36.

13. Fermand JP, Ravaud P, Chevret S, et al. High-dose therapy and autologous peripheral blood stem cell transplantation in multiple myeloma: upfront or rescue treatment. Blood 1998; 92:3131–3136.

14. Harousseau JL, Milpied N, Laporte JP, et al. Double-intensive therapy in high-risk multiple myeloma. Blood 1992; 79:3131–6.

15. Vesole D, Barlogie B, Jagannath S, et al. High-dose therapy for refractory multiple myeloma: improved prognosis with better supportive care and double transplants. Blood 1994; 84:950–956.

16. Barlogie B, Jagannath S, Desikan KR, et al. Total therapy with tandem transplant for newly diagnosed multiple myeloma. Blood 1999; 93:55–65.

17. Attal M, Harousseau JL, Facon T, et al. Single versus double autologous stem cell transplantation for multiple myeloma. N Engl J Med 2003; 349:2495–502.

18. Sonneveld P, Van Der Holt B, Segeren CM, et al. Intermediate dose Melphalan compared with myeloablative treatment in multiple myeloma. long-term follow up of the Dutch Cooperative group HOVON 24 trial. Haematologica 2007; 92: 928–35.

19. Cavo M, Tosi P, Zamagni E, et al. Prospective randomized study of single compared with double autologous stem-cell transplantation for multiple myeloma Belogna 93 clinical study. J Clin Oncol 2007; 25:234–41.

20. Goldschmidt H. Single versus double high dose therapy in multiple myeloma: second analysis of the trial GMMG-HD2. Haematologica 2005; 90(suppl 1):38 (abstract).

21. Fermand JP. High dose therapy supported with autologous blood stem cell transplantation in multiple myeloma: long-term follow-up of the prospective-studies of the MAG group. Haematologica 2005; 90(t suppl 1):40.

22. Desikan R, Barlogie B, Sawyer J, et al. Results of high dose therapy for 1000 patients with multiple myeloma: durable complete remission and superior survival in the absence of chromosome 13 abnormalities. Blood 2000; 95: 4008–10.

23. Facon T, Avet-Loiseau H, Guillerm G, et al. Chromosome 13 abnormalities identified by FISH analysis and serum $\alpha 2$ microglobulin produce powerful myeloma staging system for patients receiving high-dose therapy. Blood 2001; 97:1566–71.

24. Barlogie B, Shaughnessy J, Tricot G, et al. Treatment of multiple myeloma. Blood 2004; 103:20–32.

25. Barlogie B, Tricot G, Rasmussen E, et al. Total therapy 2 without thalidomide in comparison with total therapy 1: role of intensified induction and post-transplantation consolidation therapies. Blood 2006; 107:2633–38.

26. Moreau P, Hullin C, Garban F, et al. Tandem autologous stem cell transplantation in high-risk de novo multiple myeloma: final results of the prospective and randomized IFM 99-04 protocol. Blood 2006; 107:397–403.

27. Singhal S, Mehta J, Desikan R. Antitumor activity of Thalidomide in refractory multiple myeloma. N Engl J Med 1999; 341:1565–71.

28. Richardson PR, Barlogie B, Berenson J, et al. A phase 2 study of bortezomib in relapsed, refractory myeloma. N Engl J Med 2003; 348:2609–17.

29. Richardson PG, Sonneveld P, Schuster MW, et al. Bortezomib or high-dose dexamethasone for relapsed multiple myeloma. N Engl J Med 2005; 352: 2487–98.

30. Dimopoulos MA, Spencer A, Attal M, et al. Study of lenalidomide plus dexamethasone versus dexamethasone alone in relapsed or refractory multiple myeloma (MM): results of a phase 3 study (MM-010). Blood 2005; 106:6a–7a (abstract).

31. Weber DM, Chen C, Niesvizky R, et al. Lenalidomide plus high-dose dexamethasone provides improved overall survival compared to high-dose dexamethasone alone for relapsed or refractory multiple myeloma (MM): Results of a North American phase III study (MM-009). J Clin Oncol 2006; 24: 4275 (abstract).

32. Barlogie B, Tricot G, Anaissie E, et al. Thalidomide and hematopoietic cell transplantation for multiple myeloma. N Engl J Med 2006; 354:1021–30.

33. Attal M, Harousseau JL, Leyvraz S, et al. Maintenance therapy with thalidomide improves survival in multiple myeloma patients. Blood 2006 Nov 15; 108(10):3289–94.

34. Rajkumar V, Blaad E, Vesole D, et al. Phase III clinical trial of Thalidomide plus Dexamethasone compared with Dexamethasone alone in newly diagnosed multiple myeloma: a clinical trial coordinated by the Eastern Cooperative Oncology Group. J Clin Oncol 2006; 24:431–6.

35. Cavo M, Zamagni E, Tosi P, et al. Superiority of Thalidomide and Dexamethasone over Vincristine-Doxorubicine-Dexamethasone (VAD) as primary therapy in preparation for autologous transplantation for multiple myeloma. Blood 2005; 106:35–9.

36. Goldschmidt H, Sonneveld P, Breitkreuz I, et al. HOVON 50/GMMG-HD3 trial: Phase III study on the effect of Thalidomide combined with high-dose Melphalan in myeloma patients up to 65 years. Blood 2005; 106:28a (abstract).

37. Macro M, Divine M, Uzunban Y, et al. Dexamethasone + Thalidomide compared to VAD as pre-transplant treatment in newly diagnosed multiple myeloma: a randomized trial. Blood 2006; 108, 22a (Abstract).

38. Jagannath S, Durie B, Wolf J, et al. Bortezomib therapy alone and in combination with Dexamethasone for previously untreated symptomatic multiple myeloma. Br J Haematol 2005; 129:776–83.

39. Harousseau JL, Attal M. Bortezomib plus Dexamethasone as induction treatment prior to autologous stem cell transplantation in patients with newly diagnosed multiple myeloma. Haematologica 2006 Nov; 91(11):1498–505.

40. Oakervee HE, Popat R, Curry N, et al. PAD combination therapy (PS341, Doxorubicin and Dexamethasone) for untreated multiple myeloma. Br J Haematol 2005; 755–62.

41. Popat R, Oakervee HE, Curry N, et al. Reduced dose PAD (PS 341, Adriamycin and Dexamethasone) for previously untreated patients with multiple myeloma. Blood 2005; 106:717a (abstract).
42. Rajkumar SV, Hayman SR, Lacy MQ, et al. Combination therapy with lenalidomide plus dexamethasone for newly diagnosed myeloma. Blood 2005; 106:4050–53.
43. Wang M, Delaballe K, Giralt S, et al. Rapid control of previously untreated multiple myeloma with Bortezomib-Thalidomide-Dexamethasone followed by early intensive therapy. Blood 2005; 106:231a (abstract).
44. Barlogie B, Tricot G, Rasmussen E, et al. Total therapy incorporating Velcade into upfront management of multiple myeloma: comparison with TT2 + Thalidomide. Blood 2005; 106:337a (Abstract).
45. Palumbo A, Bringhen S, Caravita T, et al. Oral Melphalan and prednisone chemotherapy plus thalidomide compared with melphalan and prednisone alone in elderly patients with multiple myeloma: randomised controlled trial. Lancet 2006; 367:825–31.
46. Mateos MV, Hernandez JM, Gutierrez WC, et al. Bortezomib plus melphalan and prednisone in elderly untreated patients with multiple myeloma: results of a multicenter phase I/II study. Blood 2006, online.
47. Palumbo A, Falco P, Falcone A, et al. Oral Revlimid plus Melphalan and Prednisone for newly diagnosed multiple myeloma: results of a multicenter phase I/II study. Blood 2006; 108:240a (abstract).
48. Gahrton G, Svensson H, Cavo M, et al. Progress in allogeneic bone marrow and peripheral blood stem cell transplantation for multiple myeloma: a comparison between transplants performed 1983–93 and 1994–98 at European Group for Blood and Marrow Transplantation Centres. Br J Haematol 2001; 113:209–16.
49. Lockhorst HM, Segeren CM, Verdonck LF, et al. Partially T-Cell depleted allogeneic stem cell transplantation for first-line treatment of multiple myeloma: a prospective evaluation of patients treated in the phase III study HOVON 20MM. J Clin Oncol 2003; 21:1728–33.
50. Kroger N, Sayer HG, Schwerdtfeger R, et al. Unrelated stem cell transplantation in multiple myeloma after a reduced-intensity conditioning with pretransplantation antithymocyte globulin is highly effective with low transplantation-related mortality. Blood 2002; 100:3919–24.
51. Giralt S, Aleman A, Anagnostopoulos A, et al. Fludarabine/Melphalan conditioning for allogeneic transplantation in patients with multiple myeloma. Bone Marrow Transplant 2002; 30:367–73.
52. Einsele H, Shäfer HJ, Hebart H, et al. Follow-up of patients with progressive myeloma undergoing allo grafts after reduced-intensity conditioning. Br J Haematol 2003; 121:411–8.
53. Badros A, Barlogie B, Spegel E, et al. Improved outcomes of allogeneic transplantation in high-risk multiple myeloma patients after non myeloablative conditioning. J Clin Oncol 2002; 20:1295–303.
54. Kroger N, Schilling G, Einsele H, et al. Deletion of chromosomes and 13q14 as detected by fluorescence in situ hybridization is a prognostic factor in patients with multiple myeloma who are receiving allogeneic-dose reduced stem cell transplantation. Blood 2004; 103:4056–61.

55. Maloney DG, Molina AJ, Sahebi F, et al. Allografting with non myeloabaltive conditioning following cytoreductive autograft for the treatment of patients with multiple myeloma. Blood 2003; 102:3447–54.

56. Garban F, Attal M, Michallet M, et al. Prospective comparison of autologous stem cell transplantation followed by reduced allograft (IFM 99-03 trial) with tandem autologous stem cell transplantation (IFM 99-04 trial) in high-risk de novo multiple myeloma. Blood 2006; 107:3474–80.

57. Van De Donk NW, Kroger N, Hegenbart U, et al. Remarkable activity of agents bortezomib and thalidomide in patients not responding to donor lymphocyte infusions following nonmyelo-ablative stem cell transplantation in Multiple Myeloma. Blood 2006; 107:3415–16.

58. Kroger N, Zabelina T, Ayuk F, et al. Bortezomib after dose-reduced allogeneic stem cell transplantation for multiple myeloma to enhance or maintain remission status. Exp hematol 2006; 34:770–7.

59. Bruno B, Rotta M, Patrirca F, et al. A comparison of allografting with autografting for newly diagnosed myeloma. N Engl J Med 2007; 356:1110–20.

11

Promising New Agents in Phase I and II Clinical Trials in Multiple Myeloma

Xavier Leleu

*Department of Medical Oncology, Dana-Farber Cancer Institute,
Harvard Medical School, Boston, Massachusetts, U.S.A. and
Service des Maladies du Sang,
CHRU, Lille, France*

Kenneth C. Anderson

*Department of Medical Oncology, Jerome Lipper Multiple Myeloma Center,
Dana-Farber Cancer Institute and Department of Medicine, Harvard Medical School,
Boston, Massachusetts, U.S.A.*

BACKGROUND

Multiple myeloma (MM) is the second most common hematological malignancy with an incidence of 4.3 per 100,000 in the general population, and a median survival of 3–5 years (1). It is a malignancy of the plasma cells, usually immature plasmablasts that exhibit chromosomal abnormalities. These early chromosomal abnormalities, such as translocations, result in overexpression of several important oncogenes (2–4). Eventually, malignant clones carrying these mutations progress and undergo further genetic insults leading to advanced disease. Environmental factors play an equally important role in the progression of the disease (Fig. 1). The malignant plasma cells home to the bone marrow (BM) where subsequent interactions promote MM cell growth, survival, and migration, as well as the development of drug resistance. The BM microenvironment (BMM) consists of extracellular matrix proteins such as laminin, collagen, fibronectin and osteopontin (5). The complex landscape of cells in the BMM includes hematopoietic stem cells, BM stromal cells (BMSC), BM endothelial cells, fibroblasts, osteoclasts and osteoblasts. Within the BMM, multiple signaling pathways and proteins are dysregulated in MM compared to normal plasma cells (6), including PI3K/Akt, MAPK, JAK/STAT, IKK/IκB/NF-κB, and HSP90, which therefore represent novel targets in MM (Fig. 2).

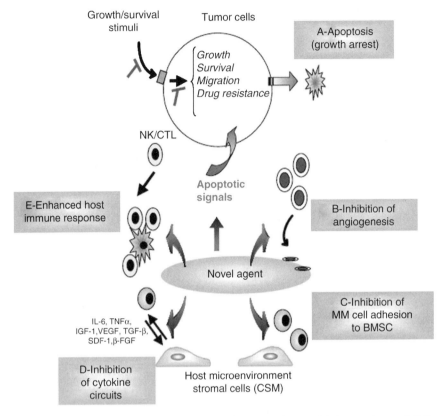

Figure 1 Novel, biologically-based therapies targeting multiple myeloma (MM) cells and the bone marrow (BM) microenvironment. Novel agents (**A**) induce G1 growth arrest and/or apoptosis in MM cell lines and patient cells resistant to conventional chemotherapy, (**B**) decrease angiogenesis, (**C**) inhibit MM cell adhesion to BMSC, (**D**) decrease cytokine production and sequelae in the BM microenvironment, and (**E**) induce host anti-MM immunity. *Abbreviations*: bFGF, basic fibroblast growth factor; CTL, cytotoxic T lymphocyte; IL, interleukin; IGF, insulin-like growth factor; NK, natural killer, SDF-1α, stromal cell-derived factor-1α; TGF-β, transforming growth factor-β; TNF-α, tumor necrosis factor-α; VEGF, vascular endothelial growth factor. *Source*: Refs. 156, 157.

Advances in our understanding of the pathogenesis of MM and the role of the BMM in the support and survival of the malignant plasma cells have resulted in the introduction of many novel targeted agents in the treatment of MM (7). The treatment of MM has evolved from the time of melphalan and prednisone in the 1960s to high-dose chemotherapy and stem cell transplantation in the 1990s to the introduction of novel, targeted therapeutic agents in the last decade (8,9). Within the past four years, three

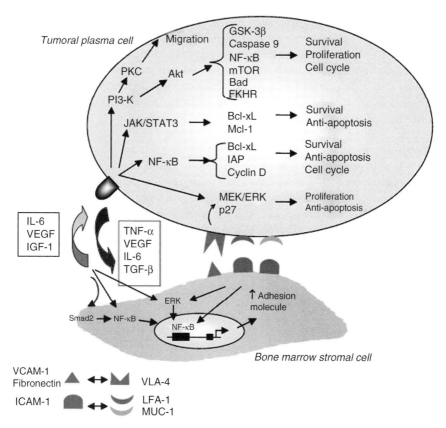

Figure 2 Interaction of multiple myeloma (MM) tumor cells and their bone marrow (BM) microenvironment cells. Binding of MM cells to BM stromal cells (BMSCs) triggers adhesion- and cytokine-mediated MM cell growth, survival, drug resistance, and migration. MM cell binding to BMSCs induces the activation of p42/44 mitogen-activated protein kinase (MAPK) and nuclear factor (NF)-κB in BM stromal cells. Adhesion-mediated activation of NF-κB upregulates adhesion molecules on both MM cells and BM stromal cells and interleukin-6 (IL-6) secretion from BMSCs. Cytokines secreted from BMSCs, such as IL-6, insulin-like growth factor-1 (IGF-1) and vascular endothelial growth factor (VEGF) upregulate IL-6 secretion from BMSCs and/or activate major signaling pathways [p42/44 MAPK, Janus kinase (JAK)/signal transducers and activators of transcription (STAT)3, phosphatidyli-nositol-3 kinase (PI3K)/Akt] and their downstream targets. *Abbreviations*: FKHR, forkhead transcription factor; GSK, glycogene synthetase kinase; ICAM, inter-cellular adhesion molecule; LFA, leukocyte function associated antigen; PKC, proteine kinase C; TGF-β, transforming growth factor-β; TNF, tumor necrosis factor; VCAM, vascular cell adhesion molecule; VLA, very late activation antigen. *Source*: From Refs. 156, 157.

novel agents were FDA approved for use in MM, bortezomib, thalidomide, and lenalidomide, leading to a paradigm shift in the treatment algorithm of MM (8,10). These agents have become the cornerstone of therapy of MM, whether in induction therapy for newly diagnosed patients or in the salvage setting for patients with relapsed and refractory disease. The success of targeted therapy in MM has led to the development and testing of over 30 new therapeutic agents in the preclinical or in early phase I and II clinical setting, making MM a model disease for the development of targeted therapeutic agents.

Herein, we will discuss novel therapeutic agents that are being tested in early phase I and II clinical trials, according to the pathways they specifically target. We will specifically discuss the preclinical evidence supporting novel therapies that target intracellular signaling pathways (Table 1), cell maintenance processes (Table 2), and cell surface receptors (Table 3). All clinical trials design and criteria are summarized in the following Internet

Table 1   Novel Agents Targeting Intracellular Signaling Pathways

Pathways	Novel agent	Company	Adm.	Description	Phase
PI3K/Akt	Perifosine	Keryx	PO	PKB inh.	II
	CCI-779	Wyeth	IV	mTOR inh.	II
	RAD001	Novartis	PO	mTOR inh.	II
	AP23573	Ariad	IV	mTOR inh.	II
MEK/ERK	AZD-6244	Astra Zeneca	PO	MEK/ERK inh.	I
	Tipifarnib/ zarnestra	J&J	PO	FTI	I/II
P38MAPK	SCIO-469	SCIOS Inc.	PO	P38MAPK inh.	II
SAPK/JNK	Aplidin®/ plitidepsin	PharmaMar	IV	Cyclic depsipeptide	II
PKC	Enzastaurin	Eli-Lilly	PO	PKC inh.	II
JAK/STAT	Atiprimod	Callisto	PO	Anti-apoptosis inh.	II
Nf-Kb	RTA 402	Reata	PO	Anti-NF-κB inh.	I
Apoptosis	Arsenic trioxyde	Cephalon	IV	Generate ROS	II
	Oblimersen	Genta	IV	Bcl-2 antisense	II
	Panzem®	EntreMed	PO	2ME2	II
Phosphatase inh.	VQD-001	VioQuest	IV	PTPase inh.	I/II

Abbreviations: Adm., route of administration; FTI, farnesil tranferase inhibitor; inh, inhibitor; IV, intravenous; mATB, monoclonal antibody; PK, protein kinase; PO, per os; PTPases, phosphatase; ROS, reactive oxygen species: sc, subcutaneous.
Source: www.myeloma.org/

site: www.clinicaltrials.gov. This list is not inclusive of all the new drugs currently in development for the treatment of MM.

NOVEL AGENTS TARGETING INTRACELLULAR SIGNALING PATHWAYS

Many agents currently being evaluated in MM exert their effects on a broad range of pathways, and for many drugs the exact mechanisms of action are still being delineated (11). Novel agents can be grouped based on their primary targets.

Targeting the PI3K/Akt Pathway

The phosphatidylinositol-3 kinase (PI3K) signaling cascade is one of two major pathways that are activated by receptor tyrosine kinases (12–14). PI3K is composed of regulatory and catalytic subunits, which when activated catalyze and further activate a wide range of downstream targets, most notably the serine/threonine protein kinase Akt (PKB). Akt has a multifaceted role in cell survival, including sequestering the FOXO family of Forkhead transcription factors from activating their proapoptotic targets, phosphorylating I-κB kinase (IKK) and thus preventing the degradation of NF-κB, and regulating the tumor suppressor gene p53. In addition, Akt regulates cell proliferation and growth by targeting the activity of glycogen synthase kinase β and preventing cyclin D1 degradation, as well as targeting mammalian target of rapamycin (mTOR). mTOR, also known as rapamycin-associated protein (FRAP), is a serine/threonine protein kinase that

Table 2 Novel Agents Targeting Cell Maintenance Processes

Cell maintenance	Novel agent	Company	Adm.	Description	Phase
Protein degradation	NPI-0052	Nereus	PO	Proteasome inh.	I
	PR-171	Proteolix	IV	Proteasome inh.	I
Transcription	SAHA	Aton	IV	HDAC inh.	I/II
	PXD101	CuraGen	IV	HDAC inh.	II
	LBH589	Novartis		HDAC inh.	II
Protein chaperoning	17AAG/ Kos953	Kosan	IV	HSP-90 inh.	I/II
	IPI-504	Infinity	IV	HSP-90 inh.	I
DNA synthesis	AVN944	Avalon	PO	IMPDH inh.	I/II

Abbreviations: Adm., route of administration; HDAC, histone acyltransferases and histone deacetylases; HSP, heat shock protein; IMPDH, inosine monophosphate dehydrogenase; inh, inhibitor; IV, intravenous; PO, per os.
Source: www.myeloma.org/

Table 3 Novel Agents Targeting Cell Surface Receptors

Cell receptors	Novel agent	Company	Adm.	Description	Phase
IL-6	CNTO 328	Centocor	IV	Anti-IL6mAbs	I/II
TNFR family	SGN-40	Seattle Genetics	IV	Anti-CD40mAbs	II
	Chir12-12	Chiron	IV	Anti-CD40mAbs	I
	HGS-ETR1	Human Genome	Sc.	TRAIL-R1/Apo2L	II
	Atacicept	ZymoGenetics	IV	TACI-Ig/anti-ligands	I/II
EGFR	Erbitux®	University of Cologne	IV	Anti-EGFR-mAbs	II
IGF1R	NVP-ADW742	Novartis	PO	IGFR tyr kin inh.	I
	CP-571871	Pfizer		anti-IGF-1RmAbs	I
VEGF	Avastin®	Genentech	IV	Anti-VEGFmAbs	II
	PI-88	Progen	SC	VEGFR inh.	II
	XL999	Exelixis	IV	VEGFR/FGFR inh.	II
	SU5416	Sugen	IV	VEGFR inh.	II
	Nexavar®	Bayer&Onyx	PO	Multikinases inh.	II
FGFR3	CHIR-258	Novartis/Chiron	PO	FGFR3 inh.	I
CD56	BB-10901	ImmunoGen	IV	CD56 inh.	I

Abbreviations: Adm., route of administration; inh, inhibitior; IV, Intravenous; mAbs, monoclonal antibody; PO, per os; sc, subcutaneous; tyr kin inh., tyrosine kinase inhibitor.
Source: www.myeloma.org/

serves as a molecular sensor which regulates cell growth and proliferation in response to nutrients, growth factors, and insulin. mTOR-dependent phosphorylation of downstream molecules is critical for the cap-dependent translation of cell cycle proteins and progression from G1 to S phase.

Recently, there has been evidence suggesting that PI3K/Akt pathway is an important target of anti-MM therapy, since Akt is constitutively activated in patient MM cells, but not in nonmalignant cells from the same patients (15,16). Importantly, many key growth factors in myeloma, such as IL-6 and IGF-1, are ligands for tyrosine kinase receptors, which activate the PI3K/Akt pathway (17). Furthermore, IL-6 overcomes dexamethasone-induced apoptosis via activation of PI3K/Akt (18). Given the importance of the PI3K/Akt pathway in tumorigenesis, several targeted therapies are currently under evaluation in MM.

Akt Inhibitor

Perifosine (NSC 639966) is an orally active alkyl-phosphocholine compound that belongs to a novel class of anti-tumor drugs which affect membrane permeability, phospholipid metabolism, and mitogenic signal transduction, specifically AKT activation (19). It does not affect upstream molecules such as PDK-1 or PI3K proteins. In MM, perifosine has demonstrated significant in vitro and in vivo activity agaist MM cell lines and patient samples, even in the presence of stromal cells that induce resistance to apoptosis. Perifosine also induced synergistic cytotoxicity with standard MM therapeutic agents used including dexamethasone, melphalan, and doxorubicin. In addition, it augmented the cytotoxicity induced by bortezomib in MM, suggesting that it may overcome resistance to bortezomib in vivo. Based on these preclinical findings, a phase II trial of perifosine with or without dexamethasone in patients with relapsed/refractory MM was initiated in early 2006 (20). Another phase II trial of the combination of perifosine with bortezomib with or without dexamethasone is currently underway.

mTOR Inhibitors

CCI-779 and RAD001 mTOR inhibitors (rapamycin analogues) and rapamycin have demonstrated in vitro and in vivo activity in MM cell lines and animal models (21,22). CCI-779 (temsirolimus) induced significant cytotoxicity in cell lines with PTEN mutation, which activates the PI3K/AKT pathway. Similarly, RAD001 (everolimus) is active at nM concentrations against a broad range of MM cells and in a SCID/NOD MM mouse model. In addition, the combination of rapamycin with other novel agents such as lenalidomide, bortezomib, and 17-AAG has demonstrated strong synergistic activity (23,24). Importantly, rapamycin inhibited angiogenesis and osteoclast activity in MM in vitro. Phase II trials of single agents CCI779 and RAD001 are being conducted in relapsed MM, with early evidence of responses and stability of disease indicating activity in vivo. A phase II trial of RAD001 in combination with lenalidomide, and another phase I/II clinical trial of CCI-779 in combination with bortezomib, are currently underway in patients with relapsed/refractory MM.

Targeting MAPK Proteins

There are three major groups of mitogen-activated protein kinases (MAPKs): the extracellular signal regulated kinase (ERK) family, the p38 MAPK family, and the c-Jun NH_2-terminal kinase (JNK) family. These families of serine/threonine kinases are activated by growth factors and other stimuli, and also regulate the production and secretion of cytokines. The MAPKs are intimately involved in the regulation of key cellular processes, such as cell cycle progression, growth, differentiation, and apoptosis; as such, they are often implicated in malignant transformation and tumor progression (25).

P38 MAPK Inhibitor, SCIO-469

P38 MAPK is a serine/threonine kinase involved in responses to environmental stress such as inflammatory cytokines, UV light, and osmotic shock. There are four known splice variants of the p38 MAPKs, and p38α has major effects on cell growth, differentiation, and apoptosis (26).

SCIO-469 is a selective p38 MAPK inhibitor (SCIOS, CA) that was first studied in clinical trials in rheumatoid arthritis. In MM, it inhibited proliferation of MM cells cocultured with bone marrow stromal cells (27). It also inhibited VEGF and IL-6 secretion by bone marrow stromal cells. The combination of SCIO-469 and bortezomib demonstrated strong synergistic activity in vitro and in vivo (28). A phase II trial of SCIO-469 alone or in combination with bortezomib is being conducted in patients with relapsed MM (29).

The MEK/ERK Inhibitors, AZD6244 and Tipifarnib

Numerous studies have shown that cytokine-induced cell proliferation is predominantly mediated through the ERK family of MAPKs (18,30,31), which are part of a large cascade of proto-oncogenes including upstream activators Ras and Raf. In MM, 30–40% of patients have mutations, which lead to constitutively active Ras, in the context of advanced stage disease (32). IL-6-dependent proliferation of MM cells is known to be dependent on ERK activation (33).

AZD6244 is a specific inhibitor of the MEK/ERK MAPK signaling pathway with promising efficacy in hepatocellular carcinoma (34). AZD6244 blocked constitutive and cytokine (IL-6, IGF-1)-stimulated ERK1/2 phosphorylation and directly inhibited proliferation and survival of human MM cell lines, either sensitive or resistant to conventional chemotherapy, as well as freshly isolated patient MM cells (35). AZD6244 overcame resistance to apoptosis in MM cells conferred by IL-6 and BMSCs, and also inhibited IL-6 secretion induced by MM adhesion to BMSCs. In addition, AZD6244 inhibited adhesion molecule expression in MM cells (i.e. integrin α4 (VLA-4), integrin β7, ICAM-1, ICAM-2, and ICAM-3). Combinations of AZD6244 and other novel and conventional agents, specifically with perifosine lenalidomide, and bortezomib, induced synergistic cytotoxic activity (35). A phase II trial is ongoing in patients with relapsed MM.

Tipifarnib (Zarnestra, formerly R115777) binds to and inhibits the enzyme farnesyl protein transferase, an enzyme involved in protein processing (farnesylation) for signal transduction. By inhibiting farnesylation of proteins, this agent prevents the activation of Ras oncogenes, inhibits cell growth, induces apoptosis, and inhibits angiogenesis (36). R115777 also induces cell death through an alternative mechanism implicating participation of Ras-independent mechanism(s) (37). R115777 with bortezomib induced synergistic cytotoxicity in MM, even in tumor cells relatively resistant to tipifarnib or in coculture with BMSC. Tipifarnib and bortezomib were also effective against MM cells adherent to fibronectin, providing evidence that the combination overcomes cell adhesion-mediated drug resistance (CAM-DR). A phase II clinical trial showed that disease stabilization was achieved in 64% of patients with advanced MM treated with Tipifarnib (38).

The SAPK/JNK Inhibitor, Aplidin

The exact role of the MAPK/JNK pathway in MM is unclear, although it is activated after chemotherapy and exhibits both oncogene and tumor-suppressor gene activities (39). JNK inactivation is one mechanism by which IL-6 protects MM cells from Fas-induced apoptosis (40,41). Several drugs induce JNK activation during MM cell apoptosis, such as proteasome inhibitor bortezomib and Akt inhibitor perifosine (19,42).

Aplidin® (plitidepsin) is a naturally occurring cyclic depsipeptide isolated from the marine tunicate *Aplidium albicans*. It exhibits very promising antitumor effects both in vitro and in vivo, and is now in phase II clinical trials for a variety of solid and hematologic tumors. Its exact mechanism of action is unclear, but Aplidin-mediated cytotoxicity is dependent on sustained activation of JNK (43). It induces apoptosis in MM cell lines and patient cells by triggering JNK, Fas and mitochondrial-mediated signaling pathways. Aplidin was well tolerated in phase I and II trials, with the major dose-limiting toxicity being adverse musculoskeletal events including increased CPK, myalgia, and weakness (44,45). Long-lasting disease stabilization following tumor shrinkage was reported in several solid tumors and non-Hodgkin's lymphoma.

Targeting PKC Proteins

The protein kinase C (PKC) family of serine/threonine kinases has a myriad of targets that are involved in a broad range of cellular events, such as proliferation, growth, and transcription (46,47).

Enzastaurin (LY 317615) is an oral PKCβ inhibitor, with downstream inhibition of Akt (48). In MM, enzastaurin has demonstrated specific inhibition of PKC isoforms and Akt activation, with associated induction of cytotoxicity and apoptosis in MM cells that are both sensitive and resistant to conventional therapies. It is active both in vitro and in vivo and overcomes the growth advantages conferred by binding of MM cells to BMSCs.

In addition, enzastaurin inhibited MM cell adhesion, as well as VEGF- and IGF-1-triggered MM cell migration and angiogenesis. Finally, enzastaurin inhibited MM growth in an in vivo xenograft model of human MM. Phase II trials are currently underway in patients with refractory or relapsed MM.

Targeting JAK/STAT Pathway

The Janus kinase (JAK) family of tyrosine kinases plays a crucial role in cytokine signaling by phosphorylating the intracellular domains of cytokine receptors and recruiting downstream factors, such as STATs (signal transducers and activators of transcription), which then migrate to the nucleus and upregulate gene transcription. STAT3 is of particular relevance in MM and other malignancies, since its binding elements are on the promoters of several antiapoptotic genes including Mcl-1, Bcl-2, and Bcl-xL (49). Importantly, IL-6 binding to its receptor and subsequent JAK/STAT3 activation is associated with MM cell survival, likely secondary to up-regulation of Mcl-1 and drug resistance (50).

Atiprimod, an orally bioavailable azaspirane, has been studied in MM in vitro (51,52). The exact mechanisms of activity of this agent are not well defined, but it was found to inhibit proliferation of MM cells via downregulation of antiapoptotic targets Mcl-1 and Bcl-2, inhibition of phosphorylation of STAT3, as well as downregulation of the expression of adhesion molecules and cytokines such as IL-6. These results were confirmed using an in vivo SCID-hu MM model in which atiprimod inhibited tumor growth in vivo. Currently, phase I/II trials are underway evaluating atiprimod in refractory or relapsed MM.

Targeting the NF-κB Pathway

Nuclear factor κB (NF-κB) family transcription factors play a central role in the pathogenesis of MM. NF-κB regulates cellular responses including immunity, inflammation, proliferation, survival, and angiogenesis (53,54). Inactive NF-κB complexes with its inhibitor, IκBα, and remains sequestered in the cytosol. A variety of stimuli trigger the phosphorylation of IκB by IKK. Phosphorylated IκB is then a target for ubiquination and proteasome-mediated degradation, which in turn releases NF-κB to translocate from the cytosol to the nucleus. Once in the nucleus, NF-κB stimulates transcription of numerous cytokines, chemokines, and cell adhesion molecules. NF-κB modulates expression of genes involved in regulation of cellular survival, proliferation, differentiation, and inflammation. It is constitutively activated in numerous hematologic malignancies, including MM (55,56), and several agents have been examined which target the NF-κB pathway directly and indirectly (57).

RTA 402 (also known as CDDO-Me) is a synthetic triterpenoid that suppresses NF-κB activity by inhibiting the activation of IKK, thereby downregulating the expression of many cancer-associated genes regulated by this transcription factor (58,59). This drug targets both constitutive and inducible NF-κB in human leukemia cell lines, as well as in tissue samples from patients. These effects also occurred in cells activated by a variety of agents including TNFα, interleukin-1β, and phorbolester. RTA 402 caused minimal toxicity in nonhuman primates when administered orally at very high doses, was well absorbed, and reached high concentrations in a wide variety of tissues. A phase 1 clinical trial is planned in patients with solid tumors, lymphoma, or MM.

Triggering Apoptotic Pathways

Almost all the therapies being evaluated in the treatment of MM exhibit in vitro apoptotic effects, and many have in vivo effects as well. They activate intrinsic, extrinsic, and mitochondrial apoptotic pathways. In this section, we will discuss arsenic trioxide, 2-methoxyestradiol, and bcl-2 antisense as the representative agents.

Arsenic trioxide (As$_2$O$_3$) is currently being used for treatment of relapsed/refractory, acute promyelocytic leukemia, and has shown promise in the treatment of MM as well (60–63). in vitro studies have suggested that it targets several different pathways. Most notably, it downregulates Bcl-2, induces caspase-9 cleavage, and induces apoptosis in both drug-sensitive and resistant MM cell lines. Furthermore, it inhibits both the JAK/STAT3 and NF-κB signaling pathways, as well as decreasing paracrine IL-6 secretion from BMSCs (64). It also up-regulates the expression of TRAIL (tumor necrosis factor-related apoptosis-inducing ligands) receptors, suggesting that combined therapy with TRAIL may be of benefit (65). Arsenic trioxide has been evaluated in clinical trials as both a single agent and in combination with other therapies (66). A phase 2, multicenter, open-label study was conducted in 24 MM patients relapsed or refractory to prior treatments. Patients received arsenic trioxide (0.25 mg/kg/day for 5 days/week) during the first two weeks of each 4-week cycle; 58% had either a > 25% reduction in serum M-protein levels or had stable disease (67). Arsenic has also been evaluated in combination with dexamethasone and melphalan. In a study of 10 patients with relapsed or refractory disease, arsenic with low-dose melphalan and ascorbic acid exhibited sustained response, and was well tolerated (68). Ascorbic acid potentiates the effects of arsenic by reducing intracellular glutathione, which functions to repair mitochondrial damage (69). Currently, phase II trials are underway to evaluate arsenic in combination with bortezomib, thalidomide, and melphalan.

Panzem®, 2-methoxyestradiol (2-ME2), an endogenous derivative of estradiol, was initially found to have significant antileukemic actions in vitro and in vivo (70). It induces apoptosis via the mitochondrial release of Smac protein and cytochrome C, which results in the inactivation of IAP (inhibitors of apoptosis) proteins, followed by activation of the caspase cascade (71).

Furthermore, it decreases VEGF and IL-6 secretion from BMSC, suggesting antiangiogenic potential. In addition, in vitro and in vivo data indicate that 2-ME2 is effective in MM cells resistant to melphalan and doxorubicin. Recently, it has been proposed that 2-ME2 at low-concentration could induce differentiation of MM cells (72,73). In Phase I/II oncology trials, orally administered Panzem has demonstrated anticancer activity in patients with solid tumors and MM, and was well tolerated in 51 patients with MM.

Oblimersen, the Bcl-2 family of proteins regulates mitochondria-dependent apoptosis. Overexpression of Bcl-2 and Bcl-xL in numerous malignancies, including MM, contributes to development of drug resistance and disease progression (74). Oblimersen sodium (previously known as G3139) is an antisense oligonucleotide that specifically binds to bcl-2 messenger RNA, decreases production of Bcl-2 protein in both human MM cell lines and patients' cells, as well as enhances the cytotoxicity of dexamethasone and doxorubicin (75,76). Combining oblimersen with other anticancer agents represents a strategy to reverse the multidrug resistance seen in MM (77). Preliminary results from these trials in patients with refractory or relapsed MM indicate that the combination of oblimersen with dexamethasone and thalidomide or vincristine–doxorubicin–dexamethasone is active and well tolerated, and may overcome chemotherapy resistance (78). Future studies will focus on the role of oblimersen in combination with novel biologic agents such as bortezomib. A randomized phase III clinical trial will compare dexamethasone plus oblimersen with dexamethasone alone in patients with relapsed or refractory MM.

Targeting Tyrosine Phosphatases

Cellular growth and development are regulated by reversible phosphorylation of tyrosine residues on target proteins. Protein tyrosine phosphatases (PTPs) catalyse removal, and protein tyrosine kinases (PTKs) addition, of phosphate. Data from various sources support a role for PTKs in transformation, and it has long been hypothesized that some PTPs will function as tumor suppressor genes. PTPs, protein tyrosine phosphatases, are a family of enzymes which play a crucial role in tumor cell formation (79) and are over-expressed in many advanced malignancies (80).

VQD-001. Sodium Stibogluconate (SSG) specifically inhibits PTPs in preclinical studies, synergizes with IFN-α to overcome IFN-α resistance in various human cancer cell lines in culture, and eradicates IFN-α-refractory tumor cells (81,82). Based on preclinical activity in animal models, VQD-001 may represent a novel therapy in MM.

Multitarget Kinase Inhibitors

Large-scale studies using gene and protein arrays on patients' samples showed patterns of predominantly involved cell signaling pathways in tumor cells. However, more than one pathway is ultimately involved in the tumor cell development. Furthermore, while the targeted pathway may be inhibited by a specific novel agent, upregulation of other pathways as compensatory mechanisms are observed in MM tumor cells. For example, the Akt inhibitor perifosine downregulates the Akt pathway, with associated activation of the MEK/ERK pathway, which mediates tumor cell survival in MM (19). Proteasome inhibitors upregulate Akt activation, providing the rationale for combining proteasome inhibitors with perifosine. Development of multitarget kinase inhibitors is ongoing to avoid resistance to novel agent, related to activation of compensatory signaling pathways.

NOVEL AGENTS TARGETING CELL MAINTENANCE PROCESSES

Targeting Protein Degradation

Proteasome Inhibitors

The ubiquitin-26S proteasome pathway, which regulates the turnover of a vast number of intracellular proteins, has become an exciting target in a variety of malignancies, most notably MM (83–86). Normally, proteins that are tagged with multiple ubiquitin molecules enter the 26S proteasome for subsequent degradation. The proper functioning of this system is crucial for cell cycle regulation, gene transcription, and signal transduction. One protein degraded by the 26S proteasome, IκBα, is an inhibitory protein, which binds to NF-κB and prevents NF-κB translocation to the nucleus. As mentioned earlier, once in the nucleus, NF-κB promotes the transcription of numerous genes involved in cell survival, proliferation, and drug resistance. Inhibition of the proteasome effectively increases the presence of IκBα and prevents NF-κB release to the nucleus.

NPI-0052. Based on the significant activity of bortezomib in MM, another proteasome inhibitor with a different structure and mechanism of activity was developed (87). NPI-0052 is an oral proteasome inhibitor that has shown significant activity in MM cells resistant to conventional and Bortezomib therapies. It inhibits NF-κB, blocks proteasome activity, and induces apoptosis in MM cells, but not BMSC; furthermore, it is active at lower concentrations than bortezomib and can be orally administered. Interestingly, NPI-0052-mediated apoptosis appears to be predominately through the caspase-8 cell death cascade. In animal tumor model studies, NPI-0052 was well tolerated and prolonged survival, with significantly reduced tumor recurrence. Interestingly, the combination of NPI-0052 and bortezomib also induced synergistic anti-MM activity, potentially due to the differences in mechanism of action between the two agents. This agent is also undergoing phase I study in MM.

PR-171 is a novel, tetrapeptide epoxomicin-related inhibitor that binds the proteasome irreversibly. PR-171 potently bound and inhibited the chymotrypsin-like subunit of the proteasome in vitro and in vivo at low concentrations. At higher concentrations, PR-171 also displayed significant inhibition of the trypsin-like and the peptidyl-glutamyl peptide hydrolyzing activities. PR-171-induced proteasome inhibition was associated with accumulation of polyubiquitinated substrates and proapoptotic Bax. Brief pulse PR-171 exposure, which simulates the in vivo pharmacokinetics of bortezomib, led to PR-171-mediated inhibition of cellular proliferation followed by induction of caspase-3-dependent apoptosis through both intrinsic and extrinsic pathways, associated with enhanced phosphorylation of SAPK/JNK. PR-171 displayed enhanced antiproliferative activity compared to bortezomib in MM cell lines and freshly isolated patient-derived CD138+ plasma cells (88). PR-171 was also a potent inhibitor of proliferation in MM cell lines resistant to bortezomib. Despite the irreversible mechanism of action, the half-life of recovery of proteasome inhibition in tissues was approximately 24 hours. PR-171 was effective in suppression of tumor growth in xenograft studies in mice when administered twice every week for three weeks. Two different phase I studies are ongoing that study different schedules with a dose of $1.2 \, \text{mg/m}^2$. In PX-171-001, PR-171 is administered QDx5 on a two-week cycle, with nine days rest; while in PX-171-002, PR-171 is administered on a four-week cycle, QDx2 weekly for three weeks with 12 days rest. Patients with MM, non-Hodgkin lymphoma, Hodgkin's disease, or Waldenström's Macroglobulinemia who have received two or more prior treatments are eligible (89).

Targeting Protein Transcription

Histones are positively charged proteins that attract and organize negatively charged DNA into nucleosomes. As such, their regulation by the opposing actions of histone acetyltransferases and histone deacetylases (HDAC) plays a key role in gene expression, cell differentiation, and survival (90,91).

HDAC Inhibitors

Several HDAC inhibitors are being tested in MM, specifically suberoylanilide hydroxamic acid (SAHA), PXD101, and LBH589 (92). *SAHA* has demonstrated in vitro and in vivo cytotoxic activity in MM cells lines and primary patient samples as well as strong antiproliferative activity when combined with other conventional and novel agents such as bortezomib (93). A phase I clinical trial of SAHA in MM is currently underway. *PXD101* is a small molecule HDAC inhibitor of the hydroxamate class, which demonstrated broad antineoplastic activity in vitro and in vivo. PXD101 has antiproliferative activity on MM cell lines, and shows additive/synergistic effects with standard agents used in myeloma, against these cell lines. PXD101 will be tested in phase II as monotherapy and in combination with standard agents for treatment of MM (94). *LBH589* is a novel cinnamic hydroxamic acid analogue of histone deacetylase inhibitor, that induces acetylation of histone H3 & H4. LBH589 induces apoptosis in MM cells resistant to conventional therapies and significant synergistic cytotoxicity in combination with bortezomib, as well as primary patient MM cells. Aggresome formation was observed in the presence of bortezomib, and the combination of LBH589 plus bortezomib induced the formation of abnormal bundles of hyeracetylated alpha-tubulin but with diminished aggresome size and apoptotic nuclei (95,96). LBH589 will be tested in phase II as monotherapy and in combination with bortezomib.

Targeting Protein Chaperoning

Heat shock proteins (HSPs) are a class of molecular chaperones that, under normal conditions, facilitate proper protein folding and regulate the turnover of important cell growth and survival proteins. When under conditions of environmental stress, HSP expression increases in an adaptive means to maintain cell homeostasis and enhance cell survival. Elevated levels of HSPs have long been noted in many malignancies, and these chaperones seem to help protect malignant cells from stressful microenvironments. as well as from otherwise lethal mutations within the tumor cells themselves (97). HSP90 plays a particularly important role in oncogenesis because many of its protein substrates (such as receptor tyrosine kinases, serine/threonine kinases, telomerase, Akt, HIF1α) are signal transducers that regulate cell growth, proliferation, and survival (98,99).

Inhibitors of Heat Shock Protein 90 (HSP90), 17-AAG, KOS-953, and IPI-504

Several HSP90 inhibitors have been tested in preclinical studies; however, only one, 17AAG, a geldanamycin derivative that binds to the N-terminal ATP-binding pocket of HSP90, has been studied in vivo and in clinical trials. In MM, 17AAG induces potent apoptosis in drug-sensitive and-resistant cells in vitro and inhibits the stress induced antiapoptotic response in MM cells. It has also been reported to act synergistically with bortezomib, HDAC inhibitors, and PI3K/Akt inhibitors (23,100,101). Phase I/II trials are currently underway for 17AAG and other HSP90 inhibitors with a more tolerable profile than 17AAG, such as KOS-953 and IPI-504 in MM. KOS-953 demonstrated stability of disease when used as a single agent, and combined with bortezomib has shown promising activity in a phase I/II trial in patients with relapsed/refractory MM (102,103).

Targeting DNA Synthesis

AVN944 (VX-944) is an oral, small molecule inhibitor of the enzyme inosine monophosphate dehydrogenase (IMPDH), which is essential for de novo synthesis of the nucleotide guanosine triphosphate (GTP). IMPDH is highly upregulated in hematologic cancers and other cancers. AVN944 inhibits cell proliferation by depleting GTP necessary for synthesis of DNA and RNA. AVN944 is orally bioavailable and well-tolerated in normal human volunteers (104). A phase I clinical trial designed to study the safety and tolerability of AVN944 in adult patients with advanced hematological malignancies, including those with leukemia, lymphoma or MM, showed no adverse side effects. Stabilization of disease after a one-month treatment cycle has been observed in half of the patients (105).

NOVEL AGENTS TARGETING CELL SURFACE RECEPTORS

Targeting IL-6

IL-6 is known to be a major growth and survival signal in MM cells whose effects are both autocrine and paracrine, since both tumor cells and BMSCs secrete IL-6 (106,107). It is augmented by direct binding between tumor cells and BMSCs, as well as by additional cytokines. Serum IL-6 levels correlate with the proliferative fraction of MM cells, and high levels are associated with a poor prognosis. IL-6 activates several major signaling cascades, including the Ras/Raf/MEK/ERK, the JAK2/STAT3, and the PI3K/Akt cascades, which mediate cell proliferation, survival, and drug resistance, respectively (108). The initial step in the activation of these pathways involves the binding of IL-6 to its low-affinity receptor (IL-6Rα/gp80) and the subsequent homodimerization of signal transducer, gp130 (109). Notably, gp130 has no IL-6 binding capacity by itself, but activation by the IL-6/IL-6R complex results in homodimerization and phosphorylation of tyrosine residues in the intracellular domain of gp130 by the JAK family of enzymes.

Anti-IL-6 Monoclonal Antibody

Treatments targeting IL-6 have focused on monoclonal antibodies (mAbs) to IL-6 and IL-6R. Anti-IL-6 mAbs have antitumor effects in animal and preclinical human studies (110). In MM, anti-IL-6 mAbs have cytostatic effects on tumor cells in vitro as well as transient, anti-MM effects in both animal models and human preclinical trials (111,112). In particular, Bataille and colleagues showed that treatment with anti-IL-6 mAbs reduced MM cell production and inhibited C-reactive protein synthesis, an acute phase reactant synthesized in the liver in response to IL-6; however, none of the patients achieved remission or improvement, as assessed by standard clinical criteria (113). *CNTO 328* is a human-mouse chimeric mAb to IL-6 that inhibits IL-6 function. A phase I study with CNTO 328 in MM patients demonstrated that the antibody was safe and had a circulating half-life of approximately 17 days (110). Another phase I trial was conducted to assess safety and pharmacokinetics of CNTO 328 in subjects with B-cell non-Hodgkin's lymphoma, MM, or Castleman's Disease. Treatment with CNTO 328 has been well tolerated at doses up to 6 mg/kg q2 weeks. No clinical immune reaction to this chimeric mAb has been observed, and early evidence of response has been observed (114).

Targeting TNF Family Receptors

The tumor necrosis factor (TNF) family includes numerous ligands, several of which have been studied in MM, including TNF-α, tumor necrosis factor-related apoptosis-inducing ligand (TRAIL/Apo2L), Fas, CD40 ligand, B-cell activating factor (BAFF/BLyS), and APRIL.

Targeting CD40

CD40 induces MM cell proliferation through activation of the PI3K/Akt pathway as well as through induction of IL-6 and VEGF secretion by stromal cells (115,116). In vitro studies using anti-CD40 monoclonal antibody induced ADCC against MM cell lines, even those resistant to conventional therapies. Two anti-CD40 agents are currently in phase I trials and demonstrated safety in preliminary reports in MM. *HCD122* (Formerly CHIR-12.12) is a novel, fully human, IgG$_1$ antagonistic monoclonal antibody targeting the CD40 receptor. HCD122 appears to be safe and well tolerated to date at doses of 1 mg/kg and 3 mg/kg weekly for 4 doses (117). *SGN-40* is a specific humanized anti-CD40 ligand. Using a dose-loading schedule, SGN-40 was administered up to 8 mg/kg without reaching a maximum tolerated dose (118).

Targeting TACI

B-lymphocyte stimulator (BLyS/BAFF), a TNF family member class II, is critical for maintenance of normal B-cell development and homeostasis. APRIL (a proliferation-inducing ligand) and BAFF are involved in a variety of tumors, including B-cell malignancies. Expression of BAFF and APRIL receptors (B-cell maturation antigen [BCMA], transmembrane activator, calcium modulator, and cyclophilin ligand interactor [TACI], and BAFF-R) was demonstrated in a majority of MM cell lines and purified primary MM cells. APRIL and BLyS are produced by MM cells and other cells within the tumor environment, resulting in the enhanced survival of malignant cells via both autocrine and paracrine loops. These factors activated NF-κB, PI3K/AκT, and MAPK pathways and induced a strong up-regulation of the Mcl-1 and Bcl-2 antiapoptotic proteins in MM cells. BAFF or APRIL was also involved in the survival of primary MM cells cultured with their bone-marrow environment, which protects against dexamethasone (DEX)-induced apoptosis (119,120).

Atacicept (formerly referred to as TACI-Ig) is a soluble receptor fusion protein comprised of the extracellular domain of TACI and the Fc portion of a human IgG, which binds to APRIL and BLyS. In a phase I study, treatment with atacicept was well tolerated. No dose limiting toxicity was observed. Disease stabilization was seen in several patients with MM (121).

TRAIL/Apo2L

TRAIL/Apo2L (TNF-related apoptosis-inducing ligand) also belongs to the TNF receptor/ligand family; it shares significant homology with CD95 (Fas) ligand and has the ability to induce apoptosis in sensitive cells through a caspase-mediated pathway. TRAIL binds to two receptors, TRAIL-R1 and TRAIL-R2, which then trimerize and ultimately trigger the activation of caspase cascade and apoptosis. TRAIL/Apo2L has been shown in MM patient and cell lines, and in xenograft mouse models to induce apoptosis selectively and overcome drug resistance. TRAIL/Apo2L also overcame the survival effect of interleukin 6 on MM cells and did not affect the survival of peripheral blood and BM mononuclear cells and purified B cells from healthy donors. TRAIL-induced apoptosis was mediated through both DR4 and DR5. The status of the TRAIL receptors did not predict TRAIL sensitivity of MM cells. NF-κB inhibitors, such as SN50 or the proteasome inhibitor bortezomib, enhance the proapoptotic activity of TRAIL/Apo2L (122). Agonists of TRAIL death receptors induce MM cell apoptosis even in the bone marrow microenvironment and thus can overcome MM drug resistance (123).

HGS-ETR1. Two human agonistic monoclonal antibodies were developed, HGS-ETR1 and HGS-ETR2. HGS-ETR1 is a human monoclonal antibody that specifically binds to the TRAIL receptor-1 protein and triggers programmed cell death, or apoptosis, in cancer cells. HGS-ETR1 mimicks the activity of the natural protein TRAIL. HGS-ETR1 and, to a lesser extent, the HGS-ETR2 mAbs induce the killing of primary MM cells in vitro and in vivo and induce the death of medullary and extramedullary MM cells. Other preclinical studies demonstrate that HGS-ETR1 enhances the tumor-killing activity of bortezomib (124). Results of the Phase 1 clinical trial demonstrate that HGS-ETR1 can be administered safely and repetitively to patients with advanced solid malignancies at doses up to and including 10 mg/kg intravenously every 14 or 28 days. A phase II clinical trial of HGS-ETR1 (Mapatumumab) in combination with bortezomib is ongoing in advanced MM.

Targeting EGF Receptor

Clinical studies have shown that HER-2/Neu is over-expressed in up to one-third of patients with a variety of cancers. These patients are frequently resistant to conventional chemotherapies. Additionally, in most patients with MM, the malignant cells over-express a number of epidermal growth factor receptors (EGFR)s and their heparin-binding growth factor ligands, HB-EGF and amphiregulin; thus this growth-factor family may be an important aspect in the pathobiology of this disease. Amphiregulin stimulates IL-6 production and growth of BM stromal cells, whereas PD169540 (a pan-ErbB inhibitor) and Iressa® (gefitinib, an ErbB1-specific inhibitor) induce apoptosis of primary MM cells and cell lines (125,126). Several small molecule inhibitors, including lapatinib (Tykerb®), and erlotinib (Tarceva®) and therapeutic antibodies, trastuzumab (Herceptin®), pertuzumab (Omnitarg™, rhuMab-2C4), cetuximab (Erbitux®, IMC-C225), panitumumab (Abenix; ABX-EGF) and ZD6474 have also been developed (127,128).

Erbitux, a therapeutic monoclonal antibody targeting EGFR, is undergoing evaluation in phase I clinical studies in solid tumors and MM (129).

Targeting Insulin-Like Growth Factor-1 Receptor

IGF-1, a critical cytokine in the pathogenesis of MM, is known to have a plethora of downstream effects, including the activation of the MAPK/ERK and PI3K/Akt signaling pathways (130). In recent studies, it has been shown to act synergistically with IL-6 and protects against dexamethasone-induced apoptosis (131). Furthermore, IGF-1 mediates MM cell growth and survival in MM cells both in vitro and in vivo. IGF-1 is a ligand for IGF receptor (IGF1R), a tyrosine kinase signaling molecule, which is universally expressed on hematologic and solid tumor cell lines, as well as patient MM cells (132). Given the pleiotropic effects of IGF-1, targeted strategies against IGFR1 may have important clinical relevance in MM, and both tyrosine kinase inhibitor (NVP-ADW742) and IGFR monoclonal antibody (CP-571871) have been developed (133).

NVP-ADW742 is a small molecule tyrosine kinase inhibitor that inhibits IGF-1R and induces cytotoxicity in MM cells, even in cell lines resistant to conventional treatments, such as dexamethasone. Importantly, systemic administration of NVP-ADW742 suppresses tumor growth, prolongs survival, and potentiates the effects of other chemotherapies in vivo (133). Both NVP-ADW742 and CP-571871 are in phase I study.

Targeting Vascular Endothelial Growth Factor

VEGF, a potent angiogenic factor, is produced both by MM cells and BMSCs (134). In addition to neovascularization, it has pleiotropic effects in MM including: induction of MM cell migration via PI3K-dependent PKCα activation; triggering proliferation and resistance to apoptotic signals via the up-regulation of Mcl-1; and increasing the secretion of IL-6 by BMSC (135–137). VEGF ligand exerts its effect after binding to high-affinity tyrosine kinase receptor molecules, which are expressed on both MM patient cells as well as cell lines. VEGF-triggered phosphorylation of its receptors activates the MAPK signaling pathway and ultimately leads to increased proliferation. Therefore, agents targeting VEGF have shown great promise in the treatment of malignancies, including humanized monoclonal antibody, selective kinase inhibitors and multi-kinase inhibitor, and oligosaccharides that inhibit heparanase. All are undergoing phase I/II clinical studies, which include MM patients.

Bevacizumab, the humanized monoclonal antibody against VEGFR bevacizumab (Avastin), was recently FDA approved as first-line therapy for metastatic colon cancer when given in combination with 5-FU (138). Given the important role that VEGF plays in the progression of MM, these agents are now being studied as potential targeted therapies. Several phase II trials of bevacizumab alone and in combination with thalidomide and with bortezomib are ongoing in relapsed or refractory MM.

PI-88 (Progen) is a mixture of highly sulfated oligosaccharides that inhibit heparanase, an extracellular matrix endoglycosidase, and the binding of angiogenic growth factors to heparan sulfate. This agent showed potent inhibition of placental blood vessel angiogenesis, as well as growth inhibition, in multiple xenograft models.

Several spectrum selective kinase inhibitors are undergoing development, *XL999 (Exelixis), SU5416, PTK787* and *GW654652*. Exelixis is a potent inhibitor of key receptor tyrosine kinases (RTKs) implicated in the development and maintenance of tumor vasculature and in the proliferation of some tumor cells. It inhibits the FGFR, VEGFR and PDGFR RTKs and exhibited excellent activity in target-specific cellular functional assays. In addition, XL999 is a potent inhibitor of FLT3. PTK787, an orally administered tyrosine kinase inhibitor that binds to the ATP-binding sites of VEGF receptors, has been shown in vitro to inhibit MM cell growth and migration, as well as inhibits paracrine interactions with IL-6 (139). SU5416, a small molecule VEGFR2, was found in phase II clinical trials to have biologic effects but minimal clinical response (140,141). Finally, the pan-VEGF inhibitor GW654652 acts on both MM cells and the BM microenvironment. GW654652 inhibits the secretion of other prominent cytokines (IL-6) and decreases MM cell proliferation even in the presence of BMSC (142).

Nexavar® (sorafenib) was approved by the U.S. Food and Drug Administration (FDA) in December 2005 for the treatment of individuals with advanced kidney cancer (143). The drug is an orally available multi-kinase inhibitor, which targets growth signaling. Nexavar is a small molecule inhibitor of tumor cell proliferation and angiogenesis targeting RAF, VEGFR-2, PDGFR, KIT, FLT-3 and RET Nexavar inhibits specifically the signaling of VEGFR-2 and PDGFR. In addition, in preclinical models the inhibition of RAF kinase, an enzyme in the RAS signaling pathway, has also been shown to have antiangiogenic effects (144–146).

Targeting the Cell Adhesion Molecules—CD56

Cell adhesion molecules (CAM) represent a large group of cell surface protein moieties with distinctive biological functions. In physiological terms they mediate cell-to-cell contact and homing and localization of MM cells in the bone marrow microenvironment. CD56/N-CAM antigen is expressed on a variety of tumor types, including MM. About 70% of MM patients have evidence of CD56 expression (147,148).

BB-10901 is a humanized monoclonal antibody that binds with high affinity to CD56 and is covalently linked to a novel cytotoxic maytansinoid DM1. Once bound to CD56, the conjugate is internalized and releases DM1. Based on preliminary results, BB-10901 has significant in vitro and in vivo anti-MM activity in a murine model. A phase I clinical study is ongoing (149).

Targeting Fibroblast Growth Factor Receptor

FGF-2 (basic FGF, bFGF) is a potent angiogenic cytokine secreted by MM cells and, to a lesser extent, BMSCs. Increased levels of FGF-2 are seen in serum, BM, and plasma cell lysates of MM patients. Studies have demonstrated that serum FGF-2 levels decrease significantly after successful MM treatment (150,151). Furthermore, paracrine interactions between FGF-2 and IL-6 contribute to increase BM neovascularization, as well as MM cell proliferation. Notably, IL-6 enhances FGF-2 expression and secretion by MM cell lines and patient cells, and stimulation of BMSCs with FGF-2 induces a time- and dose-dependent increase in IL-6 secretion. FGF-2 signaling is mediated by binding to a family of four distinct tyrosine kinase receptors (FGFR1-FGFR4), all of which are present on patient BMSCs and MM cells. Activation of FGFRs transduces signals through MAPK and PI3K pathways. Deregulation of fibroblast growth factor receptor 3 (FGFR3) by the t(4;14) translocation is known to confer a poorer prognosis and is a primary event in 15–20% of MM cases, resulting in ectopic expression of the RTK, fibroblast growth factor receptor 3 (FGFR3) (152,153). Thus, there has been interest in targeting FGFR3 by both selective small molecule tyrosine kinase inhibitors and monoclonal antibodies. Inhibition of activated FGFR3 in MM cells induces apoptosis, validating FGFR3 as a therapeutic target in t(4;14) MM and encouraging the clinical development of FGFR3 inhibitors for the treatment of these patients, who have a poor prognosis. Two types of agents were then developed, an anti-FGFR3 tyrosine kinase inhibitor and a monoclonal antibody.

PRO-001 is an anti-FGFR3 monoclonal antibody with high affinity for FGFR3, which inhibits FGFR3 autophosphorylation and downstream signaling, thereby decreasing proliferation and inducing apoptosis in t(4:14) MM cells (154). *TKI-258* is a small-molecule inhibitor of class III, IV, and V

RTKs and an inhibitor of FGFR3. It induces in vitro and in vivo activity against MM tumor cells (155). Phase I clinical trials are ongoing.

FUTURE DIRECTIONS: NOVEL DRUG COMBINATIONS

The treatment of MM has changed over the last two decades from chemotherapy with melphalan and prednisone to a new era of novel therapeutic agents. These exciting developments in the treatment of MM have raised new challenges to define the best combinations of novel agents that achieve high responses and improved survival in MM. We also need to understand the mechanisms of response and resistance to these agents and how to individualize therapy, not only based on risk factors for aggressive disease, but also on the molecular signatures of specific MM subtypes. Indeed, many agents which demonstrate strong activity in vitro do not show similar activity in vivo in clinical trials, indicating that the in vivo microenvironment plays a critical role in modulating the response to these agents. A more individualized approach using combinations of novel therapeutic agents, based on targeting specific molecular signatures or aberrant pathways, is needed to achieve higher response rates, longer remissions, and better survival rates for patients with MM.

REFERENCES

1. Jemal A, Murray T, Ward E, et al. Cancer statistics, 2005. CA Cancer J Clin 2005; 55:10–30.
2. Avet-Loiseau H, Attal M, Moreau P, et al. Genetic abnormalities and survival in multiple myeloma: the experience of the Intergroupe Francophone du Myelome. Blood 2007; 109:3489–95.
3. Shaughnessy J Jr, Zhan F, Barlogie B, Stewart AK. Gene expression profiling and multiple myeloma. Best Pract Res Clin Haematol 2005; 18:537–52.
4. Zhan F, Huang Y, Colla S, et al. The molecular classification of multiple myeloma. Blood 2006; 108:2020–8.
5. Hideshima T, Podar K, Chauhan D, Anderson KC. Cytokines and signal transduction. Best Pract Res Clin Haematol 2005; 18:509–24.
6. Federica C, Antonio P, Guido T, Mario B. Targeting signaling pathways in multiple myeloma. Curr Pharm Biotechnol 2006; 7:407–13.
7. Anderson KC. Moving disease biology from the lab to the clinic. Cancer 2003; 97:796–801.
8. Kyle RA, Rajkumar SV. Multiple myeloma. N Engl J Med 2004; 351:1860–73.
9. Kyle RA. Five decades of therapy for multiple myeloma: a paradigm for therapeutic models. Leukemia 2005; 19:910–12.
10. Kumar S, Rajkumar SV. Thalidomide and lenalidomide in the treatment of multiple myeloma. Eur J Cancer 2006; 42:1612–22.
11. Talapatra S, Thompson CB. Growth factor signaling in cell survival: implications for cancer treatment. J Pharmacol Exp Ther 2001; 298:873–8.

12. Vivanco I, Sawyers CL. The phosphatidylinositol 3-kinase AKT pathway in human cancer. Nat Rev Cancer 2002; 2:489–501.

13. Dancey JE. Molecular targeting: PI3 kinase pathway. Ann Oncol 2004; 15 (Suppl: 4):233–9.

14. Wetzker R, Rommel C. Phosphoinositide 3-kinases as targets for therapeutic intervention. Curr Pharm Des 2004; 10:1915–22.

15. Panwalkar A, Verstovsek S, Giles FJ. Mammalian target of rapamycin inhibition as therapy for hematologic malignancies. Cancer 2004; 100: 657–66.

16. Pene F, Claessens YE, Muller O, et al. Role of the phosphatidylinositol 3-kinase/Akt and mTOR/P70S6-kinase pathways in the proliferation and apoptosis in multiple myeloma. Oncogene 2002; 21:6587–97.

17. Lentzsch S, Chatterjee M, Gries M, et al. PI3-K/AKT/FKHR and MAPK signaling cascades are redundantly stimulated by a variety of cytokines and contribute independently to proliferation and survival of multiple myeloma cells. Leukemia 2004; 18:1883–90.

18. Hideshima T, Nakamura N, Chauhan D, Anderson KC. Biologic sequelae of interleukin-6 induced PI3-K/Akt signaling in multiple myeloma. Oncogene 2001; 20:5991–6000.

19. Hideshima T, Catley L, Yasui H, et al. Perifosine, an oral bioactive novel alkylphospholipid, inhibits Akt and induces in vitro and in vivo cytotoxicity in human multiple myeloma cells. Blood 2006; 107:4053–62.

20. Richardson R, Lonial S, Jakubowiak A, et al. A Multicenter Phase II Study of Perifosine (KRX-0401) Alone and in Combination with Dexamethasone (Dex) for Patients with Relapsed or Relapsed/Refractory Multiple Myeloma (MM). Blood 2006; 108:1023a.

21. Mitsiades N, McMullan C, Poulaki V, et al. The mTOR Inhibitor RAD001 (Everolimus) is Active against Multiple Myeloma Cells in vitro and in vivo. Blood 2004; 104:1496a.

22. Shi Y, Yan H, Frost P, Gera J, Lichtenstein A. Mammalian target of rapamycin inhibitors activate the AKT kinase in multiple myeloma cells by up-regulating the insulin-like growth factor receptor/insulin receptor substrate-1/phosphatidylinositol 3-kinase cascade. Mol Cancer Ther 2005; 4:1533–40.

23. Francis LK, Alsayed Y, Leleu X, et al. Combination mammalian target of rapamycin inhibitor rapamycin and HSP90 inhibitor 17-allylamino-17-demethoxygeldanamycin has synergistic activity in multiple myeloma. Clin Cancer Res 2006; 12:6826–35.

24. Raje N, Kumar S, Hideshima T, et al. Combination of the mTOR inhibitor rapamycin and CC-5013 has synergistic activity in multiple myeloma. Blood 2004; 104:4188–93.

25. Platanias LC. MAP kinase signaling pathways and hematologic malignancies. Blood 2003; 101:4667–79.

26. Olson JM, Hallahan AR. p38 MAP kinase: a convergence point in cancer therapy. Trends Mol Med 2004; 10:125–9.

27. Hideshima T, Akiyama M, Hayashi T, et al. Targeting p38 MAPK inhibits multiple myeloma cell growth in the bone marrow milieu. Blood 2003; 101:703–5.

28. Hideshima T, Podar K, Chauhan D, et al. p38 MAPK inhibition enhances PS-341 (bortezomib)-induced cytotoxicity against multiple myeloma cells. Oncogene 2004; 23:8766–76.

29. Siegel D, Krishnan A, Lonial S, et al. Phase II Trial of SCIO-469 as Monotherapy (M) or in Combination with Bortezomib (MB) in Relapsed Refractory Multiple Myeloma (MM). Blood 2006; 108:1022a.

30. Huynh H, Nguyen TT, Chow KH, Tan PH, Soo KC, Tran E. Over-expression of the mitogen-activated protein kinase (MAPK) kinase (MEK)-MAPK in hepatocellular carcinoma: its role in tumor progression and apoptosis. BMC Gastroenterol 2003; 3:19.

31. Hu L, Shi Y, Hsu JH, Gera J, Van Ness B, Lichtenstein A. Downstream effectors of oncogenic ras in multiple myeloma cells. Blood 2003; 101: 3126–35.

32. Corradini P, Ladetto M, Inghirami G, Boccadoro M, Pileri A. N- and K-ras oncogenes in plasma cell dyscrasias. Leuk Lymphoma 1994; 15:17–20.

33. Ogata A, Chauhan D, Teoh G, et al. IL-6 triggers cell growth via the Ras-dependent mitogen-activated protein kinase cascade. J Immunol 1997; 159:2212–21.

34. Huynh H, Soo KC, Chow PK, Tran E. Targeted inhibition of the extra-cellular signal-regulated kinase kinase pathway with AZD6244 (ARRY-142886) in the treatment of hepatocellular carcinoma. Mol Cancer Ther 2007; 6:138–46.

35. Yu-Tzu Tai X-FL, Iris Breitkreutz, et al. Inhibition of ERK1/2 Activity by the MEK1/2 inhibitor AZD6244 (ARRY-142886) induces human multiple myeloma cell apoptosis in the bone marrow microenvironment: a new therapeutic strategy for MM 2006; 108:987a.

36. Le Gouill S, Pellat-Deceunynck C, Harousseau JL, et al. Farnesyl transferase inhibitor R115777 induces apoptosis of human myeloma cells. Leukemia 2002; 16:1664–7.

37. Beaupre DM, Cepero E, Obeng EA, Boise LH, Lichtenheld MG. R115777 induces Ras-independent apoptosis of myeloma cells via multiple intrinsic pathways. Mol Cancer Ther 2004; 3:179–86.

38. Alsina M, Fonseca R, Wilson EF, et al. Farnesyltransferase inhibitor tipifarnib is well tolerated, induces stabilization of disease, and inhibits farnesylation and oncogenic/tumor survival pathways in patients with advanced multiple myeloma. Blood 2004; 103:3271–7.

39. Bossy-Wetzel E, Bakiri L, Yaniv M. Induction of apoptosis by the transcription factor c-Jun. Embo J 1997; 16:1695–709.

40. Chauhan D, Kharbanda S, Ogata A, et al. Interleukin-6 inhibits Fas-induced apoptosis and stress-activated protein kinase activation in multiple myeloma cells. Blood 1997; 89:227–34.

41. Xu FH, Sharma S, Gardner A, Tu Y, Raitano A, Sawyers C, Lichtenstein A. Interleukin-6-induced inhibition of multiple myeloma cell apoptosis: support for the hypothesis that protection is mediated via inhibition of the JNK/SAPK pathway. Blood 1998; 92:241–51.

42. Hideshima T, Hayashi T, Chauhan D, Akiyama M, Richardson P, Anderson K. Biologic sequelae of c-Jun NH(2)-terminal kinase (JNK) activation in multiple myeloma cell lines. Oncogene 2003; 22:8797–801.

43. Cuadrado A, Gonzalez L, Suarez Y, Martinez T, Munoz A. JNK activation is critical for Aplidin-induced apoptosis. Oncogene 2004; 23:4673–80.
44. Maroun JA, Belanger K, Seymour L, et al. Phase I study of Aplidine in a daily × 5 one-hour infusion every 3 weeks in patients with solid tumors refractory to standard therapy. A National Cancer Institute of Canada Clinical Trials Group study: NCIC CTG IND 115. Ann Oncol 2006; 17:1371–8.
45. Faivre S, Chieze S, Delbaldo C, et al. Phase I and pharmacokinetic study of aplidine, a new marine cyclodepsipeptide in patients with advanced malignancies. J Clin Oncol 2005; 23:7871–80.
46. Li S, Phong M, Lahn M, et al. Retrospective analysis of protein kinase C-beta (PKC-beta) expression in lymphoid malignancies and its association with survival in diffuse large B-cell lymphomas. Biol Direct 2007; 2:8.
47. Serova M, Ghoul A, Benhadji KA, et al. Preclinical and clinical development of novel agents that target the protein kinase C family. Semin Oncol 2006; 33: 466–78.
48. Podar K, Raab MS, Zhang J, et al. Targeting PKC in multiple myeloma: in vitro and in vivo effects of the novel, orally available small-molecule inhibitor enzastaurin (LY317615.HCl). Blood 2007; 109:1669–77.
49. Alas S, Bonavida B. Inhibition of constitutive STAT3 activity sensitizes resistant non-Hodgkin's lymphoma and multiple myeloma to chemotherapeutic drug-mediated apoptosis. Clin Cancer Res 2003; 9:316–26.
50. Brocke-Heidrich K, Kretzschmar AK, Pfeifer G, et al. Interleukin-6-dependent gene expression profiles in multiple myeloma INA-6 cells reveal a Bcl-2 family-independent survival pathway closely associated with Stat3 activation. Blood 2004; 103:242–51.
51. Amit-Vazina M, Shishodia S, Harris D et al. Atiprimod blocks STAT3 phosphorylation and induces apoptosis in multiple myeloma cells. Br J Cancer 2005; 93:70–80.
52. Hamasaki M, Hideshima T, Tassone P, et al. Azaspirane (*N-N*-diethyl-8,8-dipropyl-2-azaspiro [4.5] decane-2-propanamine) inhibits human multiple myeloma cell growth in the bone marrow milieu in vitro and in vivo. Blood 2005; 105:4470–6.
53. Bours V, Bentires-Alj M, Hellin AC, et al. Nuclear factor-kappa B, cancer, and apoptosis. Biochem Pharmacol 2000; 60:1085–9.
54. Viatour P, Merville MP, Bours V, Chariot A. Phosphorylation of NF-kappaB and IkappaB proteins: implications in cancer and inflammation. Trends Biochem Sci 2005; 30:43–52.
55. Feinman R, Siegel DS, Berenson J. Regulation of NF-κB in multiple myeloma: therapeutic implications. Clin Adv Hematol Oncol 2004; 2: 162–6.
56. Ni H, Ergin M, Huang Q, et al. Analysis of expression of nuclear factor kappa B (NF-kappa B) in multiple myeloma: downregulation of NF-kappa B induces apoptosis. Br J Haematol 2001; 115:279–86.
57. Hideshima T, Chauhan D, Richardson P, et al. NF-kappa B as a therapeutic target in multiple myeloma. J Biol Chem 2002; 277:16639–47.
58. Konopleva M, Tsao T, Ruvolo P, et al. Novel triterpenoid CDDO-Me is a potent inducer of apoptosis and differentiation in acute myelogenous leukemia. Blood 2002; 99:326–35.

59. Shishodia S, Sethi G, Konopleva M, Andreeff M, Aggarwal BB. A synthetic triterpenoid, CDDO-Me, inhibits IkappaBalpha kinase and enhances apoptosis induced by TNF and chemotherapeutic agents through down-regulation of expression of nuclear factor kappaB-regulated gene products in human leukemic cells. Clin Cancer Res 2006; 12:1828–38.

60. Bonati A, Rizzoli V, Lunghi P. Arsenic trioxide in hematological malignancies: the new discovery of an ancient drug. Curr Pharm Biotechnol 2006; 7:397–405.

61. Rousselot P, Labaume S, Marolleau JP, et al. Arsenic trioxide and melarsoprol induce apoptosis in plasma cell lines and in plasma cells from myeloma patients. Cancer Res 1999; 59:1041–8.

62. Rousselot P, Larghero J, Labaume S, et al. Arsenic trioxide is effective in the treatment of multiple myeloma in SCID mice. Eur J Haematol 2004; 72:166–71.

63. Berenson JR, Yeh HS. Arsenic compounds in the treatment of multiple myeloma: a new role for a historical remedy. Clin Lymphoma Myeloma 2006; 7:192–8.

64. Hayashi T, Hideshima T, Akiyama M, et al. Arsenic trioxide inhibits growth of human multiple myeloma cells in the bone marrow microenvironment. Mol Cancer Ther 2002; 1:851–60.

65. Liu Q, Hilsenbeck S, Gazitt Y. Arsenic trioxide-induced apoptosis in myeloma cells: p53-dependent G1 or G2/M cell cycle arrest, activation of caspase-8 or caspase-9, and synergy with APO2/TRAIL. Blood 2003; 101: 4078–87.

66. Bahlis NJ, McCafferty-Grad J, Jordan-McMurry I, et al. Feasibility and correlates of arsenic trioxide combined with ascorbic acid-mediated depletion of intracellular glutathione for the treatment of relapsed/refractory multiple myeloma. Clin Cancer Res 2002; 8:3658–68.

67. Hussein MA, Saleh M, Ravandi F, Mason J, Rifkin RM, Ellison R. Phase 2 study of arsenic trioxide in patients with relapsed or refractory multiple myeloma. Br J Haematol 2004; 125:470–6.

68. Borad MJ, Swift R, Berenson JR. Efficacy of melphalan, arsenic trioxide, and ascorbic acid combination therapy (MAC) in relapsed and refractory multiple myeloma. Leukemia 2005; 19:154–6.

69. Grad JM, Bahlis NJ, Reis I, Oshiro MM, Dalton WS, Boise LH. Ascorbic acid enhances arsenic trioxide-induced cytotoxicity in multiple myeloma cells. Blood 2001; 98:805–13.

70. Lakhani NJ, Sparreboom A, Xu X, Veenstra TD, Venitz J, Dahut WL, Figg WD. Characterization of in vitro and in vivo metabolic pathways of the investigational anticancer agent, 2-methoxyestradiol. J Pharm Sci 2007.

71. Chauhan D, Catley L, Hideshima T, et al. 2-Methoxyestradiol overcomes drug resistance in multiple myeloma cells. Blood 2002; 100:2187–94.

72. Hou J, Xiong H, Gao W, Jiang H. 2-Methoxyestradiol at low dose induces differentiation of myeloma cells. Leuk Res 2005; 29:1059–67.

73. Hou J, Xiong H, Gao WR, Jiang H. Preliminary investigation of 2-methoxyestradiol inducing differentiation of myeloma cell line CZ-1. Zhongguo Shi Yan Xue Ye Xue Za Zhi 2006; 14:65–9.

74. Chauhan D, Anderson KC. Mechanisms of cell death and survival in multiple myeloma (MM): Therapeutic implications. Apoptosis 2003; 8: 337–43.

75. Klasa RJ, Gillum AM, Klem RE, Frankel SR. Oblimersen Bcl-2 antisense: facilitating apoptosis in anticancer treatment. Antisense Nucleic Acid Drug Dev 2002; 12:193–213.

76. van de Donk NW, Kamphuis MM, van Dijk M, Borst HP, Bloem AC, Lokhorst HM. Chemosensitization of myeloma plasma cells by an antisense-mediated downregulation of Bcl-2 protein. Leukemia 2003; 17:211–19.

77. Chanan-Khan AA. Bcl-2 antisense therapy in multiple myeloma. Oncology (Williston Park) 2004; 18:21–4.

78. Badros AZ, Goloubeva O, Rapoport AP, et al. Phase II study of G3139, a Bcl-2 antisense oligonucleotide, in combination with dexamethasone and thalidomide in relapsed multiple myeloma patients. J Clin Oncol 2005; 23:4089–99.

79. Julien SG, Dube N, Read M, et al. Protein tyrosine phosphatase 1B deficiency or inhibition delays ErbB2-induced mammary tumorigenesis and protects from lung metastasis. Nat Genet 2007; 39:338–46.

80. Easty D, Gallagher W, Bennett DC. Protein tyrosine phosphatases, new targets for cancer therapy. Curr Cancer Drug Targets 2006; 6:519–32.

81. Yi T, Pathak MK, Lindner DJ, Ketterer ME, Farver C, Borden EC. Anticancer activity of sodium stibogluconate in synergy with IFNs. J Immunol 2002; 169:5978–85.

82. Pathak MK, Hu X, Yi T. Effects of sodium stibogluconate on differentiation and proliferation of human myeloid leukemia cell lines in vitro. Leukemia 2002; 16:2285–91.

83. Chauhan D, Hideshima T, Mitsiades C, Richardson P, Anderson KC. Proteasome inhibitor therapy in multiple myeloma. Mol Cancer Ther 2005; 4: 686–92.

84. Altun M, Galardy PJ, Shringarpure R, et al. Effects of PS-341 on the activity and composition of proteasomes in multiple myeloma cells. Cancer Res 2005; 65:7896–901.

85. Voorhees PM, Orlowski RZ. The proteasome and proteasome inhibitors in cancer therapy. Annu Rev Pharmacol Toxicol 2006; 46:189–213.

86. Nencioni A, Grunebach F, Patrone F, Ballestrero A, Brossart P. Proteasome inhibitors: antitumor effects and beyond. Leukemia 2007; 21:30–6.

87. Chauhan D, Catley L, Li G, et al. A novel orally active proteasome inhibitor induces apoptosis in multiple myeloma cells with mechanisms distinct from Bortezomib. Cancer Cell 2005; 8:407–19.

88. Deborah J. Kuhn QC, Voorhees PM, et al. The novel, irreversible proteasome inhibitor PR-171 demonstrates potent anti-tumor activity in pre-clinical models of multiple myeloma, and overcomes bortezomib resistance. Blood 2006; 108:987a.

89. O'Connor OA, Orlowski RZ, Alsina M, et al. Multicenter phase i studies to evaluate the safety, tolerability, and clinical response to intensive dosing with the proteasome inhibitor PR-171 in patients with relapsed or refractory hematological malignancies. Blood 2006; 108:687a.

90. Mitsiades N, Mitsiades CS, Richardson PG, et al. Molecular sequelae of histone deacetylase inhibition in human malignant B cells. Blood 2003; 101: 4055–62.

91. Mitsiades CS, Mitsiades NS, McMullan CJ, et al. Transcriptional signature of histone deacetylase inhibition in multiple myeloma: biological and clinical implications. Proc Natl Acad Sci USA 2004; 101:540–5.

92. Acharya MR, Sparreboom A, Venitz J, Figg WD. Rational development of histone deacetylase inhibitors as anticancer agents: a review. Mol Pharmacol 2005; 68:917–32.

93. Pei XY, Dai Y, Grant S. Synergistic induction of oxidative injury and apoptosis in human multiple myeloma cells by the proteasome inhibitor bortezomib and histone deacetylase inhibitors. Clin Cancer Res 2004; 10: 3839–52.

94. Sullivan D, Singhal S, Schuster M, et al. A Phase II Study of PXD101 in Advanced Multiple Myeloma. Blood 2006; 108:1023a.

95. Catley L, Weisberg E, Kiziltepe T, et al. Aggresome induction by proteasome inhibitor bortezomib and alpha-tubulin hyperacetylation by tubulin deacetylase (TDAC) inhibitor LBH589 are synergistic in myeloma cells. Blood 2006; 108:3441–9.

96. Maiso P, Carvajal-Vergara X, Ocio EM, et al. The histone deacetylase inhibitor LBH589 is a potent antimyeloma agent that overcomes drug resistance. Cancer Res 2006; 66:5781–9.

97. Bagatell R, Whitesell L. Altered Hsp90 function in cancer: a unique therapeutic opportunity. Mol Cancer Ther 2004; 3:1021–30.

98. Dai C, Whitesell L. HSP90: a rising star on the horizon of anticancer targets. Future Oncol 2005; 1:529–40.

99. Whitesell L, Lindquist SL. HSP90 and the chaperoning of cancer. Nat Rev Cancer 2005; 5:761–72.

100. Mimnaugh EG, Xu W, Vos M, et al. Simultaneous inhibition of hsp 90 and the proteasome promotes protein ubiquitination, causes endoplasmic reticulum-derived cytosolic vacuolization, and enhances antitumor activity. Mol Cancer Ther 2004; 3:551–66.

101. Rahmani M, Yu C, Dai Y, et al. Coadministration of the heat shock protein 90 antagonist 17-allylamino-17-demethoxygeldanamycin with suberoylanilide hydroxamic acid or sodium butyrate synergistically induces apoptosis in human leukemia cells. Cancer Res 2003; 63:8420–7.

102. Siegel D, Jagannath S, Mazumder A, et al. Update on Phase I Clinical Trial of IPI-504, a Novel, Water-Soluble Hsp90 Inhibitor, in Patients with Relapsed/Refractory Multiple Myeloma (MM). Blood 2006; 108:1022a.

103. Richardson P, Chanan-Khan AA, Lonial S, et al. A multicenter phase 1 clinical trial of tanespimycin (KOS-953) + Bortezomib (BZ): Encouraging activity and manageable toxicity in heavily pre-treated patients with relapsed refractory multiple myeloma (MM). Blood 2006; 108:125a.

104. Ishitsuka K, Hideshima T, Hamasaki M, et al. Novel inosine monophosphate dehydrogenase inhibitor VX-944 induces apoptosis in multiple myeloma cells primarily via caspase-independent AIF/Endo G pathway. Oncogene 2005; 24: 5888–96.

105. Takebe N, Cheng X, Wu S, et al. Phase I clinical trial of the inosine monophosphate dehydrogenase inhibitor mycophenolate mofetil (cellcept) in advanced multiple myeloma patients. Clin Cancer Res 2004; 10: 8301–8.

12

Immunotherapeutic Strategies for the Management of Multiple Myeloma

Rao H. Prabhala, Dheeraj Pelluru, and Nikhil C. Munshi

Dana-Farber Cancer Institute, Harvard Medical School and Boston VA Healthcare System, Boston, Massachusetts, U.S.A.

High-dose chemotherapy achieves significant improvement in event free and overall survival. Novel targeted therapies are achieving responses in over 90% of newly diagnosed patients with one-third of these patients achieving complete or near-complete responses. However, patients still experience disease progression and curative outcomes are rare, prompting evaluation of innovative therapeutic interventions. Based on the success of allogeneic transplant in achieving long-term disease free survival, various vaccination strategies have been evaluated to maintain remissions achieved by conventional and novel agents. Development of successful vaccine strategy in MM has been directed at two aspects. First to develop a vaccine strategy able to specifically target MM cells with therapeutic efficacy; and second to improve the immune function in MM to allow sustained robust responses to immune-based intervention (1).

Here, we will provide a brief summary of the status of the immune system in myeloma and provide a detailed account of the clinical trials performed using various vaccine strategies including idiotype (Id) based vaccinations, proteins-pulsed dendritic cells (DCs) based vaccinations as well as whole cell vaccines. Future immunotherapy strategies for the improvement of treatment of multiple myeloma and monoclonal gammapathy of undetermined significance (MGUS) will also be covered.

IMMUNE SUPPRESSION IN MYELOMA

T and B cell responses

MM is associated with dysfunction in both humoral and cellular immunity (1). A significant impairment of T cell function is observed in both patients with MM and in individuals with MGUS. Although both phenotypic and functional aberrations in CD4 and CD8 cells have been described in MM and MGUS (2–4), the biological basis for these abnormalities remains unclear. Some studies suggest that the immune abnormalities seen in myeloma might be due to impairment in the global T cell receptor (TCR) diversity by V-beta analysis, especially in patients following high dose chemotherapy (5). Although both cellular and humoral immune responses have been observed against both viral and tumor antigens (6). more than 80% of myeloma patients were unable to generate protective antibody levels against certain bacterial infections that were causing pneumonia (7,8) and poor viral antigen-specific cytotoxic T lymphocytes (CTL) responses are observed in myeloma patients (6). It is generally agreed upon that overall T cells are hyperactive and B cell-driven antibody responses are deficient in myeloma. In a study utilizing patient-specific Id protein coupled with keyhole limpet hemocyanin (KLH), the development of an anti-KLH response confirmed immune competence in myeloma patients. Moreover, induction of Id-specific immune responses including generation of CTL specifically able to kill MM cells, confirmed the ability to induce immune response to the MM-specific antigen.

Dendritic Cells

Dendritic cells are the most potent antigen-presenting cells (APCs) equipped with the necessary costimulatory, adhesion and major histocompatibility (MHC) molecules, to effectively present MM-associated antigens and induce MM-specific immune responses. A number of investigators have confirmed that the antigen presenting cells in MM patients are functional, supporting their use in clinical studies (9). The cultured DCs from myeloma patients can efficiently and rapidly endocytose different classes of myeloma proteins providing support for using myeloma protein-pulsed DCs for generating in vivo anti-myeloma immune responses (10). However, three other groups reported that DCs from myeloma patients were functionally defective. Brown et al. (3) showed that despite normal numbers of DCs in myeloma patients, DCs failed to show the up-regulation of CD80 upon stimulation in association with the progression of the disease. This might be due to persistent exposure to immune-suppressive cytokines like transforming growth factor-beta (TGF-β) and interleukin (IL)-10 in these myeloma patients. Ratta et al. (11) observed that circulating DCs in myeloma patients were decreased in number and defective in their function. In addition, CD34+ DC progenitor cells

Table 1 Idiotype-Based Clinical Trials in Myeloma

Author	Year	Vaccine	No. of Patients	Clinical responses
Bergenbrant et al. (26)	1996	Id alone repeated injections	5 I–III stage	Incomplete CR
Osterborg et al. (27)	1996	Id + GM-CSF, 6 injections	5	No clear CR
Massaia et al., Coscia et al. (30,31)	1999, 2004	Id + KLH + GM-CSF	12 HD chemo and autoSCT	Residual tumor burden was not reduced after 36 mos
Rasmussen et al. (28)	2003	Id + IL, 12 +/– GM-CSF-7 injections	6 Stage I	4/6 down tumor burden
Bertinetti et al. (29)	2006	Id + GM-CSF, 4 shots; HepB vac	3 autoSCT	No alteration in tumor burden No abs to HepB
Borrello et al. (unpublished)	2004	Tumor cell + GM-CSF-producing K562 8 injections	16 autoSCT	11/16 CR/PR
Neelapu et al. (32)	2005	Id + KLH + GM-CSF, 6 donor vaccination injections	5 alloSCT	3/5 stable CR
Munshi et al. (unpublished)	2002	Id + KLH + GM-CSF	52 w tandem autoSCT	26/52 improved

Abbreviations: alloSCT, allogeneic stem cell transplantation; autoSCT autologous stem cell transplantation; GM-CSF, granulocyte-macrophage colony-stimulating factor; HD, high dose; ID, idiotype; KLH, keyhole limpet hemocyanin.

vaccination and most of the patients showed elevated myeloma paraprotein levels in the serum.

Under allo-settings, a creative way of generating donor Id-specific marrow cells prior to BMT has been described. In this clinical trial (32), five myeloma patients and their HLA-matched sibling donors were vaccinated with Id+KLH+GM-CSF. First donors were vaccinated before collection of bone marrow. All donor blood in vitro analysis showed excellent anti--idiotype antibody responses and idiotype-specific T-cell responses. Then, marrow cells were given to recipients with appropriate pre- and post-BMT regimen. Recipients were administered an additional three booster vaccinations between three and six months post-BMT. Three out of five patients showed idiotype-specific T-cell responses by producing TNF-α following specific proliferation. Three out of five who survived exhibited only partial remission prior to BMT and Id vaccinations, and continued to maintain CR cohort 1 up to 5–8 years. In another study (unpublished as an abstract only), we had conducted three different cohort studies using a total of 50 myeloma patients. In cohort 1, eighteen patients followed by double auto BMT received three idiotype vaccines with GM-CSF and KLH. In cohort 2, 21 patients received six vaccinations, and in cohort 3, six vaccines were given before and after second transplant in 13 patients. During the post-vaccination period, most of the patients (58%) produced Th1 type of cytokines (TNF-α, IFN-γ, and IL-2) and had elevated proliferative responses in addition to DTH responses (42%)

Besides validation of feasibility from these idiotopic vaccination clinical studies, it can be concluded that idiotype itself is not the strongest immunogen, and, therefore, one has to couple it with a cytokine and other immunogens. The majority of the studies showed that anti-idiotype antibodies play a less than significant role in the generation of antimyeloma responses to eradicate tumor cells as it is difficult to produce sufficient anti-idiotype antibodies to exceed myeloma paraprotien levels in order to neutralize it. Furthermore, a number of studies indicate that cellular immunity plays a critical role in the generation of antimyeloma responses. It has been shown that CD4 T cells play an important role in idiotypic vaccinations to drive robust antimyeloma responses (33). Also, the majority of immunodominant or high avidity idiotype-specific T cells would have been removed from the circulation during thymic education in the early years due to the auto/self-antigenic nature of the idiotype. To stimulate low avidity T cells to a specific-idiotype, an ideal approach would be to vaccinate donors prior to transplantation.

DC-Based Vaccination in Myeloma

Since initial reports indicating that dendritic cells with a distinctive morphology play a critical role in immune responses, DCs have been studied

2. Better quality of DCs should be generated for clinical settings using recent advances in DC maturation protocols. Although the immature DC are efficient in uptaking and processing antigens, administration of immature DCs showed the limitation in triggering T cell responses due to their low expression of costimulatory and MHC molecules on cell surfaces.

3. Also, monocyte-derived immature DCs are not stable and may differentiate back to macrophages when IL-4 and GM-CSF are withdrawn (46) and the use of mature DC derived from peripheral blood monocytes would serve better as antigen stimulators than immature DC. Also, Yi et al. (34) examined the efficacy of DC vaccination in MM patients by administration of Id-pulsed mature DC, subcutaneously. Their studies showed promising results, demonstrating that Id-specific T-cell responses in most (80%) myeloma patients with stable partial remissions following high-dose chemotherapy.

4. Several studies suggest that Id vaccinations may have a therapeutic effect in the setting of allogeneic stem cell transplantation. Although use of tumor-derived Id as an immunogen to elicit antitumor immunity against MM is a more attractive idea, the broader use of idiotypic vaccines has been hampered by the fact that Id in the autologous setting is not only a weakly immunogenic, self-antigen, but is also patient specific so that the vaccine must be individually prepared for each patient.

FUTURE DIRECTIONS

Novel myeloma-associated antigens have been identified by screening myeloma cDNA expression libraries using the SEREX technique for eventual development of an antigen cocktail. We have identified a series of antigens using this technique as well as myeloma expression profile data and have begun to validate individual antigens such as Xbp-1 and CD138 (Bae et al., unpublished).

Several antigens on MM cells have been identified as potential targets for immunotherapeutic strategies. MUC1 is a transmembrane protein expressed on most glandular epithelial cells (47) and abundantly overexpressed in a hypoglycosylated form on the entire cell surface of many human tumors, including MM cell lines and fresh patient MM cells (48,49).

Expression of so-called cancer-testis (CT) antigens on MM cells has also been reported (50). The CT antigens, which are expressed in various malignancies but not in normal tissues except male germ-line cells, include members of the MAGE family, BAGE, GAGE, PRAME, NY-ESO-1, and Sperm protein17 (51). Due to their tumor-restricted expression pattern and their immunogenicity, CT antigens are under active evaluation for immunotherapy of cancer.

However, the clinical effectiveness of all these cellular antigens for vaccination of myeloma patients remains to be investigated. The major obstacle with these antigens is that they are all self-antigens, and even though these antigens might be expressed in a restricted fashion on normal tissues, one has to keep in mind potential toxicity. In addition, most of these antigens are shown to be upregulated in the latephase of myeloma and may be associated with only a subset of myeloma cells. This may pose a problem when using these antigens to effectively vaccinate patients because it may be too late in the disease process to obtain clinical improvement.

REFERENCES

1. Munshi NC. Immunoregulatory mechanisms in multiple myeloma. Hematol Oncol Clin North Am 1997; 11:51–69.
2. Massaia M, Bianchi A, Attisano C, et al. Detection of hyperreactive T cells in multiple myeloma by multivalent cross-linking of the CD3/TCR complex. Blood 1991; 78:1770–80.
3. Brown RD, Pope B, Murray A, et al. Dendritic cells from patients with myeloma are numerically normal but functionally defective as they fail to up-regulate CD80 (B7-1) expression after huCD40LT stimulation because of inhibition by transforming growth factor-beta1 and interleukin-10. Blood 2001; 98:2992–8.
4. Xie J, Wang Y, Freeman ME, 3rd, Barlogie B, Yi Q. Beta 2-microglobulin as a negative regulator of the immune system: high concentrations of the protein inhibit in vitro generation of functional dendritic cells. Blood 2003; 101: 4005–12.
5. Mariani S, Coscia M, Even J, et al. Severe and long-lasting disruption of T-cell receptor diversity in human myeloma after high-dose chemotherapy and autologous peripheral blood progenitor cell infusion. Br J Haematol 2001; 113: 1051–9.
6. Maecker B, Anderson KS, von Bergwelt-Baildon MS, et al. Viral antigen-specific CD8+ T-cell responses are impaired in multiple myeloma. Br J Haematol 2003; 121:842–8.
7. Zinneman HH, Hall WH. Recurrent pneumonia in multiple myeloma and some observations on immunologic response. Ann Intern Med 1954; 41: 1152–63.
8. Robertson JD, Nagesh K, Jowitt SN, et al. Immunogenicity of vaccination against influenza, *Streptococcus pneumoniae* and *Haemophilus influenzae* type B in patients with multiple myeloma. Br J Cancer 2000; 82:1261–5.
9. Raje N, Gong J, Chauhan D, et al. Bone marrow and peripheral blood dendritic cells from patients with multiple myeloma are phenotypically and functionally normal despite the detection of Kaposi's sarcoma herpesvirus gene sequences. Blood 1999; 93:1487–95.
10. Butch AW, Kelly KA, Munshi NC. Dendritic cells derived from multiple myeloma patients efficiently internalize different classes of myeloma protein. Exp Hematol 2001; 29:85–92.

11. Ratta M, Fagnoni F, Curti A, et al. Dendritic cells are functionally defective in multiple myeloma: the role of interleukin-6. Blood 2002; 100:230–7.

12. Wang S, Hong S, Yang J, et al. Optimizing immunotherapy in multiple myeloma: Restoring the function of patients' monocyte-derived dendritic cells by inhibiting p38 or activating MEK/ERK MAPK and neutralizing interleukin-6 in progenitor cells. Blood 2006; 108:4071–7.

13. Dauer M, Obermaier B, Herten J, et al. Mature dendritic cells derived from human monocytes within 48 hours: a novel strategy for dendritic cell differentiation from blood precursors. J Immunol 2003; 170:4069–76.

14. West MA, Wallin RP, Matthews SP, et al. Enhanced dendritic cell antigen capture via toll-like receptor-induced actin remodeling. Science 2004; 305: 1153–7.

15. Hermans IF, Silk JD, Gileadi U, et al. Dendritic cell function can be modulated through cooperative actions of TLR ligands and invariant NKT cells. J Immunol 2007; 178:2721–9.

16. Prabhala RH, Neri P, Bae JE, et al. Dysfunctional T regulatory cells in multiple myeloma. Blood 2006; 107:301–4.

17. Beyer M, Kochanek M, Giese T, et al. In vivo peripheral expansion of naive CD4+CD25 high FoxP3+ regulatory T cells in patients with multiple myeloma. Blood 2006; 107:3940–9.

18. Pasare C, Medzhitov R. Toll pathway-dependent blockade of CD4+CD25+ T cell-mediated suppression by dendritic cells. Science 2003; 299:1033–6.

19. Bettelli E, Carrier Y, Gao W, et al. Reciprocal developmental pathways for the generation of pathogenic effector TH17 and regulatory T cells. Nature 2006; 441:235–8.

20. Steinman L. A brief history of T(H)17, the first major revision in the T(H)1/T(H) 2 hypothesis of T cell-mediated tissue damage. Nat Med 2007; 13:139–45.

21. Dhodapkar MV, Geller MD, Chang DH, et al. A reversible defect in natural killer T cell function characterizes the progression of premalignant to malignant multiple myeloma. J Exp Med 2003; 197:1667–76.

22. Lynch RG, Graff RJ, Sirisinha S, Simms ES, Eisen HN. Myeloma proteins as tumor-specific transplantation antigens. Proc Natl Acad Sci USA 1972; 69:1540–4.

23. Yi Q, Osterborg A, Bergenbrant S, Mellstedt H, Holm G, Lefvert AK. Idiotype-reactive T-cell subsets and tumor load in monoclonal gammopathies. Blood 1995; 86:3043–9.

24. King CA, Spellerberg MB, Zhu D, et al. DNA vaccines with single-chain Fv fused to fragment C of tetanus toxin induce protective immunity against lymphoma and myeloma. Nat Med 1998; 4:1281–6.

25. Stritzke J, Zunkel T, Steinmann J, Schmitz N, Uharek L, Zeis M. Therapeutic effects of idiotype vaccination can be enhanced by the combination of granulocyte-macrophage colony-stimulating factor and interleukin 2 in a myeloma model. Br J Haematol 2003; 120:27–35.

26. Bergenbrant S, Yi Q, Osterborg A, et al. Modulation of anti-idiotypic immune response by immunization with the autologous M-component protein in multiple myeloma patients. Br J Haematol 1996; 92:840–6.

27. Osterborg A, Yi Q, Henriksson L, et al. Idiotype immunization combined with granulocyte-macrophage colony-stimulating factor in myeloma patients

induced type I, major histocompatibility complex-restricted, CD8- and CD4-specific T-cell responses. Blood 1998; 91:2459–66.

28. Rasmussen T, Hansson L, Osterborg A, Johnsen HE, Mellstedt H. Idiotype vaccination in multiple myeloma induced a reduction of circulating clonal tumor B cells. Blood 2003; 101:4607–10.

29. Bertinetti C, Zirlik K, Heining-Mikesch K, et al. Phase I trial of a novel intradermal idiotype vaccine in patients with advanced B-cell lymphoma: specific immune responses despite profound immunosuppression. Cancer Res 2006; 66:4496–502.

30. Massaia M, Borrione P, Battaglio S, et al. Idiotype vaccination in human myeloma: generation of tumor-specific immune responses after high-dose chemotherapy. Blood 1999; 94:673–83.

31. Coscia M, Mariani S, Battaglio S, et al. Long-term follow-up of idiotype vaccination in human myeloma as a maintenance therapy after high-dose chemotherapy. Leukemia 2004; 18:139–45.

32. Neelapu SS, Munshi NC, Jagannath S, et al. Tumor antigen immunization of sibling stem cell transplant donors in multiple myeloma. Bone Marrow Transplant 2005; 36:315–23.

33. Lauritzsen GF, Weiss S, Dembic Z, Bogen B. Naive idiotype-specific CD4+ T cells and immunosurveillance of B-cell tumors. Proc Natl Acad Sci USA 1994; 91:5700–4.

34. Yi Q, Desikan R, Barlogie B, Munshi N. Optimizing dendritic cell-based immunotherapy in multiple myeloma. Br J Haematol 2002; 117:297–305.

35. Gong J, Koido S, Chen D, et al. Immunization against murine multiple myeloma with fusions of dendritic and plasmacytoma cells is potentiated by interleukin 12. Blood 2002; 99:2512–17.

36. Lim SH, Bailey-Wood R. Idiotypic protein-pulsed dendritic cell vaccination in multiple myeloma. Int J Cancer 1999; 83:215–22.

37. Cull G, Durrant L, Stainer C, Haynes A, Russell N. Generation of anti-idiotype immune responses following vaccination with idiotype-protein pulsed dendritic cells in myeloma. Br J Haematol 1999; 107:648–55.

38. Titzer S, Christensen O, Manzke O, et al. Vaccination of multiple myeloma patients with idiotype-pulsed dendritic cells: immunological and clinical aspects. Br J Haematol 2000; 108:805–16.

39. Liso A, Stockerl-Goldstein KE, Auffermann-Gretzinger S, et al. Idiotype vaccination using dendritic cells after autologous peripheral blood progenitor cell transplantation for multiple myeloma. Biol Blood Marrow Transplant 2000; 6:621–7.

40. Reichardt VL, Okada CY, Liso A, et al. Idiotype vaccination using dendritic cells after autologous peripheral blood stem cell transplantation for multiple myeloma—a feasibility study. Blood 1999; 93:2411–19.

41. Reichardt VL, Milazzo C, Brugger W, Einsele H, Kanz L, Brossart P. Idiotype vaccination of multiple myeloma patients using monocyte-derived dendritic cells. Haematologica 2003; 88:1139–49.

42. Bendandi M, Rodriguez-Calvillo M, Inoges S, et al. Combined vaccination with idiotype-pulsed allogeneic dendritic cells and soluble protein idiotype for

multiple myeloma patients relapsing after reduced-intensity conditioning allogeneic stem cell transplantation. Leuk Lymphoma 2006; 47:29–37.

43. Eggert AA, Schreurs MW, Boerman OC, et al. Biodistribution and vaccine efficiency of murine dendritic cells are dependent on the route of administration. Cancer Res 1999; 59:3340–5.

44. Morse MA, Coleman RE, Akabani G, Niehaus N, Coleman D, Lyerly HK. Migration of human dendritic cells after injection in patients with metastatic malignancies. Cancer Res 1999; 59:56–8.

45. Fong L, Brockstedt D, Benike C, Wu L, Engleman EG. Dendritic cells injected via different routes induce immunity in cancer patients. J Immunol 2001; 166: 4254–9.

46. Palucka KA, Taquet N, Sanchez-Chapuis F, Gluckman JC. Dendritic cells as the terminal stage of monocyte differentiation. J Immunol 1998; 160:4587–95.

47. Ho SB, Niehans GA, Lyftogt C, et al. Heterogeneity of mucin gene expression in normal and neoplastic tissues. Cancer Res 1993; 53:641–51.

48. Treon SP, Maimonis P, Bua D, et al. Elevated soluble MUC1 levels and decreased anti-MUC1 antibody levels in patients with multiple myeloma. Blood 2000; 96:3147–53.

49. Takahashi T, Makiguchi Y, Hinoda Y, et al. Expression of MUC1 on myeloma cells and induction of HLA-unrestricted CTL against MUC1 from a multiple myeloma patient. J Immunol 1994; 153:2102–9.

50. Jungbluth AA, Ely S, DiLiberto M, et al. The cancer-testis antigens CT7 (MAGE-C1) and MAGE-A3/6 are commonly expressed in multiple myeloma and correlate with plasma-cell proliferation. Blood 2005; 106:167–74.

51. Zendman AJ, Ruiter DJ, Van Muijen GN. Cancer/testis-associated genes: identification, expression profile, and putative function. J Cell Physiol 2003; 194:272–88.

52. LeBlanc R, Hideshima T, Catley LP, et al. Immunomodulatory drug costimulates T cells via the B7-CD28 pathway. Blood 2004; 103:1787–90.

13

Novel Therapeutic Options in Primary Systemic Amyloidosis

Morie A. Gertz

Division of Hematology, Mayo Clinic, Rochester, Minnesota, U.S.A.

INTRODUCTION

Amyloid is defined in tissue sections as an amorphous deposit that binds the dye Congo red and demonstrates apple-green birefringence when viewed under polarized light. X-ray diffraction studies have shown that the binding of Congo red is due to the β-pleated sheet configuration of the amyloid protein. All amyloid deposits are extracellular, and the clinical syndrome resulting from the deposition of amyloid is termed amyloidosis. This chapter discusses amyloidosis related to immunoglobulin light-chain deposits (AL amyloidosis) and current therapies directed at the management of this type of amyloidosis (1).

DIAGNOSIS OF AMYLOIDOSIS

Amyloidosis represents 9% of all the cases of monoclonal gammopathy seen at Mayo Clinic (Fig. 1); 73% of these amyloidosis cases are the AL type. However, not all patients with amyloidosis have systemic amyloid deposition, and an appropriate diagnostic evaluation is warranted before beginning therapy to ensure that the amyloidosis is correctly classified; errors in classification have occurred (2).

The serum monoclonal (M) protein concentration in patients with amyloidosis reflects their low-tumor-burden state. Less than 15% of patients have an M protein concentration greater than 1.5 mg/dL. The most common monoclonal protein in the serum in patients with amyloidosis is

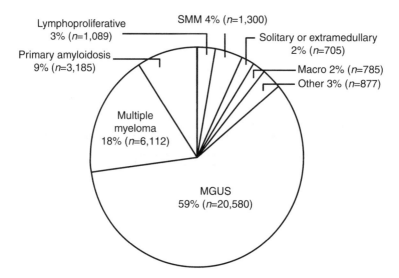

Figure 1 Cases of monoclonal gammopathy seen at Mayo Clinic, 1960–2005 ($N = 34,633$). *Abbreviations*: Macro, macroglobulinemia; MGUS, monoclonal gammopathy of undetermined significance; SMM, smoldering multiple myeloma. *Source*: From Ref. 60.

free λ monoclonal light chain (Bence Jones proteinemia). In multiple myeloma, nearly 30% of patients have a G κ monoclonal protein, but in AL amyloidosis G κ is present in less than 10% of patients. In multiple myeloma, the ratio of κ to λ light chain is 2:1, and in amyloidosis it is 1:3.6. The median M protein concentration in the urine of patients with amyloidosis is only 0.2 g/dL. For patients with AL amyloidosis, 66% have a λ light chain, 20% have κ, 1% have biclonal light chains, and 13% have no light chain in the urine. The median number of bone marrow plasma cells is 7%; only 14% of patients have greater than 20% plasma cells in the bone marrow. Most patients with amyloidosis do not fulfill criteria for multiple myeloma because they often have no bone disease, cast nephropathy, or anemia.

SUPPORTIVE CARE FOR AMYLOIDOSIS

Cardiac Amyloidosis

Therapy for amyloidosis is both supportive and specific, usually directed against the immunoglobulin light chain. The mortality associated with AL amyloidosis is best predicted by the extent of cardiac involvement at diagnosis (3), and the management of heart-related symptoms is an important aspect of supportive care.

   The cornerstone of supportive management of cardiac amyloidosis is the use of diuretics (4). However, associated orthostatic hypotension, intravascular volume contraction due to concomitant nephrotic syndrome, can often limit diuretic therapy (5). Patients with recurrent syncope often benefit from pacemaker implantation (6). Some centers now routinely place a defibrillator when considering high-dose chemotherapy followed by stem cell transplantation. Afterload reduction with angiotensin-converting enzyme inhibitors is standard in the management of heart failure (7). The high frequency of hypotension in amyloidosis, however, makes administration of therapeutic doses of angiotensin-converting enzyme inhibitors challenging. The use of calcium-channel blockers has been reported to aggravate the heart failure associated with AL amyloidosis.

Cardiac transplantation has been used to manage cardiac amyloidosis. Hosenpud et al. (8) reported on seven patients with amyloidosis who had cardiac transplantation, five of whom were still alive at a median of 32 months after transplantation. In a follow-up study of 10 patients with cardiac amyloidosis who received allograft hearts, two patients died perioperatively and seven died at a median of 32 months after transplantation, four due to recurrent amyloidosis (9). Recently, the National Amyloidosis Center in Great Britain reported the use of cardiac transplantation followed by high-dose chemotherapy and stem cell transplantation in an effort to prevent recurrent amyloid deposits. Heart transplantation followed by stem cell transplantation was performed in five patients with AL amyloidosis and cardiomyopathy (10). After a median follow-up of 95 months, three patients were well without evidence of amyloid accumulation in the heart, and two died of progressive amyloidosis 33 and 90 months after heart transplantation with relapse of the plasma cell dyscrasia.

Renal Amyloidosis

Supportive care for renal amyloid disease includes the use of diuretics. Continuous urinary protein loss due to amyloidosis ultimately results in end-stage renal disease (11). Ramipril has been reported to reduce proteinuria in patients with nephrotic syndrome (12).

Often, the disease results in the need for dialysis; median time from diagnosis of renal AL amyloidosis to dialysis is 14 months, and median survival from the start of dialysis is eight months (13). Dialysis in patients with amyloidosis is often challenging; concomitant cardiac amyloid makes dialysis difficult because of associated hypotension. The survival of patients with AL amyloidosis who are on dialysis is decreased compared with that for patients who are on dialysis as a result of primary renal disease (14). In 61 patients with amyloidosis, 18 died within a month after starting dialysis therapy; 15 of 43 patients were alive at a median of 61 months. The most important complications were subsequent cardiac and gastrointestinal tract amyloid development.

The experience at Mayo Clinic with renal transplantation in patients with primary amyloidosis has now been published (15). It is debated whether it is better to give high-dose chemotherapy followed by a renal transplant or to perform a renal transplant followed by high-dose chemotherapy (16). In general, patients who receive a kidney before beginning chemotherapy initially tolerate the transplant better, but they often are already receiving immunosuppressive therapy, usually consisting of corticosteroids and mycophenolic acid. Use of immunosuppressive therapy increases the post–stem cell transplant infection rate. Moreover, patients with amyloidosis receiving high-dose therapy may not achieve a complete response, and if a kidney has already been transplanted, prevention of recurrent amyloid can be frustrating. At present, the practice at Mayo Clinic is to start patients on reduced-dose melphalan chemotherapy, and only those who have a complete response are referred for kidney transplantation, usually from a living related donor (15).

In one report, a group of 15 patients with systemic amyloidosis had renal transplantation from 42 to 216 months after diagnosis (17). The 10 patients in whom the underlying amyloidogenic disorder had been treated first remained stable. Amyloid presence in the graft, however, was identified in 4 of the 10; in all four, amyloid fibril precursor protein concentration had not been diminished (17). Two patients with AL amyloidosis in whom chemotherapy resulted in an eradication of free light-chain production did receive renal transplantation, and both patients have normal renal function after more than four years of follow-up.

SPECIFIC THERAPY FOR AMYLOIDOSIS

Stem Cell Transplantation

Indications for Stem Cell Transplantation

At Mayo Clinic, the current approach to treatment of amyloidosis is to stratify patients on the basis of their eligibility and suitability for stem cell transplantation. Patients who have an adequate performance status on the Eastern Cooperative Oncology Group scale, no major comorbid conditions, fewer than three organs involved, and mild to moderate cardiac amyloidosis are offered treatment in a phase III clinical trial of conventional therapy with high-dose chemotherapy with or without stem cell transplantation. If patients decline participation in the trial they are given high-dose chemotherapy and stem cell transplantation (18).

The use of stem cell transplantation in AL amyloidosis is based on its known efficacy in multiple myeloma, for which survival benefit has been demonstrated in phase III studies. Amyloidosis appears to be an ideal model for stem cell transplantation because the patients with multiple myeloma who appear to have the best outcomes have the lowest tumor burden and indolent plasma cell kinetics, which are typical of patients with AL amyloidosis (19). The disease characteristics of amyloidosis, however, are very different from those of multiple myeloma. In multiple myeloma, patients have abnormal bone marrow but good organ function, and treatment-related mortality rates are 1% to 2%. Amyloidosis is characterized by minimal involvement of the bone marrow, but organ dysfunction can be widespread, which can lead to a wide range of post–stem cell transplant complications including dialysis-dependent renal, cardiac, and hepatic failure (20).

Mayo Clinic Experience

Cohort Characteristics: Stem cell transplantation has been performed in 270 patients with AL amyloidosis at Mayo Clinic since 1996. Men represented 59% of the patients, and the median age was 57 years (range, 31–75 years). The median serum albumin level was 2.8 g/dL, reflecting the high prevalence of nephrotic syndrome. Ten percent of stem cell transplant recipients had a serum creatinine level greater than 1.8 mg/dL; 75% had a creatinine value less than 1.3 mg/dL. Nineteen percent of patients had an alkaline phosphatase level greater than twice normal, which is a surrogate marker for hepatic involvement. Urine protein excretion was more than 3 g in a 24-hour collection in 54% of patients; only 6% had greater than 1 g of monoclonal light chain excretion in 24 hours. The percentage of patients with 1-, 2-, and 3-organ involvement was 48%, 38%, and 14%, respectively.

The 270 patients with AL amyloidosis received stem cell transplant at a median of 4.2 months after diagnosis, 25% within 3 months, and 75% within 7.2 months of diagnosis. All had biopsy-verified amyloidosis; liver, endoscopic, cardiac, and renal biopsy results were positive in 95% of patients. Amyloid deposits were demonstrable in the bone marrow in 75% and in subcutaneous fat in 71%. The extent of cardiac amyloid by echocardiography was less in the transplant group than in a cohort not selected for stem cell transplant. The median interventricular septal thickness was 12 mm; it was 10 mm or less in 25% and less than 14 mm in 75%. The median ejection fraction was 65%; ejection fraction was less than 70% in 75% of the patients and less than 60% in 25%.

Transplant Data: The median number of apheresis collections in the Mayo Clinic cohort was 3 (interquartile range, 2–4 aphereses). The median number of CD34$^+$ cells collected was 6.5 × 10^6/kg (range, 2.0-50.9 × 10^6/kg). The engraftment kinetics were similar to those of patients with multiple myeloma, but growth factor was not administered after transplantation because of its effects on fluid retention and its ability to precipitate congestive heart failure. A neutrophil count of 500/μL was achieved at a median of 14 days with a range of 7–116 days. Twenty-five percent of the patients had neutrophil engraftment before day 13, 75% by day 16, and 90% by day 22. Twenty thousand platelets/μL was achieved at a median of 14 days (range, 6-406 days). One-fourth of the patients had 20,000 platelets/μL by day 12, 75% by day 19, and 90% by day 28. A platelet count of 50,000/μL was achieved at a median of 18 days. Twenty-five percent of patients had platelet engraftment by day 14 and 75% by day 28. In 10% of the patients, 50,000 platelets/μL had not been achieved at day 52.

The number of CD34$^+$ cells collected and infused seems to affect the engraftment of platelets. If the number of CD34$^+$ cells infused was between three and four million, the time to engraftment was not significantly different from that in patients with more than four million CD34$^+$ cells infused. However, the time to platelet engraftment was significantly longer if the number of CD34$^+$ cells infused was between two and three million compared with more than three million.

The chemotherapy regimens used at Mayo Clinic were typical of those used in patients with multiple myeloma; 62% received melphalan at a dose of 200 mg/m^2, 26% received melphalan at 140 mg/m^2, and a small fraction received lower doses primarily because of advanced cardiac amyloid. A previous report from Mayo Clinic showed that the intensity of chemotherapy used is important for outcome and that patients receiving full-dose melphalan (200 mg/m^2) appear to have better outcomes, although this may be because patients selected for reduced-intensity therapy tend to have more advanced amyloidosis (21).

The 100-day mortality in the 270 Mayo Clinic patients was 11%, which compares favorably with other institutional reports of mortality as high as 40% (22–24). Achieving a low 100-day mortality is critical for positive outcomes and is certainly necessary if stem cell transplantation is to be compared with conventional chemotherapy with survival as an end point. The median actuarial survival for the entire group was 75 months.

With ongoing experience, the mortality rate at Mayo Clinic has successively decreased. Before 2004, 12.1% of stem cell transplant recipients died before day 100, whereas only 10 of 107 patients who received a stem cell transplant since January 1, 2004, died before day 100 (9.3%). The causes of death in the 10 patients included ventricular tachycardia (in one case the patient had a defibrillator in place), and one patient with factor X deficiency bled to death. Duration of hospitalization ranged from 0 to 78 days with a median of nine days. Eighteen percent of patients were never hospitalized, 25% were hospitalized for three days or less, and 75% for 17 days or less.

Results of Previous Trials

A report from the American Bone Marrow Transplant Registry described 107 patients from 48 transplant centers (25). The 30-day treatment-related mortality was 18%, compared with 7.4% at Mayo Clinic. The transplant registry report showed high response rates with only an 11% incidence of disease progression after stem cell transplantation. The median projected survival in the transplant registry study was 47 months. The study reported a total response rate of 34%; 33% of the patients were stable (25). In the transplant registry study, the most important predictor of survival was the level of experience of the transplant center; those receiving a stem cell transplant within the past five years fared significantly better than patients who had transplantation more than five years ago. This finding raises the question of whether stem cell transplantation for amyloidosis should be performed preferentially in specialized centers with extensive experience or can be done at centers that have extensive transplant experience in non-amyloid disease. One Eastern Cooperative Oncology Group study suggested that treatment-related mortality is not higher in multicenter cooperative group studies than in single-center studies (26).

Stem cell transplantation is not a proven therapy in the management of amyloidosis despite reports of organ remissions in 50% of patients treated with transplantation (18,27,28). A French multicenter randomized trial (MAG and IFM Intergroup) presented at the 2005 American Society of Hematology suggested that overall survival for stem cell transplantation may not be superior to that for a regimen of melphalan plus high-dose dexamethasone (29). This trial randomly assigned 100 patients to medical therapy (melphalan plus high-dose dexamethasone) or stem cell transplantation; median actuarial survival was 57 months with medical therapy and 49 months with transplantation. The transplant patients received melphalan at a dose of 140 or 200 mg/m^2, and stem cells were mobilized with filgrastim alone. The hematologic response rates for the transplant and nontransplant groups were 65% and 64%. Caution is required in interpreting these results, however; the follow-up time was short (median, 29 months) and the treatment-related mortality for the transplant group was high (24%), which makes it difficult to demonstrate a survival benefit. In fact, only 29 of the 100 patients received a stem cell transplant and were considered evaluable for response. Because of these small numbers, it would be premature to abandon transplantation as a therapy for amyloidosis.

Factors Affecting Outcome

Inherent bias is present in the patient-selection process for transplant candidacy. At Mayo Clinic, only one-fourth of patients evaluated ultimately have stem cell transplantation. In a study of 207 patients with amyloidosis at Mayo Clinic who met the eligibility criteria for stem cell transplantation but were treated conventionally, median survival was 45 months, not the oft-quoted 12 to 18 months (30). Therefore, patients selected for stem cell transplantation have an inherently better prognosis than those not selected for transplantation. However, in a case-matched control study of 63 stem cell transplant recipients and 63 conventionally treated patients matched for age, sex, cardiac function, creatinine level, urinary protein loss, and liver involvement, the stem cell transplant patients had an overall survival advantage (31).

Other factors that appear to affect survival include the absolute lymphocyte count at day 15 after stem cell transplant (32) and the number of organs involved in amyloidosis. Patients with 2-organ involvement have a median survival of 55 months, versus 25.5 months for 3-organ involvement (Fig. 2) (33). Factors reported to be statistically significant in predicting outcome include the serum creatinine level, serum troponin T, brain natriuretic peptide (BNP) level, and interventricular septal thickness. Excessive fluid accumulation during stem cell mobilization and greater than 2% weight gain is predictive of a higher mortality rate with stem cell transplantation (34). The BNP level substantially affects survival after stem cell transplantation presumably because it reflects the severity of cardiac failure (Fig. 3) (35). The median level of BNP among 117 Mayo Clinic patients was 170 pg/mL. One study showed that response to transplantation has a profound effect on survival (36). Patients who had a 50% decrease in light chain concentration had greater survival than those who did not. Of interest, another study showed that overall survival also was linked to the pretransplant free light chain level and the number of organs involved (37).

In large centers performing stem cell transplantation, treatment-related mortality has ranged from 6% to 18%, hematologic complete responses from 16% to 50%, and organ responses from 34% to 64%, although organ responses are a time-dependent variable and often can be delayed for 36 months after transplant (38).

Other Techniques

Tandem stem cell transplants have been performed in patients with amyloidosis and are feasible. The ultimate impact of tandem stem cell transplants on patients with amyloidosis remains unknown (39). One study evaluating induction therapy with 2 cycles of melphalan and prednisone

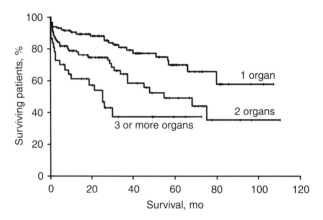

Figure 2 Survival in 270 Mayo Clinic patients with AL amyloidosis after stem cell transplantation based on number of involved organs. *Source*: From Ref. 60.

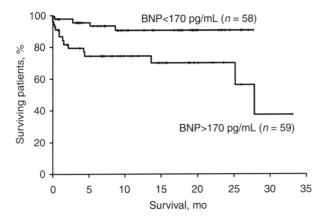

Figure 3 Effect of BNP concentration on survival in 117 Mayo Clinic patients with AL amyloidosis after stem cell transplantation ($p = 0.008$). *Source*: From Ref. 60.

before stem cell transplantation showed no effect of the induction therapy on hematologic or organ responses (40).

Nontransplant Therapy

Melphalan

For most patients with amyloidosis who are not candidates for a stem cell transplant, other forms of chemotherapy are necessary. Melphalan-based therapy combined with standard prednisone has been used in the management of amyloidosis for more than 30 years. Two prospective randomized studies have demonstrated survival advantages with melphalan-based therapy. One 3-arm study accrued 219 patients and randomly assigned them to receive colchicine (0.6 mg twice daily), standard melphalan and prednisone, or melphalan and prednisone plus colchicine (41). Half of the patients had proteinuria in the nephrotic range and 20% had heart failure. The median survival for the melphalan-containing regimens was 17 months, compared with 8.5 months for colchicine alone (41). A second prospective randomized study of 100 patients—50 receiving colchicine and 50 receiving melphalan, prednisone, and colchicine—showed a median survival of 6.7 months in the colchicine alone group, versus 12 months in the 3-drug group (42). Because of the survival advantage in the melphalan-based group and because this regimen is well tolerated, most patients should receive an initial trial of this therapy. However, a median survival of only 18 months leaves a good deal of room for improvement.

Dexamethasone

Nine consecutive patients with biopsy-proven AL amyloidosis were treated with pulsed dexamethasone for 3 to 6 cycles, followed by maintenance interferon (3–6 million units, 3×weekly) (43). Improvement in at least 1 organ with amyloid involvement was seen in 8 of 9 patients. Seven patients had nephrotic-range proteinuria and the proteinuria was decreased in 6. The median time to response was 4 months; the improvement was durable. Neither of 2 patients with heart failure improved. In a cohort of long-term survivors from Mayo Clinic, dexamethasone as a single agent was shown to be beneficial in the treatment of AL amyloidosis (44,45). A modified, milder schedule (lower dose and frequency) of dexamethasone can produce a response in 35% of patients with a median time to response of 4 months (46).

Between 1996 and 2003, 93 patients with AL amyloidosis were enrolled in a multicenter cooperative group trial of dexamethasone and α-interferon (47). Hematologic complete remissions were seen in 24% of patients, and improvement in organ dysfunction occurred in 45% of evaluable patients. The median survival was 31 months. Two-year overall survival and event-free survival were 60% and 52%, respectively. Heart failure and serum β_2-microglobulin levels were predictors of adverse outcomes. In a subset of patients eligible for stem cell transplantation, the estimated 2-year overall survival was 78%. Dexamethasone can lead to durable reversal of amyloid-related organ dysfunction (47).

Melphalan and Dexamethasone

Palladini et al. (48) have reported on the use of melphalan plus high-dose dexamethasone in the management of amyloidosis. These patients were selected on the basis of their ineligibility for high-dose melphalan plus transplant therapy. Of 46 patients, a hematologic response was seen in 31 and a hematologic complete response was seen in 15 (33%). Improvement in organ dysfunction was seen in 22 patients (48%). Advantages of this regimen included the low 100-day mortality (4%), resolution of cardiac failure in 6 of 32 patients with a median time to response of 4.5 months, and only 11% adverse effects (48).

Thalidomide

Thalidomide has been used in the management of amyloidosis, both as a single agent and combined with dexamethasone. In one study, 12 patients with amyloidosis received thalidomide; 8 had renal involvement and 4 had cardiac involvement (49). Ten patients had previous high-dose therapy with various drugs with stem cell transplantation. The median maximum tolerated dose of thalidomide was 500 mg. Four patients discontinued treatment because of toxicity. Worsening azotemia developed in 2. No patient had more than a 50% decrease in M component value. Three patients had disease progression. In a study from Mayo Clinic, significant toxicity was associated with use of thalidomide (50). Median time on thalidomide therapy was 72 days with a median dose of 50 mg (50).

The combination of thalidomide and intermediate-dose dexamethasone has been used as second-line treatment for AL amyloidosis (51). Hematologic responses were seen in 48% of patients, with complete responses in 19%. Median time to hematologic response was 3.6 months, severe adverse events were frequent (65%), and symptomatic bradycardia was common (26%) (51). Thalidomide was clearly less well tolerated in this cohort than in a group of patients with myeloma and was associated with serious adverse effects.

Lenalidomide, an immunomodulatory drug related to thalidomide, has been reported to be effective in the management of amyloidosis. In a study of 34 patients reported at the 2006 American Society of Clinical Oncology annual meeting, 8 of 13 had a measurable response, 4 to lenalidomide alone. Nine additional patients responded when dexamethasone was added (52).

Etanercept

Tumor necrosis factor alpha has been implicated in amyloid disorders; etanercept (a tumor necrosis factor blocker) has been used to treat patients with advanced amyloidosis in whom other therapies had failed (53). Of 16 patients treated with etanercept for a median of 42 weeks, 8 had objective improvement and 14 patients had subjective improvement. Only 1 patient had an adverse effect. The estimated median survival was 24.2 months. Six of 12 patients with cardiac involvement were alive at the time of publication, and the patients' performance status improved significantly. Etanercept may provide a new therapeutic option for the management of amyloidosis.

Eprodisate

Eprodisate is a sulfated glycosaminoglycan developed for the treatment of AA (secondary) amyloidosis that was submitted for a new drug application to the U.S. Food and Drug Administration in February 2006. A 2-year international multicenter randomized, double-blind, placebo-controlled, phase II–III clinical trial was designed to evaluate the efficacy and safety of the drug in patients with AA amyloidosis. A total of 183 patients were enrolled at 27 sites. If activity is seen, the potential for applying this drug to the management of AL amyloidosis exists (54).

Immunologic Therapy

The development of murine amyloid-reactive monoclonal antibodies has provided a passive immunotherapy approach to the management of AL amyloidosis (55). These antibodies against human light chain–related fibrils recognize an epitope common to the β-pleated sheet structure of AL and can improve amyloidolysis when administered to mice injected with human AL extracts. One chimeric prototype antibody has been developed and is planned for an eventual phase I and phase II clinical trial in AL amyloidosis

(56). Demonstration of therapeutic efficacy would provide a proof of principle that immunotherapy might benefit individuals with AL amyloidosis (57).

Nonchemotherapy-Based Treatment

Recently, allogeneic bone marrow transplantation was reported to be feasible for patients with amyloidosis (58). However, treatment-related mortality was high (40%). Seven of 10 patients in remission were long-term survivors. Chronic graft-versus-host disease was believed to contribute to disease control.

In another study, patients with amyloidosis underwent apheresis, and mononuclear cells were expanded ex vivo and induced to differentiate into dendritic cells (59). The dendritic cells were then exposed to M protein from patients with amyloidosis in an effort to induce antigen recognition. These dendritic cells were administered to patients at two, four, and sixteen weeks. One patient had resolution of proteinuria; in vitro T-cell proliferative response is correlated with clinical responses.

SUMMARY

The optimal therapy for AL amyloidosis is unknown. Most patients receive some form of cytotoxic chemotherapy, either high-dose with stem cell reconstitution, or dexamethasone-based therapy with oral or parenteral melphalan. A phase III clinical trial is underway to determine the optimal therapy for this disorder.

REFERENCES

1. Dumoulina M, Bader R. A short historical survey of developments in amyloid research. Protein Pept Lett 2006; 13(3):213–17.
2. Comenzo RL, Zhou P, Fleisher M, et al. Seeking confidence in the diagnosis of systemic AL (Ig light-chain) amyloidosis: patients can have both monoclonal gammopathies and hereditary amyloid proteins. Blood 2006; 107(9):3489–91 [Epub 2006 Jan. 26].
3. Falk RH. Diagnosis and management of the cardiac amyloidoses. Circulation 2005; 112(13):2047–60.
4. Parikh S, de Lemos JA. Current therapeutic strategies in cardiac amyloidosis. Curr Treat Options Cardiovasc Med 2005; 7(6):443–8.
5. Chamarthi B, Dubrey SW, Cha K, et al. Features and prognosis of exertional syncope in light-chain associated AL cardiac amyloidosis. Am J Cardiol 1997; 80(9):1242–5.
6. Mathew V, Chaliki H, Nishimura RA. Atrioventricular sequential pacing in cardiac amyloidosis: an acute Doppler echocardiographic and catheterization hemodynamic study. Clin Cardiol 1997; 20(8):723–5.

7. Nash KL, Brij SO, Clesham GJ. Cardiac amyloidosis and the use of diuretic and ACE inhibitor therapy in severe heart failure. Int J Clin Pract 1997; 51(6): 384–5.

8. Hosenpud JD, Uretsky BF, Griffith BP, et al. Successful intermediate-term outcome for patients with cardiac amyloidosis undergoing heart transplantation: results of a multicenter survey. J Heart Transplant 1990; 9(4):346–50.

9. Hosenpud JD, DeMarco T, Frazier OH, et al. Progression of systemic disease and reduced long-term survival in patients with cardiac amyloidosis undergoing heart transplantation: follow-up results of a multicenter survey. Circulation 1991; 84(Suppl. 5):III338–43.

10. Gillmore JD, Goodman HJ, Lachmann HJ, et al. Sequential heart and autologous stem cell transplantation for systemic AL amyloidosis. Blood 2006; 107(3):1227–9 [Epub 2005 Oct. 6].

11. Gertz MA, Leung N, Lacy MQ, et al. Myeloablative chemotherapy and stem cell transplantation in myeloma or primary amyloidosis with renal involvement. Kidney Int 2005; 68(4):1464–71.

12. Mayr M, Dickenmann MJ. Further evidence for the renoprotective effect of ACE inhibitors: ramipril protects against the progression of chronic renal insufficiency in non-diabetic nephropathy with nephrotic proteinuria [German]. Schweiz Med Wochenschr 2000; 130(13):491.

13. Gertz MA, Lacy MQ, Dispenzieri A. Immunoglobulin light chain amyloidosis and the kidney. Kidney Int 2002; 61(1):1–9.

14. Gertz MA, Kyle RA, O'Fallon WM. Dialysis support of patients with primary systemic amyloidosis: a study of 211 patients. Arch Intern Med 1992; 152(11): 2245–50.

15. Leung N, Griffin MD, Dispenzieri A, et al. Living donor kidney and autologous stem cell transplantation for primary systemic amyloidosis (AL) with predominant renal involvement. Am J Transplant 2005; 5(7):1660–70.

16. Merlini G, Remuzzi G. Autologous stem cell and kidney transplantation for primary amyloidosis associated with ESRD: which should come first? [editorial]. Am J Transplant 2005; 5(7):1585–6.

17. Gillmore JD, Madhoo S, Pepys MB, et al. Renal transplantation for amyloid end-stage renal failure: insights from serial serum amyloid P component scintigraphy. Nucl Med Commun 2000; 21(8):735–40.

18. Comenzo RL, Gertz MA. Autologous stem cell transplantation for primary systemic amyloidosis. Blood 2002; 99(12):4276–82.

19. Gertz MA, Lacy MQ, Dispenzieri A, et al. High-dose chemotherapy with autologous hematopoietic stem cell transplantation in patients with multiple myeloma. Expert Rev Anticancer Ther 2006; 6(3):343–60.

20. Kumar S, Dispenzieri A, Lacy MQ, et al. High incidence of gastrointestinal tract bleeding after autologous stem cell transplant for primary systemic amyloidosis. Bone Marrow Transplant 2001; 28(4):381–5.

21. Gertz MA, Lacy MQ, Dispenzieri A, et al. Risk-adjusted manipulation of melphalan dose before stem cell transplantation in patients with amyloidosis is associated with a lower response rate. Bone Marrow Transplant 2004; 34(12): 1025–31.

22. Chow LQ, Bahlis N, Russell J, et al. Autologous transplantation for primary systemic AL amyloidosis is feasible outside a major amyloidosis referral centre: the Calgary BMT Program experience. Bone Marrow Transplant 2005; 36(7): 591–6.

23. Schonland SO, Perz JB, Hundemer M, et al. Indications for high-dose chemotherapy with autologous stem cell support in patients with systemic amyloid light chain amyloidosis. Transplantation 2005; 80(Suppl. 1): S160–3.

24. Worel N, Schulenburg A, Mitterbauer M, et al. Autologous stem-cell transplantation in progressing amyloidosis is associated with severe transplant-related toxicity. Wien Klin Wochenschr 2006; 118(1–2):49–53.

25. Vesole DH, Perez WS, Akasheh M, et al. Plasma Cell Disorders Working Committee of the Center for International Blood and Marrow Transplant Research. High-dose therapy and autologous hematopoietic stem cell transplantation for patients with primary systemic amyloidosis: a Center for International Blood and Marrow Transplant Research Study. Mayo Clin Proc 2006; 81(7):880–8.

26. Gertz MA, Blood E, Vesole DH, et al. A multicenter phase 2 trial of stem cell transplantation for immunoglobulin light-chain amyloidosis (E4A97): an Eastern Cooperative Oncology Group Study. Bone Marrow Transplant 2004; 34(2):149–54.

27. Comenzo RL, Vosburgh E, Falk RH, et al. Dose-intensive melphalan with blood stem-cell support for the treatment of AL (amyloid light-chain) amyloidosis: survival and responses in 25 patients. Blood 1998; 91(10): 3662–70.

28. Seldin DC, Anderson JJ, Sanchorawala V, et al. Improvement in quality of life of patients with AL amyloidosis treated with high-dose melphalan and autologous stem cell transplantation. Blood 2004; 104(6):1888–1893 [Epub 2004 May 20].

29. Jaccard A, Moreau P, Leblond V, et al. Autologous stem cell transplantation (ASCT) versus oral melphalan and high-dose dexamethasone in patients with AL (primary) amyloidosis: results of the French Multicentric Randomized Trial (MAG and IFM Intergroup) [abstract]. Blood 2005; 106(11):127a.

30. Dispenzieri A, Lacy MQ, Kyle RA, et al. Eligibility for hematopoietic stem-cell transplantation for primary systemic amyloidosis is a favorable prognostic factor for survival. J Clin Oncol 2001; 19(14):3350–6.

31. Dispenzieri A, Kyle RA, Lacy MQ, et al. Superior survival in primary systemic amyloidosis patients undergoing peripheral blood stem cell transplantation: a case–control study. Blood 2004; 103(10):3960–3 [Epub 2004 Jan. 22].

32. Porrata LF, Gertz MA, Litzow MR, et al. Early lymphocyte recovery predicts superior survival after autologous hematopoietic stem cell transplantation for patients with primary systemic amyloidosis. Clin Cancer Res 2005; 11(3): 1210–18.

33. Gertz MA, Lacy MQ, Dizpenzieri A, et al. Amyloidosis: diagnosis and management. Clin Lymphoma Myeloma 2005; 6(3):208–19.

34. Leung N, Leung TR, Cha SS, et al. Excessive fluid accumulation during stem cell mobilization: a novel prognostic factor of first-year survival after stem cell

transplantation in AL amyloidosis patients. Blood 2005 Nov 15; 106(10): 3353–3357 [Epub 2005 Jul 21].

35. Palladini G, Campana C, Klersy C, et al. Serum N-terminal pro-brain natriuretic peptide is a sensitive marker of myocardial dysfunction in AL amyloidosis. Circulation 2003; 107(19):2440–5 [Epub 2003 Apr 28].

36. Sanchorawala V, Seldin DC, Magnani B, et al. Serum free light-chain responses after high-dose intravenous melphalan and autologous stem cell transplantation for AL (primary) amyloidosis. Bone Marrow Transplant 2005; 36(7): 597–600.

37. Dispenzieri A, Lacy MQ, Katzmann JA, et al. Absolute values of immunoglobulin free light chains are prognostic in patients with primary systemic amyloidosis undergoing peripheral blood stem cell transplantation. Blood 2006 Apr 15; 107(8):3378–83 [Epub 2006 Jan 5].

38. Leung N, Dispenzieri A, Fervenza FC, et al. Renal response after high-dose melphalan and stem cell transplantation is a favorable marker in patients with primary systemic amyloidosis. Am J Kidney Dis 2005; 46(2):270–7.

39. Quillen K, Wright DG, Seldin DC, et al. Feasibility of second autologous peripheral blood stem cell (PBSC) collection followed by a second cycle of high dose melphalan (HDM) in patients relapsing after an initial course of HDM for the treatment of AL amyloidosis [abstract]. Blood 2004; 104 (11): 391b–2b.

40. Sanchorawala V, Wright DG, Seldin DC, et al. High-dose intravenous melphalan and autologous stem cell transplantation as initial therapy or following two cycles of oral chemotherapy for the treatment of AL amyloidosis: results of a prospective randomized trial. Bone Marrow Transplant 2004; 33(4): 381–8.

41. Kyle RA, Gertz MA, Greipp PR, et al. A trial of three regimens for primary amyloidosis: colchicine alone, melphalan and prednisone, and melphalan, prednisone, and colchicine. N Engl J Med 1997; 336(17):1202–7.

42. Skinner M, Anderson J, Simms R, et al. Treatment of 100 patients with primary amyloidosis: a randomized trial of melphalan, prednisone, and colchicine versus colchicine only. Am J Med 1996; 100(3):290–8.

43. Dhodapkar MV, Jagannath S, Vesole D, et al. Treatment of AL-amyloidosis with dexamethasone plus alpha interferon. Leuk Lymphoma 1997; 27(3–4): 351–6.

44. Gertz MA, Lacy MQ, Lust JA, et al. Phase II trial of high-dose dexamethasone for previously treated immunoglobulin light-chain amyloidosis. Am J Hematol 1999; 61(2):115–19.

45. Gertz MA, Lacy MQ, Lust JA, et al. Phase II trial of high-dose dexamethasone for untreated patients with primary systemic amyloidosis. Med Oncol 1999; 16(2):104–9.

46. Palladini G, Anesi E, Perfetti V, et al. A modified high-dose dexamethasone regimen for primary systemic (AL) amyloidosis. Br J Haematol 2001; 113(4): 1044–6.

47. Dhodapkar MV, Hussein MA, Rasmussen E, et al. United States Intergroup Trial Southwest Oncology Group. Clinical efficacy of high-dose dexamethasone with maintenance dexamethasone/alpha interferon in patients with

primary systemic amyloidosis: results of United States Intergroup Trial Southwest Oncology Group (SWOG) S9628. Blood 2004; 104(12):3520–6 [Epub 2004 Aug 12].

48. Palladini G, Perfetti V, Obici L, et al. Association of melphalan and high-dose dexamethasone is effective and well tolerated in patients with AL (primary) amyloidosis who are ineligible for stem cell transplantation. Blood 2004; 103(8): 2936–8 [Epub 2003 Dec. 18].

49. Seldin DC, Choufani EB, Dember LM, et al. Tolerability and efficacy of thalidomide for the treatment of patients with light chain-associated (AL) amyloidosis. Clin Lymphoma 2003; 3(4):241–6.

50. Dispenzieri A, Lacy MQ, Rajkumar SV, et al. Poor tolerance to high doses of thalidomide in patients with primary systemic amyloidosis. Amyloid 2003, 10(4), 257–61.

51. Palladini G, Perfetti V, Perlini S, et al. The combination of thalidomide and intermediate-dose dexamethasone is an effective but toxic treatment for patients with primary amyloidosis (AL). Blood 2005; 105(7):2949–51 [Epub 2004 Nov. 30].

52. Sanchorawala V, Wright DG, Rosenzweig M, et al. A phase II trial of lenalidomide for patients with AL amyloidosis [abstract]. J Clin Oncol 2006; 24(Suppl. 20):18S.

53. Hussein MA, Juturi JV, Rybicki L, et al. Etanercept therapy in patients with advanced primary amyloidosis. Med Oncol 2003; 20(3):283–90.

54. Geerts H. NC-531 (Neurochem). Curr Opin Investig Drugs 2004; 5(1):95–100.

55. O'Nuallain B, Hrncic R, Wall JS, et al. Diagnostic and therapeutic potential of amyloid-reactive IgG antibodies contained in human sera. J Immunol 2006; 176(11):7071–8.

56. Solomon A, Weiss DT, Wall JS. Immunotherapy in systemic primary (AL) amyloidosis using amyloid-reactive monoclonal antibodies. Cancer Biother Radiopharm 2003; 18(6):853–60.

57. Solomon A, Weiss DT, Wall JS. Therapeutic potential of chimeric amyloid-reactive monoclonal antibody 11-1F4. Clin Cancer Res 2003; 9(10 Pt 2): 3831S–8S.

58. Schonland SO, Lokhorst H, Buzyn A, et al. Chronic Leukemia Working Party, Myeloma Subcommittee of the European Cooperative Group for Blood and Marrow Transplantation. Allogeneic and syngeneic hematopoietic cell transplantation in patients with amyloid light-chain amyloidosis: a report from the European Group for Blood and Marrow Transplantation. Blood 2006; 107(6): 2578–84 [Epub 2005 Nov. 17].

59. Lacy MQ, Wettstein PJ, Gertz MA, et al. Post autologous transplantation consolidation of multiple myeloma with idiotype-pulsed antigen presenting (dendritic) cells. J Clin Oncol 2002; 21(1):31a.

60. Gertz MA, Lacy MQ, Dispenzieri A, Hayman SR, Hayman SR, Kumar S. Transplantation for Amyloidosis. Curr Opin Oncol 2007; 19:136–41.

14

Novel Options of Therapy in Waldenström Macroglobulinemia

Irene M. Ghobrial

Department of Medical Oncology, Dana-Farber Cancer Institute, Harvard Medical School, Boston, Massachusetts, U.S.A.

Anne-Sophie Moreau and Xavier Leleu

Department of Medical Oncology, Dana-Farber Cancer Institute, Harvard Medical School, Boston, Massachusetts, U.S.A. and Service des Maladies du Sang, CHRU, Lille, France

Meletios A. Dimopoulos

Department of Clinical Therapeutics, Alexandra Hospital, University of Athens School of Medicine, Athens, Greece

INTRODUCTION

Waldenström macroglobulinemia (WM) is a distinct low grade B-cell lymphoma characterized by the presence of lymphoplasmacytic cells in bone marrow and a serum monoclonal IgM protein (1–3). It was first described by Dr. Jan Gosta Waldenström in 1944 when he identified two patients who developed oronasal bleeding, lymphadenopathy, anemia, and thrombocytopenia, elevated erythrocyte sedimentation rate, high serum viscosity, normal bone radiographs, and bone marrow showing predominantly lymphoid cells (3,4). The overall incidence of WM is about three per million persons per year, with 1500 new cases diagnosed per year in the United States (5,6). Unlike multiple myeloma, WM is more common in Caucasians than in African Americans (5). It is a sporadic disease with unknown etiology; however, studies have demonstrated a high familial incidence of this disease, with 18.7% of the patients having at least a first degree relative with a B-cell neoplasm (7,8). The main risk factor for the development of

WM is the presence of IgM-monoclonal gammopathy of undetermined significance (IgM-MGUS) (9), which confers a 46-fold higher relative risk to develop WM than the general population (9). The median overall survival of patients with WM is 5–6 years; however a recent study in 337 patients with symptomatic WM, demonstrated median disease-specific survival of 11.2 years (10).

WM is currently classified by the Revised European American Lymphoma (REAL) and World Health Organization (WHO) systems as a lymphoplasmacytic lymphoma (11). WM cells express pan B-cell markers including CD19, CD20, and CD22, but lack CD10, CD23, CD38, FMC7, and cytoplasmic Ig (11,12). CD5 and CD23 are expressed in 5–20% and 35% of the cases respectively (13).

The origin of the malignant clone is thought to be a B-cell arrested after somatic hypermutation in the germinal center, before terminal differentiation to plasma cells (14,15). The malignant cells have undergone VH gene somatic mutation, but not isotype class switching. Analysis of 14q32 demonstrates that WM cells lack IgH (Ig heavy chain) rearrangement. The most common cytogenetic abnormality identified using FISH analysis in patients with WM is deletion of the long arm of chromosome 6 seen in 55% of cases (16). Other cytogenetic abnormalities include trisomy 4, trisomy 5, monsomy 8, and deletion 20q (17–19). Genes dysregulated in WM include tumor suppressor gene BLIMP-1, which is localized on 6q21 and regulates the transition of mature B-cells to terminally differentiated plasma cells (20), HAS1, and XBP-1 (21–23). Further studies to define the role of these genes in the pathogenesis of WM are underway. In addition, WM is characterized by upregulation of cytokines and chemokines that induce proliferation and survival of the malignant clone. These include B-lymphocyte stimulator (BLyS), IL-6, CD40 ligand, BAFF, APRIL, and stromal derived factor (SDF-1) (24–29).

GENOMIC AND PROTEOMIC ANALYSIS OF PATIENTS WITH WM

Gene expression analysis has allowed a better understanding of the underlying molecular alterations in WM. For example, gene expression profiling of 23 samples of WM compared to cases of multiple myeloma and chronic lymphocytic leukemia (CLL) showed that WM has a homogenous expression profile similar to that of patients with CLL, with a unique subset of genes identified in WM patients, which included the MAPK pathway and IL-6 (25). Another study confirmed those observations, and showed that 4 genes discriminated WM cells from CLL cells: LEF1 (WNT/beta-catenin pathway), MARCKS, ATXN1, and FMOD (30). Other genes involved in plasma cell differentiation including PAX5, IRF4 and BLIMP1 were also dysregulated in WM (30). To further determine the molecular signatures of WM at the protein level, we performed protein expression profiling of patients with symptomatic and asymptomatic WM compared to healthy controls using antibody-based protein microarrays (31). Proteins upregulated by > 2-fold included Ras family proteins such as Rab-4 and p62DOK, as well as Rho family proteins such as CDC42GAP and ROKα. Other proteins upregulated by > 1.3-fold included cyclin dependent kinases (CDKs), apoptosis regulators, and histone deacetylases (HDACs). Three proteins were different by > 2-fold in symptomatic versus asymptomatic WM, including heat shock protein HSP90 (31).

CLINICAL PRESENTATION AND PROGNOSIS OF PATIENTS WITH WM

WM is a heterogenous disease and patients can present with a broad spectrum of symptoms and signs (2,10,32). The most common clinical presentations are related to cytopenias, specifically anemia related to replacement of the bone marrow with tumor cells. Fatigue is a very common presentation of WM that is multifactorial, due at least in part to the underlying degree of cytopenias. Patients may also present with symptoms of hyperviscosity related to elevated IgM levels including headache, blurring of vision, and epistaxis. Hepatosplenomegaly and lymphadenopathy occur in 20% of the patients, and some patients may present with B symptoms including night sweats, fever, and weight loss. Other presentation features include neuropathy, cryoglobulinemia, skin rash (Shnitzler's syndrome) (33), cold-agglutinin hemolytic anemia, and amyloidosis (1,34). Because patients with WM have a wide range of overall survival, it is important to define prognostic factors. Factors associated with poor prognosis in patients with WM include: advanced age, high β2-microglobulin (2M), cytopenias, low albumin, serum IgM monoclonal protein, and organomegaly (10,35–38). A recent study by Morel et al. (39) described the International Prognostic Staging System (IPSS) for WM, with age > 65 years, elevated β2M microglobulin at 3 mg/L, IgM monoclonal protein > 70g/L, and hemoglobin < 11.5 g/dL conferring poor prognosis. We have recently demonstrated that serum-free light-chain levels correlate with elevated β2M and cytopenias (40).

INITIATION OF THERAPY

The Third International Workshops on WM confirmed the original recommendations of consensus panels on WM that patients should receive therapy only if they have symptoms or signs related to WM or specific laboratory abnormalities, and not based only on the serum monoclonal protein level (41). The most common reason for initiation of therapy is anemia. Other causes include hyperviscosity symptoms, cytopenias, evidence of disease transformation, and significant neuropathy, adenopathy, or hepatosplenomegaly (37,41–43).

THERAPEUTIC OPTIONS

There is no standard of therapy for the treatment of WM (41). In addition, to date there are no FDA approved therapeutic agents for the specific treatment of WM (41). Most treatment options were originally derived from other lymphoproliferative disease including multiple myeloma and CLL (43). The Third International Workshop on MM updated the treatment recommendations for frontline and salvage therapy of WM (41). The panel emphasized that many factors should be considered in making the decision: the age of the patient, presence of cytopenias, and the rate of disease progression. The recommendations for upfront therapy included alkylating agents, nucleoside analogs, and the monoclonal antibody rituximab (41). For patients with relapsed disease, the use of alternate first-line agents, reuse of a first-line agent, use of combination myelotoxic chemotherapy, and the use of thalidomide as a single agent or in combination therapy were recommended (41). High-dose chemotherapy with autologous stem cell rescue in primary refractory or relapsed disease should be considered for eligible patients. However, allogeneic and "nonmyeloablative allogeneic" transplantations should be cautiously approached, given the associated high mortality and/or morbidity risks, and should be undertaken only in context of a clinical trial (41). The new response criteria recommended in the Second International Workshop of WM are summarized in Table 1. Single agents used in WM are summarized in Table 2, the combinations of alkylating agents, purine nucleoside analogues, and rituximab are summarized in Table 3, and novel therapeutic agents are presented in Table 4.

Table 1 Response Criteria Recommended by the Second International Workshop of Walderström Macroglobulinemia

Complete response (CR)	Disappearance of monoclonal protein by immunofixation; no histologic evidence of BM involvement, resolution of any adenopathy/organomegaly. Reconfirmation of CR is required after 6 weeks
Partial response (PR)	At least 50% reduction of serum monoclonal IgM concentration on protein electrophoresis and at least 50% decrease in adenopathy/organomegaly
Minor response (MR)	At least 25% reduction of serum monoclonal IgM by protein electrophoresis
Stable disease (SD)	Less than 25% reduction in serum monoclonal IgM by electrophoresis
Progressive disease (PD)	At least 25% increase in serum monoclonal IgM by protein electrophoresis. Reconfirmation by a second measurement is required after 3 weeks

Table 2   Single-Agent Therapies in Waldenström Macroglobulinemia

Study	Regimen	No. of patients	Phase of study	ORR %
Kyle (44)	Chlorambucil continuous vs. intermittent	46	III	68
Facon (89)	Chlorambucil	128	II	31
Dimopoulos (90)	Cladribine	46	II	45
Dimopoulos (49)	Fludarabine	28	II	36
Leblond (91)	Fludarabine	64	II	30
Dhodapkar (35)	Fludarabine	64	II	34
Johnson (92)	Fludarabine vs. chlorambucil	Ongoing	III	Ongoing
Gertz (50)	Rituximab	34	II	135
Treon (51)	Rituximab	29	II	48
Dimopoulos (93)	Rituximab	29	II	52

STANDARD THERAPIES USED IN WM

Alkylating Agents

Chlorambucil was the first agent used in clinical trials in WM. In a prospective randomized study by Kyle et al., there was no significant difference in the overall response rate between daily (0.1 mg/kg/day) or intermittent chlorambucil (0.3 mg/kg for 7 days, every 6 weeks). Overall responses to single agent chlorambucil varied between 31% and 92% (41,44). Reasons for these variations include small sample size, as well as different inclusion and response criteria. The main complication of chlorambucil is the risk of developing myelodysplasia and acute myelogenous leukemia (2,41). In addition, stem cell damage due to therapy may prevent collection of stem cells (41). The use of steroids in combination with alkylator therapy resulted in a partial response in 72% of patients (41).

The combination of CHOP (cyclophosphamide, doxorubicin, vincristine, prednisone) together with rituximab (CHOP-R) has been tested in patients with WM. The German Low Grade Lymphoma Study Group (GLSG) performed a randomized upfront study of CHOP-R versus CHOP in 72 patients with low-grade lymphoma (71% of who had lymphoplasmacytic lymphoma) (45). The response rate in the CHOP-R arm was 94% compared to 69% in the CHOP arm (45). A small retrospective study of 13 patients with relapsed WM who received CHOP-R was reported by

Table 3   Combination Therapies in Waldenström Macroglobulinemia

Study	Regimen	No. of patients	Phase of study	ORR %
Tam (94)	Fludara/CTX	9	II	88
Leblond (60)	Fludara/CTX	49	II	78
Weber (59)	Cladribine/CTX	37	II	84
Pertucci (95)	Melphalan/CTX/chlorambucil/ prednisolone	31	II	68
Case (96)	Carmustine/CTX/VCR/ melphalan/prednisolone	33	II	82
Annibali (97)	Melphalan/CTX/prednisone	72	II	87
Dimopoulos (98)	CTX/VCR/prednisolone	16	II	44
Leblond (99)	Fludarabine vs CAP	92	III	30 vs. 11%
Owen (11)	Fludara/rituximab	43	II	82
Tam (100)	Fludara/CTX/rituximab	5	II	80
Weber (59)	Cladribine/CTX/rituximab	27	II	94
Hensel (101)	Pentostatin/CTX/rituximab	17	II	90
Dimopoulos (61)	Dex/CTX/rituximab	??	II	??
Treon (46)	CHOP/rituximab	13	II	77
Dimopoulos (102)	CHOP/rituximab vs CHOP	72	II	94

Abbreviations: CTX, cyclophosphamide; Dex, dexamethasone; Fludara, fludarabine; VCR, vincristine.

Hunter et al. (46) and showed that 10 patients achieved a major response (77%) including 3 complete responses (CR), 7 partial responses (PR), and 2 minor responses (MR). A prospective study of CHOP-R in newly diagnosed patients with WM is ongoing in the Eastern Cooperative Oncology Group.

Purine Nucleoside Analogues

Cladribine and fludarabine have been extensively studied in WM and induced durable responses. Cladribine administered as intravenous infusion or by subcutaneous bolus injections has resulted in major responses in 40–90% of newly diagnosed patients, versus 38% to 54% in the salvage setting (2,41,43,47,48). The overall response rate with daily infusional fludarabine therapy administered mainly on 5-day schedules in previously untreated and treated WM patients has ranged from 38% to 100% and 30% to 40%, respectively (2,41,47,49). The main complications of these agents are myelosuppression and immunosuppression, especially of T cells leading

Table 4   Novel Agents in WM: Completed and Ongoing Studies

Study	Agents	No. of patients	Phase of study	ORR
Dimopoulos (64)	Thal/dex/ Clarithromycin	20	II	25
Branagan (65)	Thalidomide/ rituximab	23	II	68
Treon (103)	Lenalidomide/ rituximab		II	Ongoing
Dimopoulos (68)	Bortezomib	10	II	60
Chen (67)	Bortezomib	27	II	44
Treon (69)	Bortezomib	26	II	84.6
Treon (70)	Bortezomib/ rituximab/dex		II	Ongoing
Ghobrial (unpublished)	Bortezomib/ Rituximab		II	Ongoing
Dimopoulos (unpublished)	Bortezomib/ rituximab/dex		II	Ongoing
Hunter (71)	Alemtuzumab		II	
Gertz (74)	Genasense		I	
Patterson (76)	Sildenafil	30	II	
Rossi (78)	Atacicept		I/II	
O'Connor (79)	PR-171		I	
Treon (77)	Imatinib mesylate	30 planned	II	Ongoing
Ghobrial (unpublished)	Perifosine		II	Ongoing
Ghobrial (unpublished)	RAD001		II	Ongoing

to an increased risk of infections and a treatment-related mortality of up to 5% in some series (43). In addition, stem cell collection may also be problematic after prolonged exposure to purine nucleoside analogues. There is limited experience in the use of an alternate nucleoside analogue to salvage patients whose disease relapsed after cladribine or fludarabine therapy: three of four patients (75%) responded to cladribine following relapse to fludarabine therapy, whereas only 1 of 10 (10%) with disease resistant to fludarabine responded to cladribine (41,43).

The Monoclonal Anti-CD20 Antibody Rituximab

Rituximab has become one of the main treatment options of patients with WM. Standard rituximab (4 weekly infusions of 375 mg/m^2) has demonstrated at least a minor response in 52% of patients (50). Four weekly rituximab treatments repeated at 3 months triggered response rates of 44–48% (51,52).

Polymorphisms in the FcγRIIIA (CD16) receptor gene may affect response to rituximab in WM (53). The response to rituximab is delayed in most patients with a median time to partial response of four months and a median time to best response of 17 months (51). In addition, the IgM level may initially increase in response to rituximab, a phenomenon termed IgM flare that occurs in about 54% of patients (54,55). These levels may persist for up to four months and do not indicate treatment failure, but may necessitate plasmapheresis to reduce hyperviscosity. Some patients receive maintenance therapy with rituximab. Although the impact of this regimen on the time to progression has not been determined specifically in WM, it has prolonged time to progression in patients with other low-grade lymphomas who received rituximab maintenance compared to those who did not (56). Rituximab may also be useful in treating patients with IgM autoantibody-related neuropathies (57). The use of radioimmunotherapy such as iodine 131I-tositumomab radioimmunotherapy in WM has been limited since the high level of bone marrow involvement precludes their use. However, case reports have shown that these therapies may be effective in patients with WM who have < 25% bone marrow involvement (58).

Combinations of Alkylating Agents, Nucleoside Analogs, and Rituximab

The addition of alkylating agents to nucleoside analogs is active against WM. For example, the combination of oral cyclophosphamide with subcutaneous cladribine in 37 newly diagnosed patients achieved 84% PR or more, with a median duration of response of 36 months (59). The combination of fludarabine and intravenous cyclophosphamide in 11 previously treated patients resulted in 55% overall response. In another study of 49 patients, the combination of fludarabine plus cyclophosphamide induced 78% overall response, with median time to treatment failure was 27 months (41,60). Hematologic toxicity was commonly observed, and three patients died of treatment-related toxicities. A phase II clinical trial of 60 patients with WM treated with cyclophosphamide, rituximab and dexamethasone (DRC) demonstrated an overall response rate of 70%, with 7% complete remission (61). Treatment was well tolerated and the main toxicity observed was grade 3–4 neutropenia in 20% of the patients. The combination of rituximab, cladribine, and cyclophosphamide was tested in 17 previously untreated patients with WM and achieved at least a partial response in 94% of the patients, with complete response in 18% (41,59). The combination of rituximab and fludarabine was evaluated in 43 WM patients, with an overall response rate of 91% and CR of 7% (62). In another study, the combination of fludarabine, cyclophosphamide, and rituximab (FCR) was tested in 21 patients with WM who had at least 1–2 prior regimens of therapy; overall response rate was 52%, with 5% complete remissions (41).

NOVEL THERAPEUTIC AGENTS

The Immunomodulatory Agents—Thalidomide and Lenalidomide

In view of their success in the treatment of patients with multiple myeloma (MM), immunomodulatory agents (IMIDs) were tested in patients with WM. A study to evaluate thalidomide alone or in combination with clarithromycin and dexamethasone showed partial response in five of 20 previously untreated and treated patients (25%) who received single-agent thalidomide. Adverse effects were common and prevented dose escalation of thalidomide in 75% of patients (63,64). Thalidomide (50 mg daily) in combination with dexamethasone (40 mg orally once a week) and clarithromycin (250 mg orally twice a day) induced partial response in 10 of 12 (83%) previously treated patients (64). However, a follow-up study of 10 patients with higher doses of thalidomide (200 mg daily) showed only 20% overall response rate (41). A phase II study of the combination of thalidomide and rituximab in 23 patients triggered response in 15 patients, and stable disease in 4. No patients with stable disease or better have progressed with a median follow-up of 10 months (range 6–13 months) (65). Similarly, based on the potent activity of lenalidomide in MM and the lack of neuropathy with this agent, a phase II study of lenalidomide 25 mg daily in combination with rituximab is ongoing in patients with relapsed or relapsed/refractory WM.

The Proteasome Inhibitor Bortezomib

The prototype 26S proteasome inhibitor bortezomib (Velcade, PS-341) selectively binds to the catalytic domain of the proteasome and prevents its activity (66). Based on its activity in MM, single agent bortezomib was tested in WM in phase II trials and achieved 40–80% responses (67–69). The combination of bortezomib, dexamethasone, and rituximab was recently evaluated in untreated patients with WM. Each cycle of therapy consisted of IV bortezomib at 1.3 mg/m^2 and IV dexamethasone 40 mg on days (1, 4, 8, and 11), and Rituximab at 375 mg/m^2 (day 11). Patients received four consecutive cycles, followed by a three-month pause, and then four more cycles, each given three months apart. The interim analysis of the first 10 patients who received the first four cycles of therapy showed partial response in 50% and minor response in the other 50%, with two patients (20%) achieving an unconfirmed complete response (70). The main complications of this trial were herpes zoster reactivation in 40% (70). Another phase II trial of weekly bortezomib at 1.6 mg/m^2 in combination with rituximab is currently ongoing in patients with relapsed or relapsed/refractory WM.

Anti-CD52 Alemtuzumab-1H (Campath®)

CD52 is highly expressed on WM cells in the bone marrow, and alemtuzumab induces cytotoxicity of WM cells in vitro. A phase II study of alemtuzumab in 25 patients with relapsed WM or newly diagnosed untreated WM showed an overall response rate of 76%, including 8 (32%) partial responses and 11 (44%) minor responses (71). Hematological toxicities were common among previously treated (but not untreated) patients and included G3/4 neutropenia (39%); thrombocytopenia (18%); anemia (7%). G3/4 nonhematological toxicity for all patients included dermatitis (11%); fatigue (7%); and infection (7%). CMV reactivation and infection was commonly seen among previously treated patients. Three patients died due to therapy-related complications (71).

The Bcl-2 Inhibitor G3139

Bcl-2 regulates apoptosis and resistance to chemotherapeutic agents; it has therefore become an attractive target for anticancer therapy in a number of malignancies including WM (72). In vitro studies have shown that Bcl-2 is expressed in WM cells, and that downregulation of Bcl-2 and increased cytotoxicity in WM cells may be achieved with oblimersen sodium [(G3139) Genasense® Genta, Inc., Berkeley Heights, New Jersey, U.S.] (73). A Phase I/II clinical trial of G3139 was conducted in patients with relapsed or relapsed/refractory WM showed favorable tolerability but little activity (74).

Sildenafil Citrate

Based on the clinical observation that patients receiving sildenafil citrate had a decrease in their IgM (75), a phase II trial of single agent sildenafil citrate in patients with slowly progressing WM, who did not meet consensus eligibility for active therapy, was initiated. The purpose of the study was to delay time to progression in these patients. Thirty patients were treated on this study, and disease progression was suppressed in more than 50% of the patients. After three months of therapy, 63% showed a decrease in IgM levels and 17% showed a minor response (76). However, disease progression at six months of follow occurred in almost all the patients (76).

Imatinib Mesylate (Gleevex)

Imatinib targets the microenvironment of WM through inhibition of stem cell factor signaling through CD117, which is expressed on WM and mast cells. A phase II trial of single agent imatinib is ongoing in patients with relapsed or refractory WM (77). Imatinib is given at 400 mg daily, with dose escalation to 600 mg after one month of therapy. After three months of therapy, 6/13 (46.2%) of patients achieved MR. The main toxicities observed included cytopenias, edema, and hyperglycemia, leading to dose reductions in 31% patients and cessation of therapy in 23% patients (77).

TACI-Ig, Atacicept (ZymoGenetics, Inc., Seattle, Washington, U.S.) contains the soluble TACI receptor that binds to the cytokines BLyS and APRIL, members of the tumor necrosis factor family that promote B-cell survival. An open-label, dose-escalation Phase 1b study enrolled 16 patients with refractory or relapsed MM or active progressive WM. Sequential cohorts received one cycle of five weekly subcutaneous injections of atacicept at 2, 4, 7, or 10 mg/kg (78). Treatment with atacicept was well tolerated, and no dose limiting toxicity was observed. A biological response was observed in this heavily treated refractory population, with disease stabilization in 75% of the patients with WM (78).

The Proteasome Inhibitor PR-171

PR-171 is a novel irreversible proteasome inhibitor under investigation for the treatment of hematological malignancies. Two phase I dose-escalation studies have been initiated, aimed at determining the safety, tolerability, and clinical response to PR-17 (79). Patients with multiple myeloma, non-Hodgkin's lymphoma, Hodgkin disease, or Waldenström macroglobulinemia who received two or more prior treatments were eligible. Two different dose-intensive schedules were employed in these phase I studies. PR-171 was well-tolerated, and several subjects have achieved long-lasting SD, reduction in paraprotein levels, or symptomatic improvement (79).

Perifosine

Perifosine [KRX-0401, Keryx Biopharmaceuticals, New York, New York, U.S.] is a novel Akt inhibitor that belongs to a class of lipid-related compounds called alkylphospholipids (80). It has shown activity in phase II trials in MM (80). Our previous studies have shown that the activity of the survival protein Akt is upregulated in patients with WM compared to normal B cells, and that downregulation of Akt leads to significant inhibition of proliferation and induction of apoptosis in WM cells in vitro (81). in vivo studies of perifosine have shown significant cytotoxicity and inhibition of tumor growth in a xenograft mouse model (81). Subsequently, perifosine was shown to induce synergistic cytotoxicity with rituximab and bortezomib as well as with other conventional agents including fludarabine and cyclophosphamide (82). Based on this preclinical activity, we initiated a phase II trial of single agent perifosine in patients with relapsed or relapsed/ refractory disease using 150 mg oral daily dosing. The preliminary data of 13 patients enrolled on the study, with a median follow-up time of three months, demonstrated promising activity of this agent. The treatment was well tolerated with minimal side effects. Seven patients were evaluable at the time of analysis and all showed evidence of IgM reduction, with a median IgM reduction of 14% (0–25%). One patient whose IgM rose in the first month had a 50% reduction from the peak of IgM level at three months, indicating a delayed response. These preliminary results indicate that perifosine is a promising agent to be used in combination in future studies in WM.

RAD001

Based on the preclinical data showing increased activity of the PI3K/mTOR pathway in WM, rapamycin (mTOR inhibitor) has been studied in vitro in WM and showed significant cytotoxicity in WM cells lines, specifically when combined with bortezomib (unpublished data). A phase II trial of single agent RAD001 (orally at 10 mg daily) was initiated in aggressive, low grade lymphomas, and rare lymphomas including WM. At the interim analysis, one patient with WM showed 50% reduction of IgM protein (personal communication with Dr. Thomas Witzig). Based on this promising activity, the study is expanding to include more patients with WM.

FUTURE THERAPEUTIC OPTIONS

Agents in Preclinical Studies

The PKC Inhibitor Enzastaurin

Proteomic studies in WM demonstrated upregulation of PKCβ in malignant cells compared to normal B cells (83). Based on this, enzastaurin a novel PKC inhibitor was used to block PKC activity in WM cells. Enzastaurin (LY 317615, Eli Lilly, Indianapolis, Indiana, U.S.) induced a significant decrease of proliferation and induced apoptosis in WM cell lines and primary patient samples, without cytotoxicity on peripheral blood mononuclear cells (83). In addition, enzastaurin overcame tumor cell growth induced by coculture of WM cells with bone marrow stromal cells. Enzastaurin inhibited Akt phosphorylation and Akt kinase activity, as well as downstream p-MARCKS and ribosomal p-S6 (83). Furthermore, Enzastaurin demonstrated additive cytotoxicity in combination with bortezomib, and synergistic cytotoxicity in combination with fludarabine. Finally, in an In vivo xenograft model of human WM, significant inhibition of tumor growth was observed in the enzastaurin-treated mice, providing the framework for clinical trials of this agent in WM (83).

The Anti-CD70 Antibody SGN-70

Lymphoplasmacytic cells stimulate cell surface expression of TNF-family ligands through release of sCD27, which induces CD70 on mast cells. WM cells and cell lines highly express CD70 (84). Therefore, directly targeting CD70 using the fully humanized monoclonal antibody SGN-70 (Seattle Genetics, Inc., Bothell, Washington, U.S.) may represent a therapeutic option in WM. SGN-70 mediated significant dose-dependent ADCC against WM cell and mast cells at concentrations of 0.1–20 μg/mL (84). SCID-hu mice bearing WM cells were treated with SGN-70 (1 mg/kg, i.p., qOD), and serum IgM and sCD27 levels were measured to monitor for disease progression. SGN-70 initiated 6 weeks following tumor engraftment blocked tumor growth in 12/12 treated mice, whereas all 5 untreated mice demonstrated disease progression (84). The results of these studies provide the framework for clinical trials to examine the therapeutic potential of the SGN-70 monoclonal antibody in WM.

The Proteasome Inhibitor NPI-0052

Based on the activity of bortezomib in patients with WM, NPI-0052 (Nereus Pharmaceuticals, San Diego, California, U.S.) was tested in WM cell lines and patient samples (85). NPI-0052 induced cytotoxicity and inhibition of DNA synthesis, with an IC50 of 20–30 nM in all cell lines tested at 24 hours (85). NPI-0052 induces 50% apoptosis at 48 hrs. Similar effects were demonstrated in primary CD19 + WM cells. Import-antly, the combination of NPI-0052 and bortezomib induced significant inhibition of proliferation compared to each agent alone (85). These results provide the framework to further study the potential therapeutic role of NPI-0052 in WM.

AMD3100

WM is characterized by widespread involvement of the bone marrow (BM), and lymphadenopathy in 20% of the patients, implying continuous trafficking of WM cells into and out of the BM and lymph nodes. The normal process of B-cell homing is regulated by cytokines, chemokines, and adhesion molecules (86). One of the most extensively studied chemokines in migration is stromal derived factor SDF-1 and its receptor CXCR4. We recently demonstrated that WM cells and patient samples highly express CXCR4; and that SDF-1 induced migration of WM cells, with rapid activation of signaling pathways downstream of CXCR4 including pERK1/2, p-Akt, and pPKC (87). The CXCR4 inhibitor AMD3100 inhibited migration of WM cells, as well as their adhesion to fibronectin (87). Adhesion of WM cells to stromal cells confers resistance to apoptosis and induces proliferation. The combination of AMD3100 (Genzyme Corporation, Cambridge, Massachusetts, U.S.) with bortezomib signifi-cantly enhances the cytotoxic effect of bortezomib in the presence of stromal cells, possibly by interfering with adhesion of WM to stromal cells and thereby overcoming their protective effect (87). These studies provide the preclinical framework to study CXCR4 inhibitors in the regulation of homing and adhesion in WM.

Triterpenoids, CDDO, and CDDO-Im

2-Cyano-3,12-dioxoolean-1,9-dien-28-oic acid (CDDO) and its methyl ester derivative (CDDO-Me) and imidazolide derivative (CDDO-Im) are synthetic triterpenoids derived from oleanolic acid. In vitro studies in primary WM samples showed that CDDO-Im inhibited cell proliferation and induced apoptosis in WM cells compared to normal B cells (88). There was evidence of PARP cleavage in a dose-dependent manner, suggesting that CDDO-Im induced malignant cell death occurs through a caspase-dependent mechanism, and may have potential efficacy in WM patients (88).

Conclusion

In summary, there have been significant advances in the understanding of the pathogenesis and molecular alterations that occur in WM. Many targeted therapeutic agents and monoclonal antibodies have been tested in the preclinical setting and in early phase I and II studies. A new paradigm shift has evolved in WM utilizing novel therapeutic agents targeting the WM clone and its bone marrow microenvironment. The current challenge is to identify combinations of agents that act synergistically against WM cells in order to carry out clinical trials that achieve high remission rates and prolonged survival in patients with WM.

ACKNOWLEDGMENTS

Supported in part by NIH R21 CA126119-01, International Waldenström Macroglobulinemia Foundation (IWMF) grant, and Lymphoma Research Foundation.

REFERENCES

1. Ghobrial IM, Gertz MA, Fonseca R. Waldenström macroglobulinaemia. Lancet Oncol 2003; 4:679–85.
2. Dimopoulos MA, Kyle RA, Anagnostopoulos A, Treon SP. Diagnosis and management of Waldenström's macroglobulinemia. J Clin Oncol 2005; 23: 1564–77.
3. Treon SP, Dimopoulos M, Kyle RA. Defining Waldenström's macroglobulinemia. Semin Oncol 2003; 30:107–9.
4. Waldenström J. Incipient myelomatosis or 'essential' hyperglobulinemia with fibrinogenopenia—a new syndrome? Acta Med Scand 1944; 117:216–47.
5. Jemal A, Murray T, Ward E, et al. Cancer statistics, 2005. CA Cancer J Clin 2005; 55:10–30.
6. Herrinton L, Weiss NS. Incidence of Waldenström's macroglobulinemia. Blood 1993; 82:3148–50.
7. McMaster M. Familial Waldenström's macroglobulinemia. Semin Oncol 2003; 30:146–52.
8. Treon SP, Hunter ZR, Aggarwal A, et al. Characterization of familial Waldenström's macroglobulinemia. Ann Oncol 2006; 17:488–94.
9. Kyle RA, Therneau TM, Rajkumar SV, et al. Long-term follow-up of IgM monoclonal gammopathy of undetermined significance. Blood 2003; 102: 3759–64.

10. Ghobrial IM, Fonseca R, Gertz MA, et al. Prognostic model for disease-specific and overall mortality in newly diagnosed symptomatic patients with Waldenström macroglobulinaemia. Br J Haematol 2006; 133:158–64.
11. Owen RG, Treon SP, Al-Katib A, et al. Clinicopathological definition of Waldenström's macroglobulinemia: consensus panel recommendations from the Second International Workshop on Waldenström's Macroglobulinemia. Semin Oncol 2003; 30:110–15.
12. Remstein ED, Hanson CA, Kyle RA, Hodnefield JM, Kurtin PJ. Despite apparent morphologic and immunophenotypic heterogeneity, Waldenström's macroglobulinemia is consistently composed of cells along a morphologic continuum of small lymphocytes, plasmacytoid lymphocytes, and plasma cells. Semin Oncol 2003; 30:182–6.
13. Hunter Z, Branagan AR, Manning R, et al. CD5, CD10, and CD23 expression in Waldenström's macroglobulinemia. Clin Lymphoma 2005; 5:246–9.
14. Kriangkum J, Taylor BJ, Treon SP, Mant MJ, Belch AR, Pilarski LM. Clonotypic IgM V/D/J sequence analysis in Waldenström macroglobulinemia suggests an unusual B-cell origin and an expansion of polyclonal B cells in peripheral blood. Blood 2004; 104:2134–42.
15. Sahota S, Forconi F, Ottensmeier CH, et al. Typical Waldenström macroglobulinemia is derived from a B-cell arrested after cessation of somatic mutation but prior to isotype switch events. Blood 2002; 100:1505–7.
16. Schop RF, Kuehl WM, Van Wier SA, et al. Waldenström macroglobulinemia neoplastic cells lack immunoglobulin heavy chain locus translocations but have frequent 6q deletions. Blood 2002; 100:2996–3001.
17. Schop RF, Jalal SM, Van Wier SA, et al. Deletions of 17p13.1 and 13q14 are uncommon in Waldenström macroglobulinemia clonal cells and mostly seen at the time of disease progression. Cancer Genet Cytogenet 2002; 132:55–60.
18. Terre C, Nguyen-Khac F, Barin C, et al. Trisomy 4, a new chromosomal abnormality in Waldenström's macroglobulinemia: a study of 39 cases. Leukemia 2006; 20:1634–6.
19. Liu Y, Miyazawa K, Sashida G, Kodama A, Ohyashiki K. Deletion (20q) as the sole abnormality in Waldenström macroglobulinemia suggests distinct pathogenesis of 20q11 anomaly. Cancer Genet Cytogenet 2006; 169:69–72.
20. Turner CJ, Mack DH, Davis MM. Blimp-1, a novel zinc finger-containing protein that can drive the maturation of B lymphocytes into immunoglobulin-secreting cells. Cell 1994; 77:297–306.
21. Wu Y, Bressette D, Carrell JA, et al. Tumor necrosis factor (TNF) receptor superfamily member TACI is a high affinity receptor for TNF family members APRIL and BLyS. J Biol Chem 2000:35478–85.
22. Adamia S, Crainie M, Kriangkum J, Mant MJ, Belch AR, Pilarski LM. Abnormal expression of hyaluronan synthases in patients with Waldenström's macroglobulinemia. Semin Oncol 2003; 30:465–8.
23. Xu L, Leleu X, Hunter Z, et al. Abnormal Expression of the Plasma Cell Differentiation Factor X-Box Protein 1 (Xbp-1) in Waldenström's Macroglobulinemia. Blood (ASN, Annual Meeting Abstracts) 2005; 106:1003.
24. Elsawa SF, Novak AJ, Grote DM, et al. B-lymphocyte stimulator (BLyS) stimulates immunoglobulin production and malignant B-cell growth in Waldenström's macroglobulinemia. Blood 2005; 107:2882–8.

25. Chng WJ, Schop R, Price-Troska T, et al. Gene expression profiling of Waldenström's macroglobulinemia reveals a phenotype more similar to chronic lymphocytic leukemia than multiple myeloma. Blood 2006; 108:2755–63.

26. MacKay F, Schneider P, Rennert P, Browning J. BAFF AND APRIL: a tutorial on B cell survival. Annu Rev Immunol 2003; 21:231–64.

27. Hatzimichael E, Christou L, Bai M, Kolios G, Kefala L, Bourantas KL. Serum levels of IL-6 and its soluble receptor (sIL-6R) in Waldenström's macroglobulinemia. Eur J Haematol 2001; 66:1–6.

28. Ngo H, Leleu X, Moreau AS, Hideshima T, Anderson KC, Ghobrial IM. Analysis of chemokine and adhesion markers in Waldenström Macroglobulinemia. Blood (ASN, Annual Meeting Abstracts) 2006; 108:4653.

29. Tournilhac O, Santos DD, Xu L, et al. Mast cells in Waldenström's macroglobulinemia support lymphoplasmacytic cell growth through CD154/ CD40 signaling. Ann Oncol 2006; 17:1275–82.

30. Gutierrez NC, Ocio EM, de Las Rivas J, et al. Gene expression profiling of B lymphocytes and plasma cells from Waldenström's macroglobulinemia: comparison with expression patterns of the same cell counterparts from chronic lymphocytic leukemia, multiple myeloma and normal individuals. Leukemia 2007; 21:541–9.

31. Hatjiharissi E, Ngo H, Leontovich A, et al. Proteomic analysis of Waldenström macroglobulinemia. Cancer Res 2007; 67:3777–84.

32. Ghobrial IM, Witzig TE. Waldenström macroglobulinemia. Curr Treat Options Oncol 2004; 5:239–47.

33. Schnitzler L, Schubert B, Boasson M, Gardais J, Tourmen A. Urticaire chronique, lésions osseuses, macroglobulinémie IgM: maladie de Waldenström? Bull Soc Fr Derm Syph 1974; 81:363–7.

34. Gertz M, Kyle RA, Noel P. Primary systemic amyloidosis: a rare complication of immunoglobulin M monoclonal gammopathies and Waldenström's macroglobulinemia 1993; 11:914–20.

35. Dhodapkar MV, Jacobson JL, Gertz MA, et al. Prognostic factors and response to fludarabine therapy in patients with Waldenström macroglobulinemia: results of United States intergroup trial (Southwest Oncology Group S9003). Blood 2001; 98:41–8.

36. Dimopoulos MA, Hamilos G, Zervas K, et al. Survival and prognostic factors after initiation of treatment in Waldenström's macroglobulinemia. Ann Oncol 2003; 14:1299–1305.

37. Kyle RA, Treon SP, Alexanian R, et al. Prognostic markers and criteria to initiate therapy in Waldenström's macroglobulinemia: consensus panel recommendations from the Second International Workshop on Waldenström's Macroglobulinemia. Semin Oncol 2003; 30:116–20.

38. Dimopoulos M, Gika D, Zervas K, et al. The international staging system for multiple myeloma is applicable in symptomatic Waldenström's macroglobulinemia. Leuk Lymphoma 2004; 45:1809–13.

39. Morel P, Duhamel A, Gobbi P, Dimopoulos M, Dhodapkar M, McCoy J, et al. International prognostic scoring system (IPSS) for Waldenström's macroglobulinemia (WM) (ASN, Annual Meeting Abstracts). Blood 2006; 108:127.

40. Moreau A, Leleu X, Manning R, Coiteux V, Darre S, Hatjiharisi E, et al. Serum free light chain in Waldenström macroglobulinemia. Blood (ASN, Annual Meeting Abstracts) 2006; 108:2420.
41. Treon SP, Gertz MA, Dimopoulos M, et al. Update on treatment recommendations from the Third International Workshop on Waldenström's macroglobulinemia. Blood 2006; 107:3442–6.
42. Treon S, Gertz MA, Dimopoulos M, et al. Update on treatment recommendations from the Third International Workshop on Waldenström's Macroglobulinemia. Blood 2006; 107:3442–6.
43. Vijay A, Gertz MA. Waldenström macroglobulinemia. Blood 2007; 109:5096–103.
44. Kyle RA, Greipp PR, Gertz MA, et al. Waldenström's macroglobulinaemia: a prospective study comparing daily with intermittent oral chlorambucil. Br J Haematol 2000; 108:737–42.
45. Buske C, Dreyling MH, Eimermacher H, et al. Combined immuno-chemotherapy (R-CHOP) results in significantly superior response rates and time to treatment failure in first line treatment of patients with lymphoplasmacytoid/ic immunocytoma: results of a prospective randomized trial of the German Low Grade Lymphoma Study Group . Blood (ASN, Annual Meeting Abstracts) 2004; 104:162.
46. Treon SP, Hunter Z, Barnagan AR. CHOP plus rituximab therapy in Waldenström's macroglobulinemia. Clin Lymphoma 2005; 5:273–7.
47. Dimopoulos MA, Kantarjian H, Estey E, et al. Treatment of Waldenström macroglobulinemia with 2-chlorodeoxyadenosine. Ann Intern Med 1993; 118: 195–8.
48. Dimopoulos MA, Kantarjian H, Weber D, et al. Primary therapy of Waldenström's macroglobulinemia with 2-chlorodeoxyadenosine. J Clin Oncol 1994; 12:2694–8.
49. Dimopoulos MA, O'Brien S, Kantarjian H, et al. Fludarabine therapy in Waldenström's macroglobulinemia. Am J Med 1993; 95:49–52.
50. Gertz MA R M, Blood E, Kaminer LS, Vesole DH, Greipp PR. Multicenter phase 2 trial of rituximab for Waldenström macroglobulinemia (WM): an Eastern Cooperative Oncology Group Study (E3A98). Leuk Lymphoma 2004; 45:2047–55.
51. Treon SP, Emmanouilides C, Kimby E, et al. Extended rituximab therapy in Waldenström's macroglobulinemia. Ann Oncol 2005; 16:132–8.
52. Dimopoulos MA, Zervas C, Zomas A, et al. Extended rituximab therapy for previously untreated patients with Waldenström's macroglobulinemia. Clin Lymphoma 2002; 3:163–6.
53. Treon S, Hansen M, Branagan AR, et al. Polymorphisms in FcγRIIIA (CD16) receptor expression are associated with clinical response to rituximab in Waldenström's macroglobulinemia. J Clin Oncol 2005; 23:474–81.
54. Ghobrial I, Fonseca R, Greipp PR, et al. Initial immunoglobulin M 'flare' after rituximab therapy in patients diagnosed with Waldenström macroglobulinemia: an Eastern Cooperative Oncology Group Study. Cancer 2004; 101:2593–8.
55. Treon S, Branagan AR, Hunter Z, Santos D, Tournhilac O, Anderson KC. Paradoxical increases in serum IgM and viscosity levels following rituximab in Waldenström's macroglobulinemia. Ann Oncol 2004; 15:1481–3.

56. van Oers MH, Klasa R, Marcus RE, et al. Rituximab maintenance improves clinical outcome of relapsed/resistant follicular non-Hodgkin's lymphoma in patients both with and without rituximab during induction: results of a prospective randomized phase 3 intergroup trial. Blood 2006; 108:3295–301.

57. Renaud S, Fuhr P, Gregor M, et al. High-dose rituximab and anti-MAG-associated polyneuropathy. Neurology 2006; 66:742–4.

58. Tsai D, Maillard I, Downs LH, et al. Use of iodine 131I-tositumomab radioimmunotherapy in a patient with Waldenström's macroglobulinemia. Leuk Lymphoma 2004; 45:591–5.

59. Weber DM, Dimopoulos MA, Delasalle K, Rankin K, Gavino M, Alexanian R. 2-Chlorodeoxyadenosine alone and in combination for previously untreated Waldenström's macroglobulinemia. Semin Oncol 2003; 30:243–7.

60. Tamburini J, Levy V, Chaleteix C, et al. Fludarabine plus cyclophosphamide: results in 49 patients. Leukemia 2005; 19:1831–4.

61. Dimopoulos M, Anagnostopoulos A, Kyrtsonis M, et al. Primary Treatment of Waldenströms Macroglobulinemia (WM) with Dexamethasone, Rituximab and Cyclophosphamide. Blood (ASN, Annual Meeting Abstracts) 2006; 108:128.

62. Treon S, Branagan A, Wasi P, et al. Combination therapy with rituximab and fludarabine in Waldenström's macroglobulinemia. Blood (ASN, Annual Meeting Abstracts) 2004; 104:753.

63. Dimopoulos MA, Zomas A, Viniou NA, et al. Treatment of Waldenström's macroglobulinemia with thalidomide. J Clin Oncol 2001; 19:3596–601.

64. Dimopoulos MA, Tsatalas C, Zomas A, et al. Treatment of Waldenström's macroglobulinemia with single-agent thalidomide or with the combination of clarithromycin, thalidomide and dexamethasone. Semin Oncol 2003; 30:265–9.

65. Branagan A, Hunter Z, Santos D, Treon SP. Thalidomide and Rituximab in Waldenström's Macroglobulinemia. Blood (ASN, Annual Meeting Abstracts) 2004; 104:1484a.

66. Hideshima T, Chauhan D, Podar K, Schlossman RL, Richardson P, Anderson KC. Novel therapies targeting the myeloma cell and its bone marrow microenvironment. Semin Oncol 2001; 28:607–12.

67. Chen CI, Kouroukis CT, White D, et al. Bortezomib is active in patients with untreated or relapsed waldenstrom's macroglobulinemia: A phase II study of the National Cancer Institute of Canada Clinical Trials Group. J Clin Oncol 2007; 25:1570–5.

68. Dimopoulos MA, Anagnostopoulos A, Kyrtsonis MC, Castritis E, Bitsaktsis A, Pangalis GA. Treatment of relapsed or refractory Waldenström's macroglobulinemia with bortezomib. Haematologica 2005; 90:1655–8.

69. Treon S, Hunter Z, Matous J, et al. Phase II Study of Bortezomib in Waldenström's Macroglobulinemia: Results of WMCTG Trial 03-248. Blood (ASN, Annual Meeting Abstracts) 2005; 106:490.

70. Treon S, Soumerai JD, Patterson CJ, et al. Bortezomib, dexamethasone and rituximab (BDR) is a highly active regimen in the primary therapy of Waldenström's macroglobulinemia: planned interim results of WMCTG clinical trial 05-180. Blood (ASN, Annual Meeting Abstracts) 2006; 108:2765.

71. Hunter Z, Boxer M, Kahl B, Patterson CJ, Soumerai JD, Treon SP. Phase II study of alemtuzumab in lymphoplasmacytic lymphoma: results of WMCTG trial 02-079. J Clin Oncol (ASCO, Annual Meeting Abstracts) 2006; 24:427.

72. Frankel S. Oblimersen sodium (G3139 Bcl-2 antisense oligonucleotide) therapy in Waldenström's macroglobulinemia: a targeted approach to enhance apoptosis. Semin Oncol 2003:300–4.
73. Nichols GL, Stein CA. Modulation of the activity of Bcl-2 in Waldenström's macroglobulinemia using antisense oligonucleotides. Semin Oncol 2003; 30: 297–9.
74. Gertz MA, Geyer SM, Badros A, Kahl BS, Erlichman C. Early results of a phase I trial of oblimersen sodium for relapsed or refractory Waldenström's macroglobulinemia. Clin Lymphoma 2005; 5:282–4.
75. Treon S, Tournilhac O, Branagan AR, et al. Clinical responses to sildenafil in Waldenström's macroglobulinemia. Clin Lymphoma 2004; 5:205–7.
76. Patterson C, Soumerai J, Hunter Z, Leleu X, Ghobrial I, Treon SP. Sildenafil citrate suppresses disease progression in patients with Waldenström's macroglobulinemia. J Clin Oncol (ASCO-Annual Meeting Abstracts) 2006; 24.
77. Treon S, Jacob S, Patterson C, et al. Imatinib Mesylate (Gleevec) Is Active in Relapsed/Refractory Waldenströms Macroglobulinemia: Planned Interim Results of WMCTG Clinical Trial 05-140. Blood (ASN, Annual Meeting Abstracts) 2006; 108: 2484.
78. Rossi J, Moreaux J, Rose M, et al. A Phase I/II study of atacicept (TACI-Ig) to neutralize APRIL and BLyS in patients with refractory or relapsed multiple myeloma (MM) or active previously treated Waldenström's macroglobuline-mia (WM). Blood (ASN, Annual Meeting Abstracts) 2006; 108:3578a.
79. O'Connor O, Orlowski R, Alsina M, et al. Multicenter Phase I Studies To Evaluate the Safety, Tolerability, and Clinical Response to Intensive Dosing with the Proteasome Inhibitor PR-171 in Patients with Relapsed or Refractory Hematological Malignancies. Blood (ASN, Annual Meeting Abstracts) 2006; 108:2430.
80. Hideshima T, Catley L, Yasui H, et al. Perifosine, an oral bioactive novel alkylphospholipid, inhibits Akt and induces in vitro and in vivo cytotoxicity in human multiple myeloma cells. Blood (ASN, Annual Meeting Abstracts) 2006; 107:4053–62.
81. Leleu X, Jia X, Moreau AS, et al. Perifosine, an Oral Bioactive Novel Akt Inhibitor, Induces In vitro and In Vivo Antitumor Activity in Waldenström Macroglobulinemia. Blood (ASN, Annual Meeting Abstracts) 2006; 108:2488.
82. Leleu X, O'Sullivan G, Jia X, Moreau AS, Ngo H, Hatjiharisi E, et al. Novel Agent Perifosine Enhances Antitumor Activity of Bortezomib, Rituximab and Other Conventional Therapies in Waldenströms Macroglobulinemia. Blood (ASN, Annual Meeting Abstracts) 2006; 108:2517.
83. Moreau AS, Jia X, Ngo HT, et al. Protein kinase C inhibitor enzastaurin induces in vitro and in vivo antitumor activity in Waldenström's macro-globulinemia. Blood (ASN, Annual Meeting Abstracts) 2007; 109:4964–72.
84. Hatjiharissi E, Ho A, Xu L, et al. Preclinical In vitro and In Vivo Evidence Support a Therapeutic Role for the CD70 Directed Monoclonal Antibody (SGN-70) in Waldenströms Macroglobulinemia (WM). Blood (ASN, Annual Meeting Abstracts) 2006; 108:2490.
85. Jia X, Leleu X, Moreau AS, Hatjiharisi E, Ngo H, O'Sullivan G, et al. The Proteasome Inhibitor NPI-0052 in Combination with Bortezomib Induces

Antitumor Activity in Waldenström Macroglobulinemia. Blood (ASN, Annual Meeting Abstracts) 2006; 108:4746.

86. Lapidot T, Dar A, Kollet O. How do stem cells find their way home? Blood 2005; 106:1901–10.

87. Ngo H, Hatjiharissi E, Leleu X, et al. The CXCR4/SDF-1 Axis Regulates Migration and Adhesion in Waldenström Macroglobulinemia. Blood (ASN, Annual Meeting Abstracts) 2006; 108:2418.

88. Elsawa S, Novak A, Konopleva M, Andreeff M, Witzig T, Ansell S. Preferential Inhibition of Malignant Cell Growth by CDDO in Waldenström Macroglobulinemia. Blood (ASN, Annual Meeting Abstracts) 2006; 108:2528.

89. Facon T, Brouillard M, Duhamel A, et al. Prognostic factors in Waldenström's macroglobulinemia: a report of 167 cases. J Clin Oncol 1993; 11:1553–8.

90. Dimopoulos MA, Weber D, Delasalle KB, Keating M, Alexanian R. Treatment of Waldenström's macroglobulinemia resistant to standard therapy with 2-chlorodeoxyadenosine: identification of prognostic factors. Ann Oncol 1995; 6:49–52.

91. Leblond V, Ben-Othman T, Deconinck E, et al. Activity of fludarabine in previously treated Waldenström's macroglobulinemia: a report of 71 cases. Groupe Cooperatif Macroglobulinemie. J Clin Oncol 1998; 16:2060–4.

92. Johnson SA, Owen RG, Oscier DG, et al. Phase III study of chlorambucil versus fludarabine as initial therapy for Waldenström's macroglobulinemia and related disorders. Clin Lymphoma 2005; 5:294–7.

93. Dimopoulos M, Zervas C, Zomas A, et al. Extended rituximab therapy for previously untreated patients with Waldenström's macroglobulinemia. Clin Lymphoma 2002; 3:163–6.

94. Tam C, Wolf MM, Westerman D, Januszewicz EH, Prince HM, Seymour JF. Fludarabine combination therapy is highly effective in frontline and salvage treatment of patients with Waldenström's macroglobulinemia. Clin Lymphoma Myeloma 2005; 2:136–9.

95. Petrucci M, Avvisati G, Tribalto M, Giovangrossi P, Mandelli F. Waldenström's macroglobulinaemia: results of a combined oral treatment in 34 newly diagnosed patients. J Intern Med 1989; 226:443–7.

96. Case DJ, Ervin TJ, Boyd MA, Redfield DL. Waldenström's macroglobulinemia: long-term results with the M-2 protocol. Cancer 1991; 9:1–7.

97. Annibali O, Petrucci MT, Martini V, et al. Treatment of 72 newly diagnosed Waldenström macroglobulinemia cases with oral melphalan, cyclophosphamide, and prednisone: results and cost analysis. Cancer 2005; 103:582–7.

98. Dimopoulos MA, Alexanian R. Waldenström's macroglobulinemia. Blood (ASN, Annual Meeting Abstracts) 1994; 83:1452–9.

99. Leblond V, Levy V, Maloisel F, et al. Multicenter, randomized comparative trial of fludarabine and the combination of cyclophosphamide-doxorubicin-prednisone in 92 patients with Waldenström macroglobulinemia in first relapse or with primary refractory disease. Blood (ASN, Annual Meeting Abstracts) 2001; 98:2640–4.

100. Tam CS, Wolf M, Prince HM, et al. Fludarabine, cyclophosphamide, and rituximab for the treatment of patients with chronic lymphocytic leukemia or indolent non-Hodgkin's lymphoma. Cancer 2006; 106:2412–20.

101. Hensel M, Villalobos M, Kornacker M, Krasniqi F, Ho AD. Pentostatin/ cyclophosphamide with or without rituximab: an effective regimen for patients with Waldenström's macroglobulinemia/lymphoplasmacytic lymphoma. Clin Lymphoma Myeloma 2005; 6:131–5.
102. Dimopoulos MA, Zervas C, Zomas A, et al. Treatment of Waldenström's macroglobulinemia with rituximab. J Clin Oncol 2002; 20:2327–33.
103. Treon S, Hunter Z, Patterson C, et al. Phase II study of CC-5013 (Revlimid) and Rituximab in Waldenström's macroglobulinemia: Preliminary Safety and Efficacy Results. Blood (ASN, Annual Meeting Abstracts) 2005; 106:2443.

Index